The Neuropsychiatric Mental Status Examination

By **Michael Alan Taylor, M.D.**
Professor and Chairman
Department of Psychiatry and
  Behavioral Sciences
University of Health Sciences/
The Chicago Medical School
Chicago, Illinois

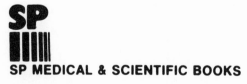

SP MEDICAL & SCIENTIFIC BOOKS

New York

SPECTRUM PUBLICATIONS, INC.
175-20 Wexford Terrace, Jamaica, N.Y. 11432

Library of Congress Cataloging in Publication Data

Taylor, Michael Alan.
  The neuropsychiatric mental status examination.

    Includes bibliographical references and index.
    1. Neuropsychiatry--Programmed instruction.
I. Title. [DNLM: 1. Mental disorders--Diagnosis--
Programmed texts. WM18 T244n]
RC341.T39   616.89'075'076   80-36794

ISBN: 0-89335-146-6 (Cloth)

ISBN: 0-89335-130-X (Paper)

For Christopher and Andrew

For Christopher and Andrew

Acknowledgments

I wish to thank the following people for their contributions to this work:

Ms. Sierra-Franco's detailed review of the program structure was of singular help to me. Whatever weaknesses remain in the design are solely my responsibility and undoubtedly exist from my resistance to respond to one of her many perceptive suggestions. Ms. Ingrid Hendricks edited an earlier revision of the manuscript and coordinated its field trials.

Ms. Sandra Mott typed and retyped multiple manuscript drafts and revisions and generally facilitated the process of writing and preparing the book. Ms. Peggy Pfeiffer and Brad Greenspan, M.D. posed for the photographs which were taken by Professor Jack DeBruin, Medical Photographer in the Department of Medical Communication at the University. Ralph Reitan, Ph.D. kindly gave his permission to use test items from his Reitan-Indiana Aphasia Screening Test. The medical students who participated in the field trials provided many insightful suggestions and were always encouraging. Ellen Taylor put up with the debris of work and hours of non-communication. She was always supportive and made life a lot easier.

Preface

There are almost as many explanations for psychiatric disorders as
there are patients with them. Each explanation is intriguing, some of
them are systematic, all of them have intellectually powerful champions.
Yet their very multitude is a scandal. It provokes the professionally
debilitating challenge: Why does every psychiatric explanation satisfy
some people and not others? Recently this question has received a
simple answer. We cannot satisfactorily explain that which we lack the
skill to describe.

To develop the fundamental skill a student must see many patients
under the direction of an experienced and involved instructor to whom he
can show his results, accept correction and advance in his abilities. But
we need a means to amplify the clinical experience, a text to supplement
the instructor in bringing forth and strengthening the vocabulary needed
to describe the phenomenology, presentations and distinctions amongst
psychiatric patients.

A "programmed text" such as this one is a satisfactory means because
it can cover rapidly many themes and variations of a vast clinical experience. It can permit the reader to progress at his own speed but bring
a sense of mastery to him as he progresses. He can check his knowledge
as he sees patients on the clinical services. This kind of text combined
with patient practice is thorough, fast and fun, but should succeed in
the important task of rapidly building for the student an authentic set of
terms and concepts suitable for both clinical work and research.

Thus, this text approximates an individual instruction method. It
supplements it but does not replace it. All phenomenological events need
to be seen to be believed, but this step by step conversation with an
author that is the strength of the programmed approach finds here a
situation that is apt for it.

This book leads to progress not because everything in it is bound to
command assent but because it uses the method of breaking complex
problems down to smaller elements, fights for clarity, strengthens its
reader through the question and answer approach and calls directly for
engagement with the teacher and the patient.

I enjoyed this book for still other reasons that emerge from the intentions
of the author. This is no "back to basics" book although there are plenty
of basics to learn. Rather this book is a piece with the "let's get down to
work" approach that has vitalized the academic psychiatric world in the

last decade. Its scholarly roots extend back to Kraepelin but reach broadly to encompass empirical work wherever it is found. It presents its information in a way that permits the reader to wrestle with it, check its reasoning and its references and to argue with the author. Here is a two-fisted "new world" style for the dissemination of information on the characteristics of psychiatric patients that is direct and unabashedly confident, but as well friendly, open to challenge, alive with vigor. It is a product of a teacher who admires his students and enjoys his subject and is prepared for the benefit of both to show how he thinks. Such an approach wins readers, respect and results. I expect this book to find a place in teaching programs that want to bring on a phenomenological interest in psychiatry. Since this is a major theme in contemporary work, it should have a large audience.

Introduction

Although much effort has been expended to develop a reliable and valid nosology of mental disorder, the process of clinical psychiatric diagnosis remains very much an art. Unfortunately, inspiration and talent, applied without effective technique and divorced from a valid data base are frequently unsuccessful. The inexperienced clinician, almost instinctively recognizing the need for technique and data, gropes for a process which will enhance recognition of signs and symptoms and which will organize these phenomena into a usable structure. The phenomenologic approach towards clinical psychiatric diagnosis is one such process. Its reliance on a structured examination, objective observation and precise definitions of clinical phenomena makes phenomenology an extremely useful tool for the evaluation and subsequent diagnosis of individuals with mental disorder.

This book is an introduction to the language, technique and concepts of the phenomenologic school. It is not intended to substitute for a well-taught course in basic psychopathology, nor can it replace hours of patient contact required to become a skilled clinician. It is a beginning.

The book is in two parts. Part I presents basic phenomenologic principles, the behaviors that comprise the major areas of concern in the mental status examination, some suggestion on how to conduct the examination and a brief exposure to behavioral relationships which lead to a clinical diagnosis. Part II builds upon Part I. It develops and reinforces the items dealing with techniques, elaborates the phenomenologic principles of diagnosis, presents diagnostic criteria which have been found to be reliable and valid in the classification of major mental disorder and presents data which aid in the delineation of those disorders.

This is a programmed book and not a comprehensive text. Reading it is not a passive experience. To gain from it, you must participate in the program. Filling in the blanks, drawing lines or circles are all part of the process of helping you learn not just from eye to brain but from hand to brain. Some items will seem absurdly simple and you will be able to rapidly go through those parts of the program. More difficult parts will take proportionately longer. Some items present new information, some review old information or present old information in new forms. The sequence is important and has been developed so the correct response to any item is either within that item or within previous items. Each page of questions or test items will be followed on the next page by the correct answers to those items. If you make an error, read back into the text until you find the items that explain the correct response. Do not skip items, for like the good mystery novel, if you read the last page first, the rest are partially ruined.

Unlike standard textbooks, this book cannot be of value if picked up for only a few moments at a time and then discarded for days or longer. Throughout the program, there are natural breaks, and pausing there will best achieve your learning goals. When starting again, a brief review of past items will help put you in the proper "set" for reading new material. To insure the correct response, always read the directions before attempting to answer.

Although many of the statements in the text are referenced, additional readings will be required to flesh out the concepts in the program and to document others further.

In my opinion, the best general English language text of adult psychiatry is the book by Slater and Roth (1969). For the reader who does not plan to specialize in psychiatry, this survey plus Woodruff, Goodwin and Guze's small, but well documented primer of Psychiatric Diagnosis (1974) should suffice.

For a more in-depth understanding of the phenomenological approach to psychopathology, Taylor and Heiser (1971) and Taylor (1972) should initially be read, followed by Hamilton's revisions of Fish's classic books. For those made of heroic stuff, Kurt Schneider's seminal work and Karl Jaspers' great General Psychopathology remain unsurpassed.

Further clinical descriptions, rich in detail and priceless in insight into the early development of clinical psychiatry, can be found in Bleuler's famous monograph (1950) on schizophrenia and in the more recent fascimilies of Kraepelin's lectures (1968) and treatises on dementia praecox (1971) and manic-depressive illness (1976) and Kahlbaum's monograph on catatonia (1973).

For a more in-depth presentation of neuropsychology, the Luria (1973) and Golden (1978) texts should suffice as an introduction to the study of higher cortical functions. A discussion of the relationships between higher cortical dysfunction and psychopathology can be found in Pincus and Tucker's (1978) Behavioral Neurology. Slater and Beard (1963), Herrington (1969) and Benson and Blumer (1975) provide detailed discussions of the behavioral manifestations of coarse brain disease.

Bibliography

Benson, D.F., Blumer, D. (Eds.): Psychiatric Aspects of Neurologic Disease. New York, Grune & Stratton, 1975.

Bleuler, E.: Dementia Praecox or the Group of Schizophrenias, (Trans. Zinkin), Int. University Press, 1950.

Golden, C.J.: Diagnosis & Rehabilitation in Clinical Neuropsychology, Springfield, C.C. Thomas, 1978.

Hamilton, M. (Ed.): Fish's Clinical Psychopathology, Signs and Symptoms in Psychiatry, Revised Reprints, Bristol, John Wright & Sons, Ltd., 1974.

Hamilton, M. (Ed.): Fish's Schizophrenia, Revised Reprints, Bristol, John Wright & Sons, Ltd., 1976.

Herrington, R.M. (Ed.): Current Problems in Neuropsychiatry: Schizophrenia, Epilepsy, the Temporal Lobe. Brit. J. Psychiat., Special Publication #4, Ashford, Kent. Headley Bros., Ltd., 1969.

Jaspers, K.: General Psychopathology, (Trans. J. Heonig and M.W. Hamilton), University Chicago Press, 1968.

Kahlbaum, K.L.: Catatonia, (Trans. Levy, Y. and Priden, T.), Baltimore, Johns Hopkins University Press, 1973.

Kraepelin, E.: Dementia Praecox & Paraphrenia, (Trans Barcley, R.M.; Ed., Robertson, G.M.), Focs. 1919 Edition, Huntington, New York, R.E. Kruger Publishing Company, 1971.

Kraepelin, E.: Lectures on Clinical Psychiatry, (Johnstone, T. Ed.) New York, Hafner, 1968.

Kraepelin, E.: Manic-Depressive Insanity and Paranoia, New York, Arno Press, 1976.

Luria, A.R.: The Working Brain: An Introduction to Neuropsychology, New York, Basic Books, Inc., 1973.

Pincus, J.H., Tucker, G.J.: Behavioral Neurology, 2nd Edition, New York, Oxford University Press, 1978.

Schneider, K.: Clinical Psychopathology, (Trans. M.W. Hamilton), New York, Grune & Stratton, 1959.

Slater, E., Roth, M.: Mayer Gross' Clinical Psychiatry, 3rd Edition, Baltimore, Williams & Wilkins, 1969.

Slater, E., Beard, A.W.: The Schizophrenia-like Psychoses of Epilepsy: 2. Psychiatric Aspects. Brit. J. Psychiat. 109:95-150, 1963.

Taylor, M.A., Heiser, J.: Phenomenology: An Alternative Approach To Diagnosis of Mental Disease. Compr. Psychiatry 12:480-486, 1971.

Taylor, M.A.: Schneiderian First Rank Symptoms and Clinical Prognostic Features in Schizophrenia. Arch. Gen. Psychiatry 26:64-67, 1972.

Woodruff, R.A., Goodwin, D.W., Guze, S.B.: Psychiatric Diagnosis, New York, Oxford University Press, 1974.

Contents

The Neuropsychiatric Mental Status Examination

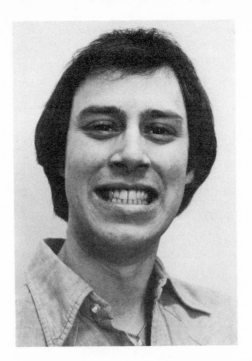

THE HUMORLESS SMILE CALLED "GRIMACE" SEEN IN CATATONIC PATIENTS

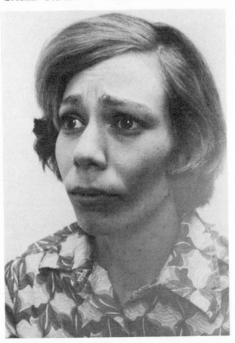

THE SAD EXPRESSION OF DEPRESSION

Part I

BASIC CONCEPTS

1.   The mental status examination is the psychiatric equivalent of the medical specialist's physical examination. It should be part of any complete medical evaluation and becomes meaningful only in the context of a complete physical and neurological examination. The mental status examination should include only observations of the patient's behavior and experiences during the examination (inter-view) period. Historical data including recent hallucinations and sui-cidal thoughts are past, not present experiences, and thus do not belong in the mental status. The goal of the mental status examination is not a psychotherapeutic interaction. It is a specialized evaluation of behavior and its goals are to establish a reasonable treater-patient relationship and a thorough evaluation of the patient's _____ _____ so that a working diagnosis can be established and a treatment plan developed, executed and monitored.

      Failure to limit the mental status examination to the patient's behavior during the interview makes evaluation of rapid behavioral changes difficult and often leads to erroneous clinical conclusions.

2.   Historical data is, of course, important and must be determined and recorded systematically. This information is then corroborated by the physical examination and the mental status evaluation. These examinations deal with the _____ status of the patient just as the historical examination deals with the patient's _____. A physician examining a patient with crushing chest pain would not be satisfied with a description of "I had no heart abnormalities last year." A physician practicing psychiatry should not be satisfied with the examination of a depressed patient who states: "I was not suicidal last year."

2

1. present behavior

2. present, past

3.   The mental status examination is based on objective observation of the patient's _____ behavior. Objective observation separates what you observe from what you believe or interpret.

Two examiners are looking at the same patient: The patient is sitting in a corner, talking to himself, masturbating in public, and constantly putting various objects he finds around him in his mouth. He appears completely unaware of the ward activities around him.

One of the examiners is quick to interpret the patient's behavior. He says, "That man's regressed." The second examiner who observes carefully sees the following behaviors: abnormal sexual behavior, orality, unusual placidity. These behaviors alert him; he shows the patient a pen and asks him to name it. The patient can't name it until he feels it. Only then does the examiner interpret his observations to suggest that the patient is suffering from Kluver-Bucy syndrome which indicates bilateral temporal lobe lesions (55). Objective _____ of _____, not past, behavior is a basic principle of the phenomenological mental status.

4.   Observations during the mental status exam should separate form (process) from the content of behavior. What a person is talking about, the subject matter, is content. How a person is talking, the fluency and accuracy of his speech, the grammatical correctness of his language is _____.

5.   The form of signs and symptoms is often diagnostic. On the other hand, the _____ of signs and symptoms is rarely of such diagnostic importance because it reflects individual experience and cultural learning rather than disease process. A bushman with a brain tumor might hallucinate an antelope whereas a Madison Avenue ad man with a similar tumor might hallucinate a bevy of models. Although the content is interesting, it is the fact that these two gentlemen see things that are not real (hallucinate) which is of prime importance and which indicates a pathological process.

6.   A patient said she heard her mother's voice coming from her radio, telling her that she was a bad girl and should kill herself. Circle the words and/or phrases that indicate the form of this experience.

7.   A patient said he clearly saw little men running through the streets screaming and waving knives at passersby. He said he was terrified and when the little men approached him, he ran away. Circle the words and/or phrases indicating the form of this experience.

8.   A patient said he felt metal worms crawling under his skin, up his arms and into his face and head. Circle the words and/or phrases indicating the form of this experience.

9.   Historical data can also be separated by form and content but the mental status includes only _____ _____.

3. present, observation, present

4. form

5. content

6. A patient said she(heard)her mother's(voice)(coming from her radio,) telling her that she was a bad girl and should kill herself.

7. A patient said he (clearly saw)little men running through the streets screaming and waving knives at passersby. He said he was terrified and when the little men approached him, he ran away.

    Although not stated, it is implied that this experience is perceived as occurring <u>outside</u> of the patient. This, too, is part of the form of this hallucination.

8. A patient said he(felt)metal worms(crawling under his skin,)up his arms and into his face and head.

9. present behavior

10.   In addition to relying heavily on objective _____ and separating behavior into _____ and _____, the phenomenologist's mental status as much as possible utilizes precise terminology.

11.   Precise terminology is necessary for accurate diagnosis. Often psychiatrists disagree about the meaning or usage of common psychiatric terms. Some use the term "paranoid" to mean delusional, others to mean suspicious or frightened and some as a synonym for schizophrenia. By avoiding such terms as "paranoid" and using instead more _____ terminology, phenomenologists try to reduce areas of confusion and disagreement. The use of precise terminology is as important for the psychiatrist as it is for the internist. Just as the internist would not be satisfied with a description of heart sounds as "odd" or "abnormal," so, too, the psychiatrist should not be satisfied with descriptions as "bizarre behavior," "incoherent speech," "paranoid."

12.   The phenomenologic mental status is based on three principles: objective _____, the separation of the _____ and _____ of behavior, and _____ terminology.

13.   Below are some words and phrases. Circle those suggesting behavior form:
"I don't think I'm well"   "A clear voice"
"A voice from inside my head"   "It says 'kill yourself'"

14.   Below are some words and phrases. Circle the words suggesting behavior content:
"A clear voice"   "The smell of burning flesh"
"Little men with knives"   "My father's voice"

15.   Below are some words and phrases. Circle the words suggesting behavior form:
Visual hallucination   "A green gas"
"A voice from outside my head"   "I'm upset about my job"

16.   The following statements are true about the phenomenological mental status except one (circle your answer).

a.   Precise terminology of objective observation is essential for a proper examination.

b.   What the patient is talking about is not nearly as diagnostically important as how he is talking.

c.   Only behaviors during the examination are recorded as part of the mental status.

d.   The identity of a hallucinated voice, e.g., who it is, is important.

In the following sections, I will describe the major areas of the mental status; how to examine and elicit psychopathology, and how to distinguish different signs and symptoms.

10. observations, form, content

11. precise

12. observation, form, content, precise

13. "I don't think I'm well" _____   ("A clear voice")
     ("A voice from inside my head")   "It says 'kill yourself'"

14. "A clear voice" _____   ("The smell of burning flesh")
     ("Little men with knives")   ("My father's voice")

15. (Visual hallucination) _____   "A green gas"
     ("A voice from outside my head")   "I'm upset about my job"

16. d. This is not true because it deals with content.

INTERVIEW CONSIDERATIONS

17.   As all the patient's _____ behaviors are important
for consideration in the mental status examination, the patient's
general appearance is the first behavioral area to be evaluated.

18.   The examiner should, whenever possible, greet the patient out
of the examining room and walk with him to the area selected for
the interview. The examination begins when you first see the patient, not when you sit down. How the patient greets you, how the
patient walks and moves are all part of the first behavioral area of
the mental status examination, the patient's _____.

19.   Inexperienced examiners often express the misconception that
they must remain impersonal with patients. The unresponsive "blank
screen" approach to interviewing is not appropriate to the mental status examination. When should you first begin evaluating the
patient? _____

20.   It is often helpful to explain your reasons for speaking with the
patient and what you are going to do and not do. Patients have
the right to be informed about their condition and treatments, and
of your opinions concerning their illness. Within the limits of good
judgment, you should uphold this right.

21.   Often the best approach for obtaining the information you need
in a mental status examination is to engage the patient in a "conversation". No matter how structured an interview, the maintenance
of a _____al atmosphere will increase your chan-
ces of success (i.e., obtaining enough information to make a working diagnosis and treatment plan). In our society, normal conversation between strangers or acquaintances has certain rules. The
inexperienced examiner often suspends these rules during a mental
status examination. It is surprising how frequently an initial "Hello,
I am Dr. So and So" is ignored in favor of a more clinical but less
effective opening such as "What's today's date?"

22.   A good mental status examination, while _____ in atmosphere, should not be haphazard. Some structuring is important.

8

17. present

18. general appearance

19. When you first see the patient

20. No answer required

21. conversation

22. conversational

23.   Your examination questions and actions should proceed in a logical pattern, yet remain responsive to the specific needs and behaviors of the patient. Your examination goals of establishing a working _____ and developing a treatment _____ and
follow-up monitoring of treatment should always be kept in mind.

24.   When you first meet a patient, who is standing sedately in the
hall, a pleasant "hello" is a fine opening. However, for the patient
who is standing on top of a table and cursing the devils about him,
a "Hello, I'm Dr. So and So, how are you?" does not direct the quality of your statements to the global behavior of the patient. Below are some descriptions of patient's global behavior. Draw lines
between each description and the appropriate opening statement.

"Hello, I'm Dr. Jones."   Elderly woman, sitting on
                                       the floor, crying.

"What's the matter?"   An elderly man, lying in
                                       bed, reading.

"I'm Dr. Jones. Let's sit   Middle aged man rushes to
down and we can talk   you and starts offering one
about this."   complaint after the other.

"Stop that. Sit down. I   A young man, standing in
want to talk with you."   the hall, starts beating him-
                                       self with his hands on his
                                       chest and head.

25.   Circle those words or phrases consistent with a good mental
status examination:

1. conversational atmosphere
2. unresponsive "blank screen" approach
3. the examination begins when you first see the patient
4. questions asked in logical pattern
5. unstructured without sequence
6. examination goal is to establish a working diagnosis and treat-
    ment plan

26.   Patients with psychiatric illnesses often ask direct and personal
questions. Although responses to personal questions must be limited, patients do have the right to know something about the person
examining and testing them, and truthful responses to questions
about your education, experience or professional role (e.g., student,
resident) are often helpful in maintaining a good relationship with
the patient. Such questions are part of any normal conversation.
In addition to their direct questioning of the examiner, patients
often say or do things that are quite humorous. When it is obvious
that you are not making fun of their illness, do not be afraid to laugh.
If humor and responses to questions help achieve the goals of the
examination, they are appropriate. Write a sentence explaining
the goals of a mental status examination.

23. diagnosis, plan

24. "Hello, I'm Dr. Jones".   Elderly woman, sitting on the floor
                                 crying.

    "What's the matter?"   An elderly man, lying in bed, reading.

    "I'm Dr. Jones. Let's sit——Middle aged man rushes to you and
    down and we can talk   starts offering one complaint after
    about this."   the other.

    "Stop that. Sit down. I——A young man, standing in the hall,
    want to talk with you".   starts beating himself with his hands
                                 on his chest and head.

25. 1. conversational atmosphere
     2. unresponsive "blank screen" approach
     3. the examination begins when you first see the patient
     4. questions asked in logical pattern
     5. unstructured without sequence
     6. examination goal is to establish a working diagnosis and treat-
        ment plan

26. The goals of the mental status examination are to establish a rea-
    sonable treater-patient relationship so that a thorough diagnostic
    evaluation can be made (a working diagnosis) and a treatment plan
    developed.

GENERAL APPEARANCE, MOTOR BEHAVIOR AND CATATONIA

27.   In the mental status examination, the first behavioral area to be evaluated is the patient's _____ _____.

28.   General appearance includes observations of body type, sex, age, race, nutrition, health, and personal hygiene. Your general impressions of the patient's manner and state of consciousness are included here. Below are a number of statements. Circle those related to general appearance.

Short and stocky   Unkempt
Hostile and suspicious   Sleepy and dazed
Says he hears voices   Owns a dress shop
Alert   Born in 1928

29.   An individual's state of consciousness refers to his degree of arousal or cortical activation. It is determined early in the examination and is included in the behavioral area: _____ _____.

30.   Cortical activation or _____ results from activity which begins in brain stem structures and is projected through the thalamus to the cortex (48).

31.   The degree of arousal or cortical _____ will determine the clinical state (levels) of consciousness.

32.   The different states of cortical activation can produce different states (levels) of _____ . These include: a) alertness; b) lethargy; c) semicoma; and d) coma.

27. general appearance

28. (Short and stocky)   (Unkempt)
    (Hostile and suspicious)   (Sleepy and dazed)
    Says he hears voices   Owns a dress shop
    (Alert)   Born in 1928

29. general appearance

30. arousal

31. activation

32. consciousness

33.   Clinical items such as those below become important as their presence or absence increases or decreases the probabilities of different disorders. Draw lines between appropriate items in the two columns:

Short and stocky   Body type
Unkempt   Manner
Hostile & suspicious   Full cortical activation
Alert   Altered level of arousal
Sleepy and dazed   Personal hygiene

34.   Draw lines between appropriate items in the two columns:

Comatose   Awake and appropriate answers all questions

Alert   Keeps on falling asleep, occassionally fails to respond to examiner's questions

Lethargic   Unresponsive to questions unless examiner shakes patient and shouts

Semicomatose   Unresponsive even to painful stimulation

35.   A patient's manner, or attitude, is also part of general appearance behaviors and can provide clues as to the reliability of the information you are trying to obtain. Cooperative/uncooperative, friendly/suspicious, open/guarded, submissive/haughty, are descriptive terms of some of the more common patient attitudes.

36.   The general appearance of a patient includes state of _____ or cortical _____ and attitude or _____. In addition, general descriptions such as an author would use to describe a character in a book should be utilized when recording your mental status examination findings.

37.   Below are two brief descriptions of a patient's general appearance. Such details often have diagnostic importance because they either increase or decrease the probability of a variety of mental conditions. Examine the two descriptions and see if all the general appearance items are covered. Review the general appearance items listed and after each description circle those items, if any, which are missing in each example:

   A. The patient is a 32-year-old, cooperative, white, ecto-morphic man (thin, small boned, small framed, little muscle mass) who appears thin, stoop-shouldered and dazed. He is unkempt, has nicotine-stained fingers and he moves in a slow, absent-minded fashion.

       age, race, sex, body type, state of consciousness, manner, nutrition, health, personal hygiene

   B. The patient is a short, stocky, hirsute, long armed, muscular 42-year-old woman, whose greasy sweat, frozen face and general bradykinesia (decreased movement) suggest recent use of neuroleptics.

       age, race, sex, body type, state of consciousness, manner, nutrition, health, personal hygiene

14

33. Short and stocky————————Body type
    Unkempt   Manner
    Hostile & suspicious————Full cortical activation
    Alert ———————————Altered level of arousal
    Sleepy and dazed ———————Personal hygiene

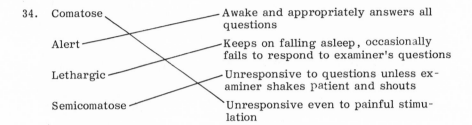

34. Comatose   Awake and appropriately answers all
                              questions

    Alert   Keeps on falling asleep, occasionally
                              fails to respond to examiner's questions

    Lethargic   Unresponsive to questions unless ex-
                              aminer shakes patient and shouts

    Semicomatose   Unresponsive even to painful stimu-
                              lation

35. no answer required

36. consciousness, activation, manner

37. A. The patient is a 32-year-old, cooperative, white ectomorphic
       man (thin, small boned, small framed, little muscle mass) who
       appears thin, stoop-shouldered and dazed. He is unkempt,
       has nicotine-stained fingers and he moves in a slow, absent-
       minded fashion.

       age, race, sex, body type, state of consciousness, manner,
       nutrition, health, personal hygiene

       None circled because all items are described

    B. The patient is a short, stocky, hirsute, long-armed, muscular
       42-year-old woman, whose greasy sweat, frozen face, and gen-
       eral bradykinesia (decreased movement) suggest recent use of
       neuroleptics.

       age, (race,) sex, body type, (state of consciousness, (manner,)
       nutrition, health, (personal hygiene)

15

38.   Obvious patient characteristics (e.g., age, sex) are often vital in developing an accurate diagnosis. If you do not consciously state the obvious, you will often omit the key to the diagnosis. In Item 37.B the facial hair and stocky body build of the patient were clues suggesting her depression was secondary to adrenal hyperplasia. Proper treatment (in this case surgery) would not have been possible without proper observations leading to an accurate

_____ .

39.   Look at the photograph at the right. Although you cannot comment on manner and state of consciousness, 1) describe the patient; and 2) what would you say to begin an interview with this patient?

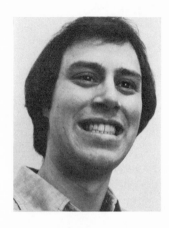

40.   Look at the photograph at the right. Describe the patient's general appearance.

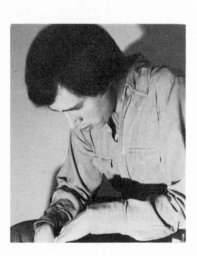

41.   Following an examination and description of the patient's ____ _____ _____ , you should observe the patient's motor behavior. Motor behavior, like the items of general appearance, is observed _____ .

38. diagnosis

39. 1) A young white male, staring fixedly into space. He has an exaggerated smile (grimace) without warmth. Remainder of general appearance items cannot be evaluated from this photograph.
   2) "Mr. Jones, what are you doing? Can you look at me? I'd like
   to speak with you."

40. A young, slim, mesomorphic (average build) white male who sits
   slumped over in a dejected manner staring at the floor. He appears
   neat and clean. (Further comments about level of consciousness,
   manner and cooperativeness will require additional observation.)

41. general appearance, initially upon meeting the patient

42.   Whenever possible, you should meet your patient in a location away from the place of examination so you have to walk with the patient. Carefully watch the patient's gait and note any abnormalities. If there is a problem, ask the patient if he is aware of it and to what he attributes his difficulty in walking.

43.   In addition to observations of gait, the examination should include comments upon: abnormal movements, frequency of movement, rhythm or coordination and motor speed. How would you begin examining these motor behaviors without disrupting your initial attempts to establish a relationship with the patient?

44.   The increase in frequency of motor behavior is termed agitation. Pacing, hand wringing, head rubbing, constant shifting of body position, are all examples of increased _____ of motor behavior or _____.

45.   Any intense mood (anxiety, depression, anger) may be expressed in the motor behavior of agitation or _____ _____
_____.

46.   The motor expression of an intense mood is termed _____.
Pacing, hand wringing, head rubbing, shifting body positions are all examples of this increased frequency of motor behavior.

47.   General restlessness, shifting body position, hand rubbing or playing with one's fingers are examples of _____.

48.   Agitation is the motor expression of an intense mood. Circle those words or phrases descriptive of agitation:

Impassive	Restless	Pacing
Foot tapping	Guilt	Hand rubbing
Immobile		

49.   Because of chronic ingestion of neuroleptic compounds, many psychiatric patients exhibit constant foot tapping, jerky pacing, pelvic thrusts and/or repetitive oral movements such as lip smacking, or moving the tongue in and out of the mouth. These increased movements are manifestations of a coarse brain disease and have been given the global term tardive dyskinesia (6,20). It should not be confused with agitation which is the motor manifestation of an _____ _____.

50.   Agitation can also be confused with the small, jerky hand, head and shoulder movements characteristic of chorea. Agitation can be distinguished from choreiform movement because it is under partial voluntary control and because it is the motor expression of an
_____ _____.

51.   The increased frequency of activities (as opposed to frequency of motor behavior or agitation) is termed hyperactivity. When the frequency of activities is decreased, it is termed hypo_____.

52.   Increased frequency of motor behavior is termed _____.
Increased frequency of activities is termed _____ and is usually goal directed.

18

42. No answer required

43. I would meet the patient away from the examination area and walk with him as I observe and perhaps discuss his motor difficulties, if any.

44. frequency, agitation

45. increased frequency of motor behavior

46. agitation

47. agitation

48. Impassive   (Restless)   (Pacing)
    (Foot tapping)   Guilt   (Hand rubbing)
    Immobile

49. intense mood

50. intense mood

51. activity

52. agitation, hyperactivity

19

53.   A patient who talks to several people, one after the other, who goes from one place to another in quick succession, is said to be _____active.

54.   A patient who sits for long periods in a corner chair, rarely moving or responding to surrounding action, is said to be _____ active.

55.   In its extreme form, hyperactivity will lead to multiple activities that are never completed and which appear purposeless (non-goal directed). This is called an excitement state. In contrast, _____ _____, or decreased frequency of activities, in its extreme form is called a stuporous state (37, 40 pp. 26-29, pp. 36-40, pp. 79-80).

56.   In extreme hypoactivity or _____, a patient may stay motionless for hours, staring fixedly or following the examiner about the room with his eyes, unresponsive even to severe pain stimulation (general analgesia) (37, 40 pp. 36-40, pp. 79-80).

57.   In extreme hyperactivity or _____, a patient may continually rush about until exhausted. Patients have been known to suffer cardiovascular collapse and even death as the result of extreme _____ (37,40).

58.   Pacing, hand wringing, head rubbing, is not goal directed. It is termed _____.

59.   Draw a line between the term in column A and its description(s) in column B. A term can be used more than once.

A	B
Hyperactivity	Restlessness
Hypoactivity	Dancing, singing, cleaning, washing and telephoning in rapid succession
Agitation	Pacing the halls
	Spree buying, yelling at passersby, writing one dozen letters, moving the furniture out of the house
	Sitting in the same position for hours

60.   It is difficult to distinguish severe agitation from a state of excitement or severe _____ because in excitement the patient impulsively interrupts one activity to begin another, thus losing apparent goal direction.

61.   When a patient exhibits extreme hyperactivity or _____ or extreme hypoactivity or _____, the diagnosis of Catatonia must be considered (37,40 p. 36).

62.   Catatonia is a syndrome (2,37) which, in 25 to 50 percent of cases (2,40 p. 36,53,74) is associated with major affective or mood disorder. In addition to specific motor behaviors to be considered, catatonia is characterized by periods of extreme hyperactivity and hypoactivity, also termed _____ and _____.

53. hyper

54. hypo

55. hypoactivity

56. stupor

57. excitement, hyperactivity

58. agitation

59. Hyperactivity   Restlessness

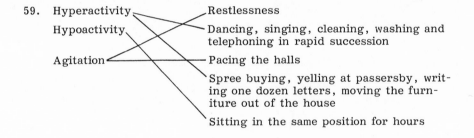

Hyperactivity   Restlessness

Hypoactivity   Dancing, singing, cleaning, washing and telephoning in rapid succession

Agitation   Pacing the halls

Spree buying, yelling at passersby, writing one dozen letters, moving the furniture out of the house

Sitting in the same position for hours

60. hyperactivity

61. excitement, stupor

62. excitement, stupor

63.   Mutism is a state of verbal unresponsiveness. In association with stupor or excitement, mutism is characteristic of _____. However, other specific motor behaviors should be present before the diagnosis of _____ is made.

64.   A flat, expressionless face without eye blinking is most characteristic of catatonia. Grimacing and other fixed facial postures can occur (37). Look at the photographs below. Check the facial expressions consistent with catatonia.

1   **2**   **3**   **4**

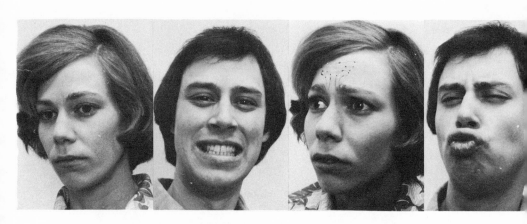

65.   The photograph of face #3 should not be checked in answer to question 64. This is the typical facial expression in major depression. Two outstanding characteristics of a depressed face are: 1. the Omega sign; and 2. Veraguth's folds (33,58). The Omega sign is a furrowing between the eyebrows that looked to an imaginative clinician of long ago like the Greek letter Ω (Omega). Veraguth described eyelid folds which formed an upward angle at the inner canthus of the eye.

63. catatonia, catatonia

64. photographs 1, 2, and 4

    1 - blank look

    2 - grimace

    4 - schnauzkrampf (German. literally: snout cramp)

      Note: Number 3 does NOT belong in this category as it is
      the expression typical of major depression.

65. No answer required.

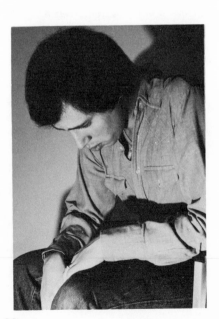

A posture characteristic of
depressive stupor.

66.   Catatonic patients, although often verbally unresponsive or
_____, can be accurately diagnosed because of the odd
positions they assume. This is called posturing.

67.   The tendency of catatonic patients to remain in postures for long
periods is called catalepsy.

68.   Patients often allow an examiner to place them in odd postures
despite instructions to the contrary. The initial resistance these
patients offer prior to slowly allowing themselves to be postured,
reminded early clinicians of a bending candle, thus the term waxy
flexibility. Below are photographs of a catatonic "patient" in several different postures. Since he is maintaining these postures for
prolonged periods, he demonstrates

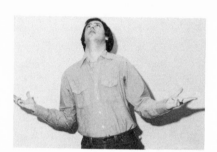 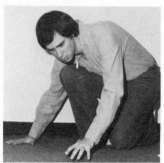

69.   When a patient positions his body or body parts in an odd way,
he is said to be _____.

70.   When a patient remains in the same position or odd posture for
a prolonged period of time, he is said to have _____.

71.   An odd body position is a _____. A prolonged body
position is _____.

66. mute

67. no answer required

68. catalepsy

69. posturing

70. catalepsy

71. posturing, catalepsy

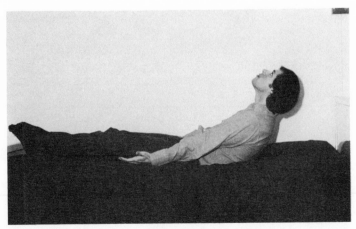

"Psychological Pillow" is a Catatonic Posture

25

72.   Patients in catatonic stupor can remain motionless or cataleptic for hours. They stare fixedly, and even when subjected to pain stimulation, they remain immobile (general analgesia). They are also mute or verbally _____.

73.   Some cataleptic patients (in a prolonged posture) resist the examiner's attempts to move their limbs. The patients exert an amount of force equal to that of the examiner: when the examiner pushes the patient's arm lightly, the patient resists to the same extent. When the examiner pulls the patient's arm vigorously, the patient resists with equal strength. This phenomenon is called Gegenhalten and is a sign of _____.

74.   Draw lines between appropriate items in the two columns:

Posturing   Severe hyperactivity

Excitement   Psychological pillow

Waxy flexibility   Slow resistance as patient allows examiner to place him in odd posture

Stupor   Increased motor frequency due to intense affect

Agitation   Severe hypoactivity often associated with generalized analgesia

75.   Draw lines between appropriate items in the two columns:

Catalepsy   The furrowed brow of depression

Omega sign   The patient resists being moved with strength equal to that applied

Gegenhalten   Spending hours in one position

Veraguth folds   The sad eyes of depression

Grimacing   A facial posture

76.   Draw a line between the matching items in the two columns:

Severe hypoactivity Frantically going from task to task until exhausted

Agitation   Immobile and unresponsive

Severe hyperactivity Rocking, pacing, hand wringing

72. unresponsive

73. catatonia

74. Posturing   Severe hyperactivity
    Excitement   Psychological pillow
    Waxy flexibility ——— Slow resistance as patient allows examiner
                                     to place him in odd posture
    Stupor   Increased motor frequency due to intense
                                     affect
    Agitation   Severe hypoactivity often associated with
                                     generalized analgesia

75. Catalepsy   The furrowed brow of depression
    Omega sign   The patient resists being moved with strength
                                     equal to that applied
    Gegenhalten   Spending hours in one position
    Veraguth folds ——— The sad eyes of depression
    Grimacing ——— A facial posture

76. Severe hypoactivity   Frantically going from task to task until
                                     exhausted
    Agitation   Immobile and unresponsive
    Severe hyperactivity   Rocking, pacing, hand wringing

77.   The motor signs of catatonia remain some of the most fascinating phenomena observed in psychiatric patients. Echo phenomena are part of the catatonic syndrome. Echolalia refers to the patient's constant repeating of the last phrase or sentence of the examiner. Echopraxia refers to the patient's copying of the interviewer's motor behavior. In the examination of a patient suspected of having catatonia, the examiner, by raising his arm above his head without comment, can often stimulate the patient to respond in a similar fashion, i.e., exhibiting _____. The examiner can also ask "When I touch my nose you touch your chest." If, despite repeated corrections, the patient also touches his nose, mimicking the examiner's movement, he is exhibiting _____. The obvious repetition of your sentences is an example of _____.

78.   Catatonic patients will often respond to light pressure, even when instructed to the contrary. If you lightly press the patient's hand and arm upward and the patient responds to the pressure despite your instructions not to lift his arm, you have demonstrated the phenomenon of Mitgehen (German for "going with"). The cooperation to light pressure by the examiner followed by a slow return to a previous position is termed Mitmachen (German for "making with"). These phenomena can be considered forms of automatic obedience to light pressure and are known by the German terms _____ _____ and _____.

79.   Place a check mark in the appropriate box to indicate into which mental status section each behavior item best fits. Check each item only once.

	General Appearance	General Motor Behavior	Catatonia
Body type			
Echopraxia			
Mitmachen			
Agitation			
Age & Sex			
Catalepsy			
Gait			
Dress			

77. echopraxia, echopraxia, echolalia

78. Mitgehen, Mitmachen

79.

	General Appearance	General Motor Behavior	Catatonia
Body type	√		
Echopraxia			√
Mitmachen			√
Agitation		√	
Age & Sex	√		
Catalepsy			√
Gait	√	√(Accepted)	
Dress	√		

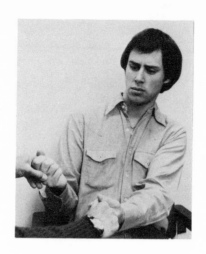

GEGENHALTEN

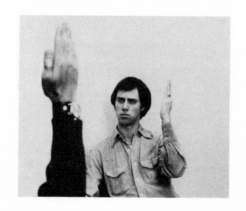

ECHOPRAXIA

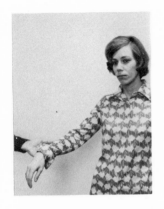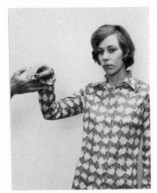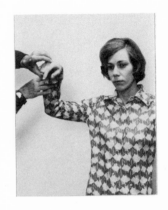

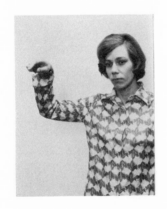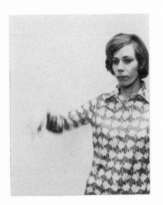

MITMACHEN

31

80.　　　Beside each major grouping of behaviors, place the numbers of the appropriate items listed below to indicate into which mental status section each behavior item best fits. Use each item only once. General appearance _____ ; General motor behavior _____ _____ ; Catatonia _____ .

1. Race
2. Hypoactive
3. Mitgehen
4. Echopraxia
5. Agitation

6. Personal Hygiene
7. Gegenhalten
8. Hyperactive
9. State of Consciousness

81.　　　In demonstrating automatic obedience (Mitgehen, Mitmachen) a patient will allow himself to be placed into postures with _____ _____ pressure from the examiner.

82.　　　You are speaking with a patient and suddenly without comment you raise your left arm high in the air. The patient copies your movement. You then also raise your right arm in the air and again the patient repeats the movement. This is an example of _____ _____ .

83.　　　You must tell the patient he should not respond when you want to demonstrate _____ obedience. Otherwise you cannot be sure that the response is not simply the result of a very cooperative patient trying to please you.

84.　　　When observing catatonic patients over prolonged periods of time, psychiatrists have noted striking non-goal directed, repetitive motor behaviors termed stereotypes. These patients may also exhibit stereotype of speech in which they repeat phrases and sentences in an automatic fashion, similar to a scratched record. On the other hand, when the patient's speech is a repetition of your speech, it is termed _____ .

85.　　　A patient standing next to your desk automatically moves your paperweight back and forth from one spot to another. You have observed a behavior termed _____ .

86.　　　Occasionally, the non-goal directed repetitive motor behavior of catatonics is mistakenly called obsessive compulsive behavior. We know, however, that the correct term is _____ .

87.　　　The patient with obsessive compulsive behavior knows the behavior is "foolish" but feels great anxiety until the compulsion to perform the behavior is obeyed. The patient with automatic repetitive behavior or _____ has no such awareness of the "foolishness" of his behavior.

80. General appearance: 1) Race; 6) Personal hygiene; 9) State of consciousness

General motor behavior: 2) Hypoactive; 5) Agitation, 8) Hyperactive
Catatonia: 3) Mitgehen; 4) Echopraxia; 7) Gegenhalten

81. light

82. echopraxia

83. automatic

84. echolalia

85. stereotype

86. stereotype

87. stereotype

88.   Draw lines between matching items in the two columns:

Stereotype   The patient repeats your movements

Echopraxia   Non-goal directed, automatic, repetitive move-
                      ment

Mitgehen   The patient repeats your words

Echolalia   Despite your verbal instructions to the contrary,
                      the patient allows you to move his arms with
                      light pressure

89.   Draw lines between matching items in the two columns.

Mitmachen   Despite your verbal instructions to the contrary,
                      the patient lets you posture his arm and when
                      released, slowly moves it back to its original
                      place

Stupor   Maintaining a posture for long periods

Catalepsy   Severe hypoactivity

Gegenhalten   When you attempt to move a patient's arm, he
                      resists with a force equal to yours

90.   Draw lines between appropriate items in the two columns:

Veraguth folds   Furrow between the eyebrows

Omega sign   Upward angle of inner canthus of eye in
                      depression

Waxy flexibility   Assuming odd body positions

Posturing   Gradual resistance but allowing placement in
                      odd body postures

91.   Draw lines between appropriate items in the two columns:

Excitement   Increased non-goal directed motor activity--
                      an expression of intense affect

Agitation   Extreme hyperactivity

Mitgehen   The patient repeats your words

Echolalia   Automatic obedience

92.   You are asked to examine a 27-year-old white male patient whom
you find lying in bed, eyes open, staring fixedly at the ceiling.
As you approach, the patient quickly shuts his eyes and the nurse
says "You see, I told you he was faking!" Knowing better, you
proceed to examine the patient and find that he has no fever, has
stable vital signs, and no focal neurological signs. When you check
his chart, you note that his laboratory tests are also within normal
limits and that no systemic cause has been found for his mutism,
immobility, and unresponsiveness. In testing the patient for response to painful stimuli, you observe general analgesia and conclude
that he is in a state of _____.

34

88. Stereotype —— The patient repeats your movements

Echopraxia —— Non-goal directed, automatic, repetitive movement

Mitgehen —— The patient repeats your words

Echolalia —— Despite your verbal instructions to the contrary, the patient allows you to move his arm with light pressure

89. Mitmachen —————— Despite your verbal instructions to the contrary, the patient lets you posture his arm and when released, slowly moves it back to its original place

Stupor —— Maintaining a posture for long periods

Catalepsy —— Severe hypoactivity

Gegenhalten —————— When you attempt to move a patient's arm, he resists with a force equal to yours

90. Veraguth folds —— Furrow between the eyebrows

Omega sign —— Upward angle of inner canthus of eye in depression

Waxy flexibility —— Assuming odd body positions

Posturing —— Gradual resistance but allowing placement in odd body postures

91. Excitement —— Increased non-goal directed motor activity-- an expression of intense affect

Agitation —— Extreme hyperactivity

Mitgehen —— The patient repeats your words

Echolalia —— Automatic obedience

92. stupor

   Catatonia is not acceptable here as not all stuporous patients are catatonic and not all catatonic patients are stuporous, i.e., immobility with general analgesia is not always present in catatonia.

35

93.   Continually harassed by the medical staff who are now greatly
impressed with your knowledge, you are asked to see a 23-year-old
black woman who was hospitalized because of a "violent" episode in
which she ran about the streets screaming, talking to people in a
confused manner, and finally collapsing into an unresponsive mute
condition. Again, "physical" examination and laboratory tests are
within normal limits.
     When you see the patient, she is standing next to her bed, one
arm raised above her head. The other arm is placed on her heart.
According to the nurse she has remained this way for a long time
and you conclude these are examples of _____ and
_____. She does not answer your questions and stares
fixedly ahead. You tell her to remain where she is and not to move;
then, with your index finger, you apply light pressure to her back
and she begins to walk forward. You again tell her, in an author-
itative voice, not to move, but with continued light pressure she
moves forward. You conclude she also exhibits _____
_____.
     Not yet satisfied, you apply light pressure to her raised arm
and although you tell her to resist, she allows you to move her arm
into a new position. When you remove your index finger, she remains in the new posture for a few moments and then slowly returns
to her former posture. You note this example of _____
and make a diagnosis of _____.

94.   You are now the talk of the entire hospital and colleagues are
desperately trying to find a chink in your armor by asking you to
see their most perplexing patients. One such patient is a 17-year-
old male who has enraged the staff by constantly mimicking what
they say and do. When you observe him doing this, you note the
automatic quality of his copying of the speech and motor behavior
of others, and you suggest to the staff that the patient is not a
"little brat" but may have catatonia and that he is exhibiting echolalia and echopraxia. They laugh at you, convinced they've finally
got you. Undaunted, you approach the patient, introduce yourself,
explain that you are going to examine him (he, of course, repeats
your words), and then you take hold of his arm and try to move
it but you feel equal resistance. If you pull hard, he resists strongly; if you pull weakly, his resistance is equally weak. You note
this example of _____ and then are surprised when
the patient suddenly sticks out his lips in a snout-like position
and then falls to his knees in a praying attitude. He remains in
this posture for 10 minutes at which time you take hold of his arm
and after some initial resistance, you feel a sudden give and then
lessening resistance as you place the arm in awkward positions
which the patient maintains. You tell your colleagues that you have
demonstrated _____; that
the patient is in a prolonged posture or _____ state and
that the diagnosis is indeed the syndrome of _____.

AFFECT

95.   For a complete mental status examination you must first examine
a patient's _____ _____ and _____
_____. You should next make careful note of his affect.
Affect is the emotional tone underlying all behaviors.

36

93. posturing, catalepsy, automatic obedience, mitmachen, catatonia.

94. Gegenhalten, waxy flexibility, cateleptic, catatonia

95. general appearance, motor behavior

96.   Affect has range, amplitude, stability, appropriateness of mood, quality of mood, and relatedness. Mood is only one facet of _____
_____ .

97.   Mood and affect are not synonymous terms. Normal mood refers to relatively transient expressions of sadness, happiness, anxiety, anger, and apathy. Mood is but a part of an individual's _____ _____ which is a more global function.

98.   The mnemonic device SHAAA may help you recall the different transient expressions of mood. They are _____ , _____ , _____ , _____ , and _____ .

99.   Relatively transient expressions of sadness, happiness, anxiety, anger, and apathy are termed _____ . The different types of mood expressed refer to the quality of mood.

100.   In mental illness, the quality of _____ may become constant despite changes in the patient's immediate surroundings. Patients with affective disorders can express a constant mood of sadness, elation, or irritability (18,40 pp. 22-24, 58,71).

101.   The variability of emotional expression over a period of time is the range of affect. Normal _____ of _____ can be compared to the variations and resonances in music. The variability of emotional expression or _____ of _____ can be constricted in mental disease.

102.   If a person essentially expresses only one mood over a period of time, regardless of what is taking place around him, his _____ _____ of affect is said to be _____ , i.e., there is little variability.

103.   If a person expresses only sadness, his affective range is _____ . If a person expresses only euphoria, his affective range is _____ . In both instances, although the quality of mood is different, the variability over time is the same.

104.   The amplitude of emotions can be graded by the amount of energy a person is expending in expressing a mood. The different qualities of mood, the transient expressions of emotions are associated with differing degrees of amplitude. Thus, the quality of anger can be associated with mild amplitude and is expressed as annoyance or irritability, or it can be expressed with great amplitude as anger and rage. List the different qualities of mood.

105.   Amplitude of affect states nothing about range of affect, which refers to the _____ of emotional expression.

106.   In many patients, affectivity, although intense (with great amplitude) can be constricted in range. The psychomotor epileptic, for example, can shout and rage with great force, never varying his mood until overcome by exhaustion. His range of affect is severely _____ but the amplitude of his affect is intense.

96. affect

97. affect

98. sadness, happiness, anxiety, anger, apathy

99. moods

100. mood

101. range, affect, range, affect

102. range, constricted

103. constricted, constricted

104. sadness, happiness, anxiety, anger, apathy

105. variability

106. constricted

107.   Normal changes in mood occur relatively slowly during the course
of the day and are well modulated. Rapid shifts during the time of
a mental status exam are pathological. Shifts in mood quality (e.g.,
anger to sadness) and in amplitude (e.g., mild to intense) refer to
the stability of affect. List the different qualities of mood. Can
affect be restricted in range and be of high intensity?

108.   Instability of affect termed lability, is most characteristic of
mania (18, 40 pp. 22-24, 71) and various coarse brain syndromes
(14,15,23). Draw a line between appropriate items in each column.

Constricted range of affect	Relatively constant expression of one mood
Decreased intensity of affect	Moods shift rapidly and frequently during a short period of time
Labile affect	Expression of little emotional energy

109.   Mood appropriateness refers only to the interview situation and
is determined in part by the examiner's own mental state and empathic understanding of the patient's behavior. What you judge to
be appropriate becomes the standard by which you evaluate the patient's behavior. Inappropriateness of mood (laughing in a sad situation) is not a pathognomonic sign (decisive indicator of a specific disorder) and may be simply the reflection of normal anxiety as
well as serious illness. Look at the descriptive phrases below and
using your empathy ("put yourself in the patient's shoes") check
those indicating inappropriateness of mood.

The patient screams in terror at a hallucinated voice.

In discussing the recent death of his parents, a patient
bursts into tears.

When asked about the events leading to her hospitalization,
a patient became angry and said she'd been wrongfully
locked up after a fight with her husband.

110.   You may hear colleagues use the term "inappropriate affect."
However, what they really mean is inappropriate _____.

111.   The most difficult facet of affect to describe and rate is relatedness. Relatedness refers to the patient's ability to express warmth,
to interact emotionally and to establish rapport with the examiner.
Schizophrenics are notoriously unable to respond in this manner
and often appear cold and unfeeling (12,13,41,42). You might feel
you are addressing a computerized voice or taped answering machine rather than a person. When a patient can express warmth and
can establish rapport with you, his affect is said to be _____.
When this rapport is missing and the patient appears cold and unfeeling, his affect is said to be _____.

107. sadness, happiness, anxiety, anger, apathy (SHAAA)
     yes

108. Constricted range of affect ————— Relatively constant expression
                                         of one mood

     Decreased intensity of affect ╲   ╱ Moods shift rapidly and freq-
                                     ╲   ╱   uently during a short period
                                      ╲ ╱   of time
                                       ╳
                                      ╱ ╲
     Labile affect ╱   ╲ Expression of little emotional
                                       energy

109. No checks. If you believed in the reality of frightening voices, you
     too would be terrified. Crying at a recent loss is appropriate. If
     you believed you'd been wrongfully locked up, you too would be
     angry. Remember, your empathy will determine appropriateness of
     mood.

110. mood

111. related, unrelated

112.   Draw a line between appropriate items in the two columns:

Relatedness   A strong mood, such as rage, fear

Affect of increased   Ability to express warmth, concern,
intensity   love

Quality of mood   Emotions of anger, happiness, sadness

Inappropriate mood   Sudden explosive laughter without
                                apparent reason

113.   Lack of relatedness is often called flatness of affect or emotional
blunting. Although considered crucial for the diagnosis of schizophrenia by most authors (12,13,41,42,65,70) the determination of
emotional _____ is difficult.

114.   The global impression of emotional blunting can be separated
into component parts which are more easily evaluated during a mental status examination. This method has been found to be reliable
(reproducible) and when used in a rating scale, helpful in diagnos-
ing patients with major mental illness (3). Decreased intensity of
affect and the lack of mood variations, or _____ affect,
are characteristic of emotional blunting.

115.   In addition to _____ range and _____ intensity of
affect, patients with emotional blunting often present with an expressionless face and unblinking eyes and speak in an unvarying
monotonous voice.

116.   Emotionally _____ individuals are often seclusive, a-
voiding social contact, and indifferent to their surroundings (hospital staff, visitors, relatives, physical environs).

     "How do you like it here in the hospital?"

     "Did you enjoy your visit with your family?"

     These are questions which will often produce apathetic respon-
ses.

117.   Emotionally blunted individuals have a _____ range
and a _____ intensity of affect. They have an _____
face, _____ eyes and they speak in an _____
voice.

118.   Emotionally blunted individuals often are indifferent and express
little affection for their family and friends. This emotional indifference leaves them unconcerned for their present situation and without plans or desires for the future. For example, when asked how
they feel about being in the hospital, or how they would feel if they
had to remain hospitalized for many months, patients respond, "Well,
I suppose I'll have to," "It's o.k. being here," "Well, I don't like it,
but what can I do?" What is the characteristic affective range and
amplitude associated with these responses? What is the characteristic quality of mood?

112. Relatedness ——— A strong mood, such as rage, fear

   Affect of increased ——— Ability to express warmth, concern,
   intensity   love

   Quality of mood ——————— Emotions of anger, happiness, sadness

   Inappropriate mood ——— Sudden explosive laughter without
                           apparent reason

113. blunting

114. constricted

115. constricted, decreased

116. blunted

117. constricted, decreased, expressionless, unblinking, monotonous
     (or unvarying)

118. constricted, decreased, apathy

119.   Circle the words or phrases associated with emotional blunting:

Apathetic mood   Profound sadness

Labile affect   Constricted affective range

Grandiose euphoric mood   Expressionless face

Monotonous voice   Friendliness

120.   Check the words or phrases associated with emotional blunting.

1. Spending all day in bed away from people
    but not sad   _____

2. Appearing content to be hospitalized and
    having no future plans   _____

3. Joking with the hospital staff   _____

4. Greeting all the visitors to the ward
    with a big "Hello"   _____

5. Crying over the recent death of a
    friend   _____

6. Shallow laughter without humor   _____

121.   Once again, you are asked to see a patient. When you first see
her, she is standing in the hall next to the nurses' station, speaking rapidly to several nearby people. When she sees you, she rushes to meet you, vigorously shakes your hand, laughs, begins to
ask you all sorts of questions, but soon interrupts herself to in-
struct the porter who is cleaning the floor, and a nurse who is beginning to administer medications. You note this example of _____
_____ and then interrupt her to tell her you'd like to speak with
her. She suddenly becomes angry and shouts at you for your bad
manners. The medication nurse tells her to stop shouting. This
results in the patient bursting into long gales of laughter. Later,
in writing your report, you state that her affective range was not
_____ and her mood amplitude was _____. Her
moods varied from _____ to _____ and, although appropriate in quality, were certainly not within the normal limits of intensity. Her rapid shifts in mood is termed _____ of affect.

44

119. (Apathetic mood)   Profound sadness

      Labile affect   (Constricted affective range)

      Grandiose euphoric mood   (Expressionless face)

      (Monotonous voice)   Friendliness

120. 1. Spending all day in bed away from people   √
          but not sad

     2. Appearing content to be hospitalized   √
         and having no future plans

     3. Joking with the hospital staff

     4. Greeting all the visitors to the ward
         with a big "Hello"

     5. Crying over the recent death of a
         friend

     6. Shallow laughter without humor   √

121. hyperactivity, constricted, increased, irritability to euphoria, lability

45

122.   Another patient is first seen sitting quietly outside your office. Even though you say hello and ask her to come in, she remains seated, staring ahead until you repeat your introduction upon which she slowly gets up and moves to a chair next to your desk. There are deep furrows between her eyebrows. Her eyes have a sunken appearance, and the inner angle of the upper lids appears to rise. Throughout the interview, the patient remains seated, head bowed. Her only movements are the constant rubbing together of her hands. She speaks in a monotonous, slow, plodding fashion, is often close to tears and, despite an attempt at humor on your part, cannot even manage a smile. She says she feels like crying but cannot. She says she feels like a bad person, and that somehow her present condition is deserved and that people would be better off if she were dead. You find yourself feeling sad for her and concerned about her pained expression. Later, in writing your report, you state that she exhibited _____ motor behavior. Because of her hand rubbing, you feel she showed mild motor _____. Her facial expression, marked by an _____ sign and _____ folds was sad.

In describing her affect, you state that her affective range was _____; she showed stability of affect and her mood was one of constant _____. Do you feel her mood was appropriate?

———————

123.   Write the numbers of the items listed below that best fit the following mental status area:

General Appearance _____

General Motor Behavior _____

Affect _____

Catatonia _____

1.	Stereotype	7.	Echolalia, echopraxia
2.	Age, sex, race	8.	Quality of mood
3.	Nutrition	9.	Lability
4.	Relatedness	10.	Mitmachen
5.	Coordination	11.	Range of affect
6.	Catalepsy	12.	Agitation

122. hypoactive, agitation, Omega, Veraguth, constricted, sadness

Do you feel her mood was appropriate? _yes_ Her profound sadness is consistent with her ideas of guilt.

123. General appearance 2. Age, sex, race; 3. Nutrition

General Motor Behavior 5. Coordination; 12. Agitation

Affect 4. Relatedness; 8. Quality of mood; 9. Lability;
11. Range of affect

Catatonia 1. Stereotype; 6. Catalepsy; 7. Echolalia, echopraxia
10. Mitmachen

124. Place a check mark in the appropriate box to indicate into which mental status section each behavior item best fits.

	General Appearance	General Motor Behavior	Catatonia	Affect
Hesitant gait				
Stupor				
Grimacing				
Manner				
Semicomatose				
Blunting				
Posturing				
Body type				
Waxy flexibility				
Agitation				

125. Label each clinical item with the appropriate term:

Mute man lying in bed, staring at ceiling, averting gaze, general analgesia _____

Mood shifts rapidly and unexpectedly from anger to laughter and then sadness _____

Mute woman standing in hall with hands held above her head and clasped in prayer-like manner _____

Woman rushes about hospital ward, talking to every staff member, greeting all visitors and doing some cleaning. She tries to help other patients but moves on to other tasks before finishing. _____

LANGUAGE FUNCTION (THOUGHT PROCESS)

126. You should evaluate a patient's thought process only after you have evaluated the mental status behavioral areas of _____, _____ _____ and _____. Thought processes are inferred from a person's speech.

127. Thought process is form and differs from thought content. The form of speech is characterized by its rate, pressure, rhythm, idiosyncrasy of word usage, tightness of associational linkage and forms of associational linkage. What the patient is talking about is thought _____.

128. The way associations are linked together is part of the form of thought processes and can be of diagnostic importance. What the patient is talking about, thought _____, reflects cultural and personal life and experience, and with few exceptions, is rarely of diagnostic importance.

48

124.

	General Appearance	General Motor Behavior	Catatonia	Affect
Hesitant gait		✓		
Stupor		✓(acceptable)	✓	
Grimacing			✓	
Manner	✓			
Semicomatose	✓			
Blunting				✓
Posturing			✓	
Body type	✓			
Waxy flexibility			✓	
Agitation		✓		

125. Mute man lying in bed, staring at ceiling, averting gaze, general analgesia   <u>stupor</u>

Mood shifts rapidly and unexpectedly from anger to laughter and then sadness   <u>lability of affect</u>

Mute woman standing in hall with hands held above her head and clasped in prayer-like manner   <u>posturing</u>

Woman rushes about hospital ward, talking to every staff member, greeting all visitors and doing some cleaning. She tries to help other patients but moves on to other tasks before finishing.   <u>hyperactivity or excitement</u>

126. general appearance, motor behavior, affect.

127. content

128. content

129.   Circle the words or phrases suggestive of the form of thought process.

Racing thoughts   "I am worried about my job."
"He talks too much."   "He speaks jibberish. It makes
                            no sense.
"My son is 12 years   "I see lights in the sky."
old."

130.   Circle the words or phrases suggestive of the content of thought.

"He jumps from topic to topic, I can't follow him"

"My boss fired me"

"I hear voices coming from the radiators"

His speech is fast, then slow, then fast again

"I think I am the cause of all this trouble in the U.S."

"It's my mother's fault"

131.   Thought content may be diagnostically helpful when it reflects mood. Grandiose ideas of wealth, great power, or high birth are often associated with a manic state (40 pp. 19-22,71). Ideas of guilt, worthlessness, and hopelessness are often associated with its opposite, a major _____ (40 pp. 75-98, 58).

132.   Unlike the thought content that reflects an altered quality of _____, strange or "bizarre" ideas are never diagnostic and can occur in many conditions (14,15,18,23).

133.   Asking a patient to interpret several proverbs is a poor test of thought processes (5,56). The answers are never diagnostic and are so culture-dependent as to be useless in a phenomenologic mental status. An examination of the rate, rhythm and pressure of speech, the idiosyncratic usage of words, and the tightness and form of associational linkage are far better guides to the presence or absence of thought process disorder. Write a sentence summarizing the difference between thought process form and content.

134.   Although the rate of speech may reflect cultural patterns, severe deviations can be readily observed in mentally ill patients. The rate of speech can be rapid or _____.

135.   Slow and/or hesitant speech is characteristic of depressions, altered states of consciousness and certain coarse brain disease in which the ability to select and/or express the proper words is defective (aphasia) (9,16,40 pp.77-80,43,58). Would you be correct if you said that observations on the rate of a person's speech deals with form, not content? _____

50

129. Racing thoughts   "I am worried about my job."

    "He talks too much!"   "He speaks jibberish. It makes no sense."

    "My son is 12 years old."   "I see lights in the sky."

    "Racing thoughts" suggests the rate of speech and thought.

    "He talks too much" suggests pressure of speech.

    "He speaks jibberish. It makes no sense" suggests a breakdown in linkage or word usage.

130. "He jumps from topic to topic, I can't follow him"
    "My boss fired me"
    "I hear voices coming from the radiators"
    His speech is fast, then slow, then fast again
    "I think I am the cause of all this trouble in the U.S."
    "It's my mother's fault"

    "He jumps from topic to topic, I can't follow him" suggests a breakdown in linkage.

    "His speech is fast, then slow, then fast again" suggests dysrhythmic speech.

131. depression

132. mood

133. Thought process form is how a person is talking; thought content is what he is talking about.

134. slow

135. yes

136.   Rapid speech is characteristic of anxiety states. When rapid speech is also pressured, it is a cardinal sign of mania (40 pp. 31-32, 41). Patients with pressured speech talk continuously, as if compelled; it is very difficult to interrupt them. As thought processes are inferred from speech, patients who have rapid and pressured speech often comment that their thoughts are _____ .

137.   The rate of thoughts can only be reported by the paitent, but may be inferred from the _____ of _____ .

138.   Pressured speech refers to the drive to talk. In its marked form, the patient's drive to _____ is so great that it becomes difficult to stop or interrupt him. Rapid, pressured speech is a cardinal sign of _____ .

139.   The rhythm of speech is not infrequently disrupted by various illnesses. Scanning speech (where word sounds are stretched, producing a slow, sliding cadence) is typical of multiple sclerosis (43), mumbled hesitant speech is often heard in patients with Huntington's chorea (50), while staccato (or abrupt, clipped) speech (both fast and slow) is often a sign of psychomotor epilepsy (15). Once again, it's not what the patient is saying, but _____ he is saying something that is diagnostically important.

140.   Draw a line between appropriate items in the two columns:

Rapid/pressured speech	Worlds are stretched out in sliding cadence
Staccato speech	Overtalkativeness, intrusive speech
Scanning speech	Words are clipped and abrupt
Mumbled speech	Speech sounds as if person had water or marbles in his mouth

141.   Scanning speech can be observed in patients with multiple sclerosis. Mumbled, hesitant speech can be observed in patients with Huntington's chorea. Staccato speech can be observed in psychomotor epilepsy. These are examples of dysfunction of the _____ of speech.

142.   The idiosyncratic use of words is often a sign of severe mental illness. A word seemingly invested and given meaning by a patient is called a neologism (new words). Some neologisms (e.g., glob, rutophobile, thoe) result from the patient's inability to utilize the proper sounds of speech (9,16,17).

136. racing (too fast)

137. rate, speech

138. talk, mania

139. how

140. Rapid/pressured speech — Words are stretched out in sliding cadence

Staccato speech — Overtalkativeness, intrusive speech

Scanning speech — Words are clipped and abrupt

Mumbled speech — Speech sounds as if person had water or marbles in his mouth

141. rhythm

142. no answer required

143.   Circle the words or phrases indicating the use of a neologism:

"I can't rutton this shirt"

"Can you give it to him when I say that you will?"

"The orroble hit him"

"I ban't rit it"

144.   Neurologists call new words resulting from a patient's inability to utilize proper sounds of speech a form of phonemic paraphasia. We also use the term _____ .

145.   Phonemic refers to sound, paraphasia to a form of language disorder. Phonemic paraphasia is the disorder of the sound formation of language (9,16,17). Write a sentence defining the phonemic paraphasia termed neologism.

146.   Another form of paraphasia is word approximation, the use of substitute words resulting from a difficulty in finding and/or in naming an object. Difficulty in using the sounds of language can produce another form of paraphasia termed _____ paraphasia.

147.   Some patients use known words but give them private meanings. It is difficult to tell where private words end and substitute words or _____ _____ begin. Perhaps both should be designated by the term paraphasia.

148.   New words or _____ and substitute words or _____ _____ are examples of paraphasia. Psychiatrists also refer to these phenomena as formal thought disorder. Formal thought disorder is considered a sign of severe brain dysfunction.

149.   In the sentences: "I need to sign some papers. May I use your writer?" the word "writer" is used instead of pen. This is an example of a _____ or word _____ .

150.   In the beginning, you may find it hard to "hear" word approximations. Your brain will translate "writer" into "pen." You may therefore believe that if a word or phrase is understandable to you, it is not an example of a paraphasia. Train yourself to listen to what patients say. Do not translate. Do not interpret. Ask the patient: "What did you call this?" And be alert for other word approximations during the rest of your examination. Circle the words or phrases indicating a paraphasia and indicate whether the paraphasic response is a neologism, a word approximation, or a private usage.

"I was going to the buying place when I became sick. I was quite inbisposed but the helper, the, you know, the treating person wouldn't put me in the bospirab. I was very industrial."

143. "I can't (rutton) this shirt"   (for "button")
"Can you give it to him when I say that you will?"
"The (orroble) hit him"   (for "automobile")
"I (ban't rit) it"   (for "can't give)

144. neologism

145. The formation of a new word due to the inability to utilize proper speech sounds.

146. phonemic

147. word approximations

148. neologisms, word approximations

149. paraphasia, approximation

150. "I was going to the (buying place) when I became sick.
I was quite (inbisposed) but the (helper,) the, you know, the (treating person) wouldn't put me in the (bospirab.) I was very (industrial.")

buying place - word approximation - store
inbisposed - neologism - indisposed
helper/treating person - word approximation - Doctor
bospirab - neologism - hospital
industrial - private use of word - upset

151.   A patient was shown this figure [ ] and was asked to name it. The answer "box" instead of "square" is a subtle form of _____ or word approximation. Many "normal" people demonstrate this particular word approximation.

152.   Studies of the speech patterns and word usages of psychiatric patients and patients with coarse brain disease have demonstrated that the speech of these two groups is strikingly similar (4,13,16,22). Patients with mental illness often demonstrate aphasia (4,22,73,75). List the paraphasias you have learned.

153.   After evaluating a patient's _____, _____ and pressure of speech as well as the presence of any paraphasias, the tightness and form of thought linkage should next be examined.

154.   The terms "incoherent," "illogical," and "irrelevant" are occasionally used to describe the speech of patients. These terms are not used in the phenomenologic mental status exam because they are not precise and only imply that the patient spoke oddly and that you didn't quite understand it. Evaluating the _____ of associations and the _____ of associational linkage is more precise and diagnostically important.

155.   Eugen Bleuler believed (13) that the apparent disruption of meaningful connections between words or phrases, termed loosening of associations, was a pathognomonic sign of schizophrenia. Was he commenting upon the content or the form of speech?

156.   To the phenomenologist, the apparent disruption of meaningful connections between words or phrases, termed _____, is not a pathognomonic sign of schizophrenia.

157.   Mild looseness of associations, or the apparent disruption of _____ between words or phrases, is frequently observed in severely anxious individuals and extreme loosening such as flight of ideas is often seen in mania (40 pp. 14-15).

158.   The disruption of meaningful connections between words and phrases, termed _____ _____, can be graded as word salad, when the loosening occurs between words and consecutive words seem unrelated in meaning, or as fragmentation, when the loosening occurs between phrases and sentences.

159.   It takes a great deal of practice to train your ear to distinguish the different varieties of thought process disorders from the jumbled speech of many patients. I will illustrate many of these disorders, but only the constant clinical practice can master the technique. Below is a quote from a patient. Is it an example of fragmentation or word salad?

    "I, or what, what, the shy, he, me, she, she, she, she, cold, it."

151. paraphasia

152. neologism (phonemic), word approximation, private use of words

153. rate, rhythm

154. tightness, form

155. form: tightness of linkage

156. loosening of associations

157. meaningful connections

158. loosening, associations

159. word salad

160.   Is the following quote from a patient an example of word salad or fragmentation?

> "Then going over the world... then coming down... I'm going to meet... riding and riding down... How's it coming, Johnny?... Now, now, going home, going home."

161.   Draw a line between the appropriate items in the two columns:

Word salad	Consecutive words without meaning
Word approximation	"You're a conseparate!"
Fragmentation	"I'm sick. I think I have a heat (fever)."
Neologism	Consecutive phrases unrelated in meaning

162.   The form of linkage of thoughts is the structural arrangement in which associations are linked. The disruption of meaningful connections between words or phrases is termed _____ _____.

The next several items will use small squares (☐) to represent associations. They will illustrate several types of disorders of the form of thought linkage. The psychiatric literature is crammed with terms and concepts of thought disorder. I will discuss only some of them.

163.   Below is an illustration with squares of fragmented speech; each square represents a phrase or sentence. Notice that there is a sequence in the associations, but that some associations are missing, leaving spaces between associations.

The arrow represents the general direction (or flow) of associations which, in this example, are goal directed. In the above example, if each square represented a word, we would have an example of _____ _____.

164.   In circumstantial speech, even though the associations follow one another (linkage is tight), extra nonessential associations are added before the goal is eventually reached. On the other hand, speech in which associations do not follow, in which each word is unconnected in any meaningful way from the preceeding and following words is termed _____ _____.

160. fragmentation

161. Word Salad ————— Consecutive words without meaning
    Word approximation   "You're a conseparate!"
    Fragmentation   "I'm sick. I think I have a heat (fever)".
    Neologism   Consecutive phrases unrelated in meaning

162. loosening of associations

163. word salad

164. word salad

165.   In response to the question, "What kind of work do you do?", a patient replies, "I've been working all my life... it's been hard, but I've never been without a job. Oh yes, we've had to cut corners, but there's always been food on the table. Now, take this present job---been at it two years now; pay's O.K., but I don't like the boss--- you know the type, they think they own the world; think just because they give you a measly salary that they can ask you to do anything. Well, they can't. I'm the doorman, but I'm not cleaning up for anyone!"

If you're still awake, picture each sentence in one of our little squares with each square numbered in sequence-- an arrow representing the general flow of associations and the goal that the patient is trying to reach (in this case, the answer to the question). Write the answers to the following questions:

Is the above an example of word salad?   _____

Does the patient reach the goal? (Does
he tell the questioner his work?)   _____

Did the patient need all those details
to reach the goal?   _____

166.   Circumstantial speech is characteristic speech of chronic epileptics, alcoholics, borderline retardates, of persons with senile brain changes, and of some passive-agressive and obsessive-compulsive personalities (8,9,17 pp. 25-59). It can be pictured thus:

where all the EVEN associations are nonessential

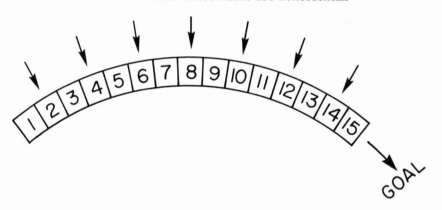

Write a sentence defining circumstantial speech

165. Is the above an example of word salad?   No

Does the patient reach the goal? (Does
he tell the questioner his work?)   Yes

Did the patient need all those details to
reach the goal?   No

166. Circumstantial speech refers to tightly linked associations, but with
extra, non-essential associations interspersed. The speech takes a
circuitous route before reaching its goal.

167.   In tangential speech, or talking past the point, although the linkage is tight, the answering associations bypass the goal by going off on a tangent; thus the goal is never reached. This speech is often observed in schizophrenia and in coarse brain disease. Tangential speech can be pictured thus:

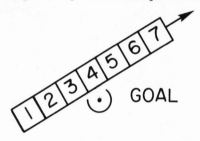

Write a sentence defining tangential speech.

168.   In response to the question, "What kind of work do you do?" a patient answers:

A. "Well, I've been working all my life." (speech stops)

Q. "Yes, but what kind of work do you do?"

A. "Never been without a job" (speech stops)

Q. "I understand that, but I'm interested in the type of work that you do   What is it?"

A. "Yes... yes. Can you imagine being out of work? I watch the news and a lot of people are out of work." (Same content, still no answer after another three minutes)

Again, picture each sentence in one of our little numbered squares, the arrow and the goal. Write the answers to the following questions:

Did the patient reach the goal?

Are the associations meaningful connections or disrupted one from the other? (loosening)

169.   Please note that the content in items 166 and 168 is similar but that the _____ is different.

170.   Draw a line between the appropriate items in the two columns:

Paraphasia   Tight but extra nonessential linkages that finally reach goal

Circumstantial speech   Consecutive phrases unrelated in meaning

Tangential speech   Tight linkages bypassing goal

Fragmented speech   Work approximations

167. Tangential speech refers to tightly linked associations which bypass the goal by going off on a tangent.

168. Did the patient reach the goal?   No
Are the associations meaningful connections or disrupted one from the other? (loosening)   No

If you answered yes to the second part, look again at the associations: working all life--a lot of people out of work. These associations do connect meaningfully, but they bypass the goal, never reaching it.

169. form

170. Paraphasia   Tight but extra non-essential linkages that finally reach goal

Circumstantial speech   Consecutive phrases unrelated in meaning

Tangential speech   Tight linkages bypassing goal

Fragmented speech   Word approximations

171.   Some patients' thought linkage may sound generally tight, but
many associations, particularly at the end of the thought, are repeated in an automatic manner. This form of speech (a verbal
stereotype) was first described by Karl Kahlbaum (37) as characteristic of catatonia, and is called verbigeration.

In response to the question, "What kind of work do you do?"
a patient answered:

"I do work, work... I do do, you the work, I do, I do I do I,
I, do."

The above speech can be pictured thus:

1	2	3	3	1	2	2	4	5	3	1	2	1	2	1	2

Did the patient reach the goal?

172.   A verbal sterotype called _____ is often associated
with the syndrome of _____ .

173.   The automatic repetition of associations, particularly at the end
of thoughts is termed _____ .

174.   Neurologists refer to automatic repetition of phrases, particularly
at the end of thoughts as palilalia (9). Psychiatrists call the same
phenomenon _____ .

175.   In item 171, the patient answered, "I do work, work... I do do,
you the work, etc..." the introduction of the word "you" after "do
do" is an association made by sound rather than by the meaning of
the words. This is termed a clang association and is typically observed in manic states (40 pp. 14-15), although it can also be
observed in patients with phonemic paraphasia (16,17). Another
form of phonemic paraphasia is _____ .

176.   The recognition of different forms of thought process disorder
has led to attempts to relate specific forms with specific illnesses or
syndromes. Thus, verbigeration has been related to _____
and clang associations to _____ states.

171. Did the patient reach the goal?   No

172. verbigeration, catatonia

173. verbigeration

174. verbigeration

175. neologism

176. catatonia, manic

177.　　　　The following table summarizes the observed relationships between the thought disorders we have examined and several major psychiatric conditions. These thought disorders are not pathognomonic (the tabled relationships are not absolute) but the presence of any one is suggestive of the condition in which it is more frequently observed.

	Mania	Catatonia	Schizophrenia	Chronic Mild-Moderate Coarse Brain Disease
Verbigeration		X	X	X
Clang associations	X			X
Tangential speech			X	X
Fragmented speech	X	X	X	X
Word salad			X	X
Word approximations			X	X
Neologisms			X	X
Circumstantial speech	X			X

　　　　Fragmented speech is the least discriminating of these thought disorders and the experienced phenomenologist will rarely use this concept. Write the definitions of the thought disorders listed in the above table.

178.　　　　Eugen Bleuler considered thought blocking to be a basic sign of schizophrenia (12,13). Thought blocking describes the sudden absence of all thoughts and mental activity. The patient simply stops and goes "blank" (altered awareness) for several moments in a manner similar to a petit mal absence in epilepsy. In psychotherapy, when a patient stops talking at an emotionally-laden moment, the term blocking is also used. The latter phenomenon, however, is not the same as thought _____ where the patient is unaware of an "absence" which appears clinically similar with that observed in _____ _____ epilepsy.

179.　　　　While describing her problems with her mother, a patient suddenly stopped talking. Her psychotherapist remarked upon this abrupt cessation of speech upon which the patient blushed, admitted her difficulty and began to relate an incident that occurred between her and her mother a number of years before.

Is this the blocking of thought associated with schizophrenia?

Is this the blocking of thought associated with petit mal epilepsy?

Explain your answers.

177. Verbigeration: a verbal stereotype in which the patient repeats associations in an automatic manner, particularly at the end of a thought.

Clang association: association by the sound of words rather than their meaning.

Tangential speech: tightly linked associations going off on a tangent bypassing the goal.

Fragmented speech: the loss of meaningful connections between words, phrases, or sentences.

Word salad: the loss of meaningful connections between words.

Word approximations: the use of words or phrases without precise meaning, a paraphasia.

Neologisms: new words formed by the improper use of the sound of words; a phonemic paraphasia.

Circumstantial speech: tightly linked associations but with extra, nonessential associations interspersed. The speech takes a circuitous route before reaching its goal.

178. blocking, petit mal

179. Is this the blocking of thought associated with schizophrenia? No
Is this the blocking of thought associated with petit mal epilepsy? No

Because patient was aware of her "block" which was related to a specific emotional thought.

180. Derailment is a term describing the sudden switch from one line of thought to a new parallel line of thought. Derailment often occurs after an episode of thought blocking or sudden _____ _____ and can be pictured thus:

```
B
L
┌─┬─┬─┬─┬─┬─┬─┐   O
│1│2│3│4│5│6│7│   C
└─┴─┴─┴─┴─┴─┴─┘   K
                  I   ┌─┬─┬─┬─┬─┬─┬─┐
                  N   │A│B│C│D│E│F│G│
                  G   └─┴─┴─┴─┴─┴─┴─┘
```

181. When asked the question, "What kind of work do you do?", a patient answered: "I'm a carpenter, I do...," the patient suddenly stopped speaking and stared past the examiner's shoulder. After a few moments, the examiner touched the patient's arm and asked, "What's happening to you now?" upon which the patient focused on the examiner and said: "I read that thousands of people are un-employed now...." The sudden cessation of mental and motor activity exhibited by this patient is called _____.
The disrupted thought associations on a parallel course following the blocking episode is called _____.

182. The apparent sudden cessation of mental and motor activity of _____, the disruption of one train of thought and the commencement of another parallel train of thought, or _____, although often associated, can occur separately.

183. When asked: "What kind of work do you do?" a patient responds, "I am a line man, you know, the weather man can't be blamed for the weather." This is an example of _____. Draw a slash line where there is a switch in associations.

184. Draw a line between the appropriate items in the two columns:

Clang associations   "How high am I, I fly, I fly, Look, look at the sky?"

Derailment   "It is indisdispu utable, able, a ble, a blbe"

Blocking   "My brother works in a paper factory, he is a puncher...
                            The problem in the town is that most people work at the factory and with all the layoffs..."

Verbigeration   Similar to a petit mal absence
(palilalia)

180.   absence of thought

181.   blocking, derailment

182.   blocking, derailment

183.   derailment
       you know/the weather

184.   Clang association ———— "How high am I, I fly, I fly, look, look at the
                                sky!"

       Derailment   "It is a indisdispu utable, able a ble, a blbe"

       Blocking   "My brother works in a paper factory, he is
                                a puncher...the problem in the town is
                                what most people work at the factory and
                                will all the layoffs..."

       Verbigeration   Similar to a petit mal absence
       (palilalia)

185.   Write the appropriate name next to each diagram of disordered thought form linkage:

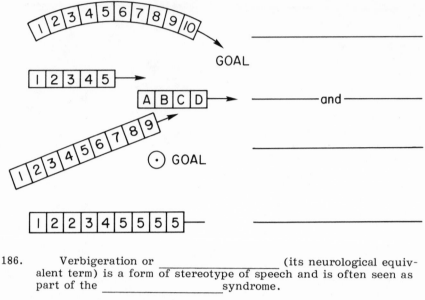

GOAL _____

_____ and _____

⊙ GOAL _____

_____

186.   Verbigeration or _____ (its neurological equivalent term) is a form of stereotype of speech and is often seen as
part of the _____ syndrome.

187.   Circumstantial speech is often observed among patients with
mania. Associations by the sound rather than the meaning of
words or _____ associations are also observed in
mania.

188.   Draw a diagram using our small numbered squares, arrow and
goal, to illustrate the following:

Circumstantial speech

Tangential speech

Verbigeration/palilalia

Word salad

Fragmented speech

185. Circumstantial
Blocking and Derailment
Tangential
Verbigeration or palilalia

186. palilalia, catatonic

187. clang

188.

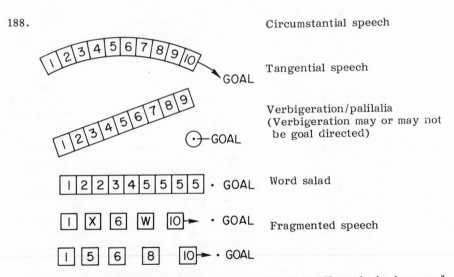

Circumstantial speech

Tangential speech

Verbigeration/palilalia
(Verbigeration may or may not
be goal directed)

Word salad

Fragmented speech

(Please note that fragmented speech and word salad differ only in degree of
loss of meaningful connection between associations (i.e., the tightness of
linkage has broken down)

71

189.   Many patients with mania exhibit signs and symptoms of
catatonia (40 p.36,71,74). Stereotype of speech or _____
can also be observed among manic patients.

190.   The repetition of stock words and phrases, i.e., words or
phrases automatically placed into the flow of speech, is termed
perseveration. Perseveration is a type of formal thought disorder
and is observed in schizophrenics and in patients with coarse brain
disease (9,13,14,17,22,23).

    Other formal thought disorders I have discussed are shown
below. Match them with the examples of speech presented in the
column on the right.

Tangential speech   That prune has many folds in it,
                               you know, canals, grooves

Verbigeration/palilalia   What is my opinion? Well, I might
                               have thought about it a long time
                               and you know there are many things
                               to consider, some this way, some
                               that.

Neologism   The weather button is dangerous.

Word approximation   He is organaniziningizinginging.

Derailment   What is my opinion. Well......

Private use of words   I grottled it.

Blocking   I was going to the store, I have
                               a bad leg and it hurts.

191.   When asked "What kind of work do you do?", a patient responds:
"I'm a brick layer, been doing it for years, been doing it all my
life, or about. Been a brick layer a long time. I work down on
Mulberry. A long time. We're doin' an office building...25 stories.
It takes a long time to put up a building." In this example of
speech, the linkage is tight, but certain stock phrases and words
("a long time") are continually repeated. Even when the subject
is changed, the patient continues to repeat the same phrases automatically "plugged" into the new topic. In very mild forms these
phrases, termed _____ may be a culture-bound speech
pattern: "You know!"

192.   The constant repetition or return to the same topic, rather
than phrase, is called perseveration of theme. Perseveration of
theme can be observed in many depressed patients (40 pp. 75-98,59).
On the other hand, perseveration of associations or the automatic
use of "plugged in" or "_____" words is a significant
indicator of coarse brain disease.

193.   If in the diagram below the number 2 indicates repetition of
the same phrase ([2]) what thought disorder does the diagram
represent? _____

| 1 | 2 | 3 | 4 | 2 | 5 | 6 | 2 | 7 | 2 | 8 |──► · GOAL

189. Verbigeration or palilalia

190. Tangential speech   That prune has many folds in it, you know, canals, grooves

Verbigeration/palilalia   What is my opinion? Well, I might have thought about it a long time and you know there are many things to consider, some this way, some that.

Neologism   The weather button is dangerous.

Word approximation   He is organanizining izinginging.

Derailment   What is my opinion. Well......

Private use of words   I grottled it.

Blocking   I was going to the store, I have a bad leg and it hurts.

191. perseveration

192. stock

193. perseveration

73

194.   Rambling speech is an example of a thought process associated
with coarse brain disease (14,66). It has been heard by almost all
party goers, businessmen at long luncheons, skid row passersby,
in short, by anyone who has heard the speech of an intoxicated
individual. The diagram below pictures rambling speech.

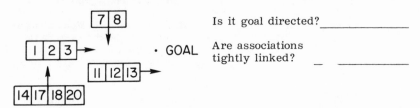

Is it goal directed?_____

Are associations
tightly linked?   _ _____

195.   Non-goal directed, fragmented (loosely linked) speech, or
_____ speech, is characteristic of acute coarse brain
disorders, particularly intoxications (14,66). Since it is often
associated with slight to severe speech slurring (depending on
the dryness of the martinis), _____ speech is not difficult
to recognize. A staggering gait, or ataxia, is another bedfellow
of _____ speech.

196.   Rambling speech suggests an _____ rather than a
chronic process. Drivelling speech, another manifestation of
_____ brain disease, is more characteristic of long
standing dysfunction (9,14,16,17,22,23).

197.   Unfortunately, our imaginations are not up to diagramming
drivelling speech. Goal? 7 X A 3 9 B B is one possibility.
Although associations appear tightly linked, syntax appears
preserved and there are no startling stereotypes (verbigeration)
or perseverations (stock words). In drivelling speech, as in
classical double-talk, sentences (and some words) simply make
little sense, the meaning of the speech is lost. When asked, "What
kind of work do you do?", a patient replied: "Never let it be
reduced that I've not been gaiting the bob. Partially layered and
down, I'm not sure. Twenty-five or twenty-six, that's the work.
I've had one grunch but the left over there is not the man I saw."
When you hear a patient's response that you know is in English
but which seems, nevertheless, to be in another unrecognizable
language, suspect _____ and listen carefully.

198.   When the syntax of speech is preserved but the words make no
sense, neurologists say an individual has jargon agrammatism
(16,17). Psychiatrists call this phenomenon _____.

199.   There are times when a patient's response, if taken out of
context, shows no evidence of thought disorder, but in context it
is totally unrelated to the examiner's question. The term for this
is non-sequitur (Latin for "does not follow"). When "flight of
ideas" (to be discussed) are not present, non-sequitur responses
are a form of thought disorder observed in schizophrenia as well
as coarse brain disease with aphasia (9,16,17). To the question
"How old are you?" a patient responds, "It could be, but I'm not
estranged." This illustrates the _____.

194. Is it goal directed? __No__

     Are associations
        tightly linked? __No__

195. rambling, rambling, rambling

196. acute, coarse

197. drivelling

198. drivelling

199. non-sequitur

200.   Draw a line between appropriate itmes in the two columns:

Non-sequitur   Automatic repetition of words and
                                      phrases, particularly at the end
                                      of associations.

Drivelling/jargon   Totally unrelated response
agrammatism

Perseveration of   Double-talk
association

Verbigeration/palilalia   Repetition of stock words in
                                      generally goal-directed speech

201.   Draw a line between the appropriate items in the two columns:

Tangential speech   Typical of acute intoxications

Rambling speech   Non-goal directed, tight associations;
                                      observed in schizophrenia and in
                                      coarse brain disease

Derailment   Circuitous but eventually goal
                                      directed

Circumstantial speech   Often associated with blocking

202.   Draw a line between matching items in the two columns. Not
all items in either column need be matched.

Clang associations   Word approximations & neologisms

Blocking   Apparent sudden cessation of mental
                                      and physical activity

Paraphasia   Associations by sound rather than
                                      by meaning

Fragmented speech   Double talk

Perseveration of   Use of stock words and phrases;
associations   associated with coarse brain disease

203.   Draw a line between items in the two columns:

Drivelling/jargon   "That's my situation. Situations
agrammatism   change and it can't be helped. My
                                      situtation is my problem, I've got
                                      to situation myself just right."

Verbigeration/palilalia   "Well, it's not that either, but with
                                      the totally generated it can't be
                                      helped."

Perseveration of   "When was I last well? Hell you
association   ding-dong, you bell, I'm well."

Clang association   "Its approxximalalal al al al."

76

200.

Non-sequitur — Automatic repetition of words and phrases, particularly at the end of associations

Drivelling/jargon agrammatism — Totally unrelated response

Perseveration of association — Double-talk

Verbigeration/palilalia — Repetition of stock words in generally goal-directed speech

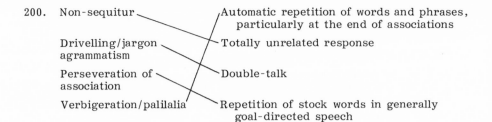

201.

Tangential speech — Typical of acute intoxications

Rambling speech — Non-goal directed, tight associations; observed in schizophrenia and in coarse brain disease

Derailment — Circuitous but eventually goal directed

Circumstantial speech — Often associated with blocking

202.

Clang associations — Word approximations & neologisms

Blocking — Apparent sudden cessation of mental and physical activity

Paraphasia — Associations by sound rather than by meaning

Fragmented speech — Double talk

Perseveration of association — Use of stock words and phrases; associated with coarse brain disease

203. Draw a line between items in the two columns:

Drivelling/jargon agrammatism — "That's my situation. Situations change and it can't be helped. My situation is my problem, I've got to situation myself just right."

Verbigeration/palilalia — "Well, it's not that either, but with the totally generated it can't be helped."

Perseveration of association — "When was I last well? Hell you ding-dong, you bell, I'm well."

Clang association — "Its approxiximalalal al al al."

204.   Draw a line between items in the two columns:

Derailment   "That's rypitcal of him"

Neologisms   "I don't understand a drum of what
                                    they're doing."

Word approximations   "He was going to tell me and I just
                                    never got to go."

Private usage of words   "I was at the engine station on
                                    time but the cars, the engine never
                                    showed up."

205.   Identify each of the examples of formal thought disorder:

"He callously disregarded my wishes. The
situation is callous and I'm very upset.
To callously disregard one is not the way   _____
to act."

"How can I tell about which I am in the
middle of. You don't really think this
is the beginning, or the end, or for   _____
that matter any of it."

"I was having this trouble sleeping, the
light you know was difficult to read by."   _____

"Stop it! Stop it! Do you think am
generated?"   _____

"What's the point of all this probeout?"   _____

206.   Draw a line between appropriate items in the two columns:

Word salad   The paraphasia of using "new" words

Neologisms   Answer unrelated to question

Word approximations   Severe form of drivelling speech

Non-sequitur   The paraphasia that consists of
                                    using incorrect words with similar
                                    meaning to the correct choice

204. Draw a line between items in the two columns

Derailment — "That's rypitcal of him"

Neologisms — "I don't understand a drum of what they're doing."

Word approximations — "He was going to tell me and I just never got to go."

Private usage of words — "I was at the engine station on time but the cars, the engine never showed up."

205. "He callously disregarded my wishes. The situation is callous and I'm very upset. To callously disregard one is not the way to act."   Perseveration/stock words

"How can I tell about which I am in the middle of. You don't really think this is the beginning, or the end, or for that matter any of it."   Drivelling

"I was having this trouble sleeping, the light you know was difficult to read by."   Derailment

"Stop it! Stop it! Do you think am generated?"   Private usage of words

"What's the point of all this probeout?"   Neologism

206. Word salad — The paraphasia of using "new" words

Neologisms — Answer unrelated to question

Word approximations — Severe form of drivelling speech

Non-sequitur — The paraphasia that consists of using incorrect words with similar meaning to the correct choice

79

207.   You have now become familiar with many different forms of
thought disorder. Although there are numerous other terms and
several other forms of disordered thinking, a presentation of the
total is beyond the scope of this book. I do, however, want to
describe one more form of thought disorder: Flight-of-ideas.
Flight-of-ideas has been described as the cardinal thought disorder
of mania (40 pp. 14-15,71). In flight-of-ideas, the patient jumps
from topic to topic, lines of thinking are fragmented and multiple
lines of thought are common. Associations often appear in response
to an external stimulus until interrupted by new stimulated lines
of thought. Severe flight-of-ideas can be pictured with the
following diagram:

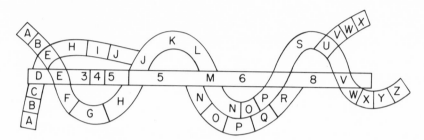

Careful examination of the confused impression of the diagram should
isolate segments which fit the definition of several previously described disorders of thinking.
    If we isolate the association line:

| I | | 3 | 4 | 5 | | 6 | | 8 |→

    This sequence has missing associations, but it is generally goal
directed. If the associations were phrases or sentences, this would
be an example of _____ speech. If we isolate the
associational line:

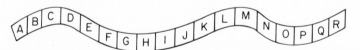

    We can see tight associations taking a circuitous route and an
example of _____ speech.

80

207. fragmented, circumstantial

208.　　Each of the following is consistent with flight-of-ideas except: (circle answer)

　　Circumstantial speech

　　Fragmented speech

　　Neologisms

　　Jumping from topic to topic

209.　　Alas, all is not simple in psychiatry! You saw in item 207 that flight-of-ideas becomes a combination of _____ speech and _____ speech. Since fragmented speech is a traditional example of _____ of _____, the possibility exists that flight-of-ideas and loosening of associations may be variants of the same disordered thought process. The elaboration of this problem is well beyond the digestive tracts of many of us and obviously beyond the scope of this book.

210.　　Place an M next to the terms associated with Motor behavior, a T next to the terms associated with Thought process and an A next to the terms associated with Affect:

Relatedness_____	Mood_____	Apathy_____
Perseveration of association_____	Echopraxia_____	Gegenhalten_____
Non-sequiturs_____	Verbigeration_____	Paraphasia_____
Catalepsy_____	Tardive dyskinesia_____	Drivelling_____

208. (Neologisms)

209. circumstantial, fragmented, loosening, associations

210. Relatedness A   Mood A   Apathy A

    Perseveration of   Echopraxia M   Gegenhalten M
    association T

    Non-sequiturs T
                         Tardive   Drivelling T
    Catalepsy M   dyskinesia M

83

211.   Place a check mark in the appropriate box indicating the most typical relationships (more than one checked category for any thought disorder is possible):

	Mania	Schizophrenia	Acute Coarse Brain Disease	Chronic Coarse Brain Disease
Drivelling				
Flight-of-ideas				
Rambling				
Perseveration				
Non-sequiturs				
Derailment				
Clang associations				
Paraphasia				
Tangential speech				
Circumstantial speech				
Blocking				
Verbigeration				

Write the definition of the thought disorders listed above.

84

211.	Mania	Schizophrenia	Acute Coarse Brain Disease	Chronic Coarse Brain Disease
Drivelling		√		√
Flight-of-ideas	√			
Rambling			√	
Perseveration		√		√
Non-sequiturs		√	√	√
Derailment		√		√
Clang associations	√			
Paraphasia		√	√	√
Tangential speech		√		√
Circumstantial speech	√			√
Blocking		√		√
Verbigeration	√	√		√

Although the relationships in this table are not absolute, please note that the pattern of thought disorder is similar for schizophrenia and coarse brain disease. Any interpretation of this similarity will undoubtedly be predetermined by the bias of the viewer.

Drivelling: Associations appear tightly linked and syntax appears preserved but the meaning of speech is lost. It is double-talk.

Flight-of-ideas: Jumping from topic to topic, often in response to external stimuli. Multiple lines of thought can occur.

Rambling: non-goal directed, fragmented speech.

Perseveration: The repetition of stock words and phrases automatically placed into the flow of speech.

Non-sequiturs: Patient's response is totally unrelated to the examiner's questions.

Derailment: The sudden switch from one line of thought to a new parallel line of thought.

Clang associations: association by the sound of words rather than meaning.

Paraphasia: The use of words or phrases without precise meaning; new words formed by the improper use of the sound of words (neologism).

Tangential speech: tightly linked associations which bypass the goal going off on a tangent.

Circumstantial speech: tightly linked associations but with extra non-essential associations interspersed. The speech takes a circuitous route before reaching its goal.

Blocking: Sudden absence of all thoughts and mental activity.

Verbigeration: a verbal stereotype in which the patient repeats associations, particularly at the end of a thought, in an automatic manner.

212.   What a person is talking about is helpful in reaching a diagnosis when the content reflects an intense mood. Once you have established the _____ of a patient's speech, or how he is speaking, you should determine whether the thought content is helpful in the diagnostic process.

213.   Feelings of hopelessness, worthlessness, helplessness, guilt and thoughts of suicide are often expressed in thought content. They reflect the presence of a sad mood (40,58,65). During the mental status exam, you must determine whether these feelings are present. The following questions can induce the patient to explain his mood.

   1.   "How does the future look?"---"Do you think your difficulties will improve?"

   2.   "Do you think your family needs you?"---"Are you a worthwhile person?"

   3.   "Do you think you can do anything about all this?"

   4.   "Have you let people down?"---"Are you a bad person?"

214.   Thoughts of suicide can be determined by asking the patient the following series of questions:

   1.   "Well, with all this going on, you must feel pretty badly. Do you ever get the feeling you'd like to go to sleep and not wake up?"

   2.   "Do you ever get the feeling you'd be better off dead?"

   3.   "Did you ever wish you could just end it all?"

   4.   "Did you ever think of harming yourself?...Of killing yourself? ...Have you tried?...Do you feel that way now?"

215.   The presence of ideas of hopelessness, worthlessness, helplessness, guilt and suicide reflect the presence of a _____ _____.

216.   The details of what a person is hopeless about or guilty about is the thought content. This content becomes diagnostically importan because it reflects an intense mood of sadness. The fact that a pa tient feels profound sadness and thus feels guilty is diagnostically more important than the detail of the guilty idea. For example, a patient said "I'm a terrible person, I masturbated when I was youn and now my family's being punished for it. I've let them down. They should kill me." The patient expressed the details of mastur bation and resulting family punishment. These details could easily have been finding money in the street and not returning it and re sulting trouble in the world. It's the feeling of guilt, manifested by these details, which is of primary concern in the diagnostic ex- amination.
        List the types of feelings associated with a sad mood.

212. form

213. No answer required

214. No answer required

215. sad mood

216. hopelessness, worthlessness, helplessness, guilt, suicide

217.   A patient responded "Yes" to the question, "Do you ever get the feeling you'd like to go to sleep and not wake up?" This response suggests he has thoughts of _____.

218.   List the thought content being evaluated by each of the following questions:

1. "How does the future look?" _____

2. "Do you think you can do anything about all this?" _____

3. "Did you ever wish you could just end it all?" _____

4. "Did you ever think of harming yourself?" _____

5. "Do you think your family needs you?" _____

219.   Questions relating to feelings of hopelessness, worthlessness, helplessness, guilt, and suicide determine the presence of ideas which reflect a _____ _____.

220.   Past thought content belongs in the historical part of your evaluation of the patient. In the mental status examination, you want to determine the _____ content.

221.   Next to each of the following descriptions, indicate which thought disorder it best illustrates:

Q. "Why did you come to the hospital?"
A. "I don't like that food."   _____

"Don't frazzle it away."   _____

"It's not because of, well you see,
the one that he was interested in
not being part of the drive."   _____

"I renigated it."   _____

Q. "Where do you live?"
A. "I live with my mother."
Q. "Yes, but where do you live?"
A. "I would rather not be there."
Q. "Yes, but what is your address?"
A. "Some people would say that I
live downtown."   _____

88

217. suicide

218. "How does the future look?" _hopelessness_
"Do you think you can do anything about all this?" _helplessness_
"Did you ever wish you could just end it all?" _suicide_
"Did you ever think of harming yourself?" _suicide_
"Do you think your family needs you?" _worthlessness_

219. sad mood

220. present

221. Non-sequitur
Private use of word - "frazzle" (a paraphasia)
Drivelling/jargon agrammatism
Neologism - "renigated" (a paraphasia)
Tangential speech. The answers follow but never reach the goal.

222.	Next to each of the following descriptions, indicate which thought disorder it best illustrates:

Q. "Do you like it here?"
A. "Well, as you know, I've been here over a week now. I came in on Friday and today is Wednesday. My brother brought me here. There are some patients who I know from last time and, of course, many of the staff - so that when you consider how sick I was at the beginning and now it really isn't so bad. It's o.k."

_____

"He was rejuvennerated ated ated"

_____

"I've been here over a week and the time I was in the army sarge"

_____

"It's a tough life. Real tough, but I think I can tough it out. You know I've been around and I've grown tough-skinned."

_____

223.	Next to each of the following descriptions, indicate which thought process disorder it best illustrates:

"You might be right, bright boy...
flight boy. What a sight!"

_____

"I don't know...We were so young...What time is it?...eh?...What went wrong?"

_____

"We went in a driver, you know, a road machine."

_____

"I'm a persistently active person. I have always persistently done my job...never give up. Perseveration, fortitude, persistance is what it takes to get ahead."

_____

"Why did I do it? How come you ask so many questions? Are you a Doctor? Doctors make a lot of money. I'd like to be rich. The idle rich you know!"

_____

90

222. Circumstantial speech (question is answered after much unnecessary information)
Verbigeration/palilalia (stereotype of speech)
Derailment (occurs after the word "week")
Stock words (perseveration) "tough"

223. Clang associations (bright - flight - sight)
Rambling speech (never reaches a goal, loosening between associations)
Word approximations (driver and road machine for car)
Stock word/perseveration - persistently
Flight-of-ideas (jumps from topic to topic)

224.   Next to each of the following descriptions, indicate which thought
disorder it best illustrates:

"What happened in the Army is my business.
I'll mind my business, you mind yours. Are
you sure you work here? Your're awful nosy!
I don't like questions. I'd rather be outside.
I like the out of doors. It's raining now but
it will be nice tomorrow. After the rain falls
the sun must shine. In any cloud there's a
silver lining."

_____

Q. "What happened to you before you were
brought here?"
A. "I came here about a week ago. I don't
think I should be here."

Q. "Well, what happened before you were
brought here that made people think
you should be hospitalized?"
A. "My sister-in-law is responsible. If it
weren't for her they wouldn't have
come for me."

_____

224. Flight-of-ideas (jumps from topic to topic)
Tangential speech (talks around the point but the answer never reaches the goal)

DELUSIONS (APOPHANY)

225.   To review: The phenomenologic mental status requires you to evaluate a patient's general _____, _____ _____, _____, and _____ _____. Your next task is to examine for apophany or delusional behavior or ideas. Apophany comes from the Greek and means "to become manifest." Phenomenologists apply the global term apophany to the category of phenomena characterized by false or arbitrary ideas developed without adequate proof. The term "delusion" is incomplete in describing behavior form and needs equalifying terms to have more precise meaning. The term "paranoid" has been used to mean everything from a suspicious mood, to delusions of persecution, to schizophrenia and will not be used in this text.

226.   Although apophanous phenomena are frequently observed in severely ill psychiatric patients, they are not pathognomonic of schizophrenia, and are frequently found in patients with affective disorders (18,31,33,40 pp. 19-22, pp. 84-85, 65,71) and coarse brain disease (14,15,16,21,23). Ideas of persecution which are apophanous are not pathognomonic of schizophrenia. Apophanous is a global term applied to the category of phenomena characterized by _____ or arbitrary ideas developed without adequate proof.

227.   There are several standard definitions of the term "delusion": "a fixed false belief, not in keeping with one's own cultural environment" (32) and "the making of a relationship without adequate proof" (35) are two of the more common ones. Write a sentence defining the use (or application) of the term apophanous.

228.   Apophanous phenomena are experiences in which the patient misconnects events, objects, experiences, and endows them with personal significance. They include: delusional mood or atmosphere, delusional ideas, autochthonous ideas and delusional perceptions. Although we will discuss the form of these phenomena individually, each will be characterized by _____ or _____ ideas developed without _____.

94

225. appearance, motor behavior, affect, thought processes

226. false

227. Apophanous is a global term applied to a category of phenomena characterized by false or arbitrary ideas developed without adequate proof.

228. false, arbitrary, adequate proof

229.   During the course of a mental status examination, many patients will reveal delusional ideas when detailing or explaining recent personal history. They will relate the nature of plots against their lives; electric waves coming from the wall; their great power; their special relationship with God; great sins they have committed.... Whenever the examiner suspects a patient's statements to be ____ _____ the next question, in essence, should be: "How do you know?"

230.   When false or arbitrary ideas are accepted as real by patients, they may readily reveal these ideas because they feel them to be obvious to everyone. Some patients who are aware that other people might think them crazy will be reluctant to reveal strange, but to them true, ideas. Once again, a conversational approach is often the best method of eliciting _____ phenomena.

231.   If during a conversation with a friend about the weather, your friend said, "There are radioactive machines in the wall", you would not calmly continue your discussion of the weather. You'd be surprised, concerned, curious. When a patient tells you such strange things, be surprised, concerned and curious. Say: "That's very unusual...How can you tell there are machines in the wall?...Who would do such a thing?...Why would anyone want to harm you?... Tell me more about this, I'm very interested in what you just said..." Don't put the patient on trial, don't argue, don't convey the feeling of: "Ho hum, so what else is new?" Questions should continue (as long as the patient is willing to discuss the matter) until you can determine the _____, not just the content of the apophanous phenomenon.

232.   Perhaps the mildest form of apophany is termed an apophanous or delusional mood, sometimes also termed delusional atmosphere. This experience is the "feeling" that something is wrong, that things are not right and are sinister. ("Something is going on out there, I don't know what it is, but I feel it and I'm afraid.") It is akin to, but more severe than, the feeling of being watched or the common experience of self-consciousness felt by sensitive persons when entering a noisy room full of people who, for a moment, become quiet to observe the newcomer. Delusional atmosphere or _____ can be observed in almost any serious psychiatric condition, and does not have diagnostic specificity.

233.   Some patients will describe a sinister atmosphere which surrounds them. This is a _____ _____. Others will relate events in such a way that you'll suspect its presence. It is perfectly proper for you to help the patient verbalize his delusion, as you would any psychopathology. Say: "You must have been frightened or suspicious...Did you feel that people were watching you...?" This approach suggests concern; it shows that you know about such things, and are interested in helping.

234.   Frequently, patients with severe mood disorders or perceptual disorders, i.e., hallucinations, will misconnect experiences in a personal manner. From their disordered mood or perceptual errors, ideas are made manifest. The phenomenon is termed an apophanous or _____ idea.

229. apophanous

230. apophanous

231. form

232. mood

233. delusional mood (apophanous mood)

234. delusional

235.   When delusional ideas develop from other psychopathology, i.e.,
an altered mood, a hallucination, the ideas are secondary in sequence
of occurrence and are sometimes called secondary delusional ideas.
As with all apophanous phenomena, secondary delusional ideas are
arbitrary and develop without _____.

236.   A depressed patient states that he is a terrible person, full of
evil, that he is being punished for his sins and that he is the cause
of all the many deaths in the hospital. This patient is expressing
ideas which follow from his terribly painful mood. These ideas,
particularly his responsibility for hospital deaths, are misconnec-
tions of events to his person and are examples of_____
_____ _____. Write a sentence
explaining why his delusional idea that he is responsible for hospital deaths is secondary.

237.   A patient states that people are going to kill him because he
overheard their conversation. When he ran away, he heard them
yell at him, threatening to shoot him. He says he frequently hears
them threaten him. Here too, the patient's idea that he is going
to be killed developed from a hallucination. Another example of

_____ _____ _____.

238.   When an apophanous or delusional idea develops from some previous psychopathology, it is referred to as a _____
delusional idea. When the delusional idea forms without obvious
development from previous psychopathology, it is termed a primary
delusional idea.

239.   An apophanous idea which appears in the patient's mind without obvious development from previous psychopathology is a ____
_____ _____. When it ap-
pears suddenly and full formed, it is also termed an autochthonous
delusional idea.

240.   Autochthonous delusional ideas occur _____ and are
_____ formed.

241.   Ideas that do not develop from any obvious psychopathology are
called _____ delusions. But ideas that develop from
previous psychopathology such as a disordered mood or perceptual
error are _____ delusions.

242.   An autochthonous delusional idea is one form of _____
delusional idea.

243.   Sudden, fully-formed, primary delusional ideas or _____
ideas are similar to the "Eureka" phenomenon. The patient suddenly
"knows" the idea is true but can't explain why, or from where the
idea came. For example, one patient said that he was sitting at home
eating breakfast when: "It suddenly dawned on me that my family
wanted to murder me. I can't understand why I never thought of
it before, but at breakfast it just came to me."

98

235. adequate proof

236. secondary delusional ideas
It is secondary because it develops from other psychopathology,
i.e., depressed mood

237. secondary delusional ideas

238. secondary

239. primary delusional idea

240. suddenly, fully

241. primary, secondary

242. primary

243. autochthonous

244.   Clinical psychiatry is not yet an exact science. Ultimately, the examiner must decide using his clinical judgment, whether an autochthonous idea is a personalized misconnection of events and therefore a primary _____ _____, or whether the autochthonous idea is simply a phobic or obsessional thought.

245.   Some primary delusional ideas develop slowly over time. Some primary delusional ideas develop suddenly and fully formed. The latter phenomenon is called _____.

246.   A patient said "The FBI is after me." When asked how he knew this he said he knew because his garbage was not picked up and he had difficulty unlocking his apartment door. He thought these events odd and after giving them some thought he concluded that the FBI had done it. This delusional idea is _____ because it does not develop from other psychopathology. It is not _____ because it developed over time, i.e., it was not sudden and fully formed.

247.   The late Kurt Schneider, a German psychiatrist, described (60) certain primary delusional ideas which, instead of developing from a disordered mood or perceptual error, developed from perceptions of real stimuli. Schneider termed these primary delusional ideas delusional perceptions. Delusional perceptions are considered primary because they do not develop from any other obvious _____.

248.   Delusional perceptions develop from perceptions of real stimuli, _____ delusional ideas develop fully formed in the patient's mind.

249.   Secondary delusional ideas often develop from unreal perceptions ---perceptions without real stimuli, i.e., hallucinations. The apophanous phenomena that develops from a real perception is termed _____ _____.

250.   Circle the examples of secondary delusional ideas:

"The FBI is after me. I can hear their radio cars talking from my TV set."

"The FBI is after me. I saw agents creeping about my apartment last night. When I chased them, they disappeared."

"The FBI is after me. I was walking down the street last week and I suddenly knew it. I just knew it."

"The FBI is after me. I passed a store window and the dummies were all undressed. That was the signal that gave me the idea."

Note: In today's world, the statement "The FBI is after me" should not automatically be greeted with skepticism. Would you commit someone as "crazy" for saying that there were "bugs" in the Democratic Headquarters in Washington and machines in the walls of the White House? Always ask the question "How do you know?" and evaluate the patient's responses to determine the form of their idea. In the above item, "The FBI is after me" was the content; you were identifying the form of secondary delusional ideas.

100

244. delusional idea

245. authchthonous

246. primary, autochthonous

247. psychopathology

248. authchthonous

249. delusional perceptions

250. "The FBI is after me. I can hear their radio cars talking from my TV set."

"The FBI is after me. I saw agents creeping about my apartment last night. When I chased them, they disappeared."

"The FBI is after me. I was walking down the street last week and I suddenly knew it. I just knew it."

"The FBI is after me. I passed a store window and the dummies were all undressed. That was the signal that gave me the idea.

251.   Circle the examples of primary delusional ideas:

"The FBI is after me. I can hear their radio cars talking from my TV set."

"The FBI is after me. I saw agents creeping about my apartment last night. When I chased them, they disappeared."

"The FBI is after me. I was walking down the street last week and I suddenly knew it. I just knew it.

"The FBI is after me. I passed a store window and the dummies were undressed. That was the signal that gave me the idea."

252.   Write a sentence defining the difference between a primary and a secondary delusional idea.

253.   Circle the examples of secondary delusional ideas:

"I feel dead. I want to cry but I cannot...My guts are rotting. My brain is full of garbage. I am being punished."

"The voice tells me it is God and I am the annointed; I am Christ; I am all powerful."

"God is my lover. We have been having sex together for over a year. I can feel him inside of me, lying on top of me. He talks to me. I have a special purpose, I am God's lover."

254.   The term "persecutory delusions" refers only to _____. It doesn't tell you whether the delusions are primary or secondary, autochthonous, or delusional perceptions.

255.   In severe depressions, the content of delusions often revolves around past sins, nihilistic ideas, somatic illness, terrible personal history, or future events (31-33,40 pp. 75-98,58,65). In mania, the content of delusion is often "grandoise," dealing with great personal power, great wealth, high birth (18,31-33, 40 pp. 22-24, 65,71). Persecutory delusional ideas can occur in individuals with depression, mania and schizophrenia (12,13,18,31-33,41,42,58,65, 71). Although the content of these apophanous ideas is helpful, their form is of major importance. The fact that they are apophanous is significant. Their content is not. Write a sentence defining an autochthonous idea and a delusional perception.

256.   Some patients give no initial hint of apophanous phenomena; but with skilled interviewing, they will reveal multiple delusional ideas. Some patients won't tell you their "crazy" ideas, but will readily tell you about the trouble with their neighbors, co-workers or family members. Several questions directed to these relationships will often reveal abundant apophanous phenomena.

Write a sentence defining apophanous phenomena.

251. "The FBI is after me. I can hear their radio cars talking from my TV set."

"The FBI is after me. I saw agents creeping about my apartment last night. When I chased them, they disappeared."

"The FBI is after me. I was walking down the street last week and I suddenly knew it. I just knew it." This is the primary delusional idea termed: autochthonous.

"The FBI is after me. I passed a store window and the dummies were all undressed. That was the signal that gave me the idea." This is the primary delusional idea termed: delusional perception.

252. A secondary delusional idea develops from other psychopathology; a primary delusional idea does not develop from other psychopathology.

253. "I feel dead. I want to cry but I cannot...My guts are rotting. My brain is full of garbage. I am being punished."

"The voice tells me it is God and I am the annointed; I am Christ. I am all powerful."

"God is my lover. We have been having sex together for over a year. I can feel him inside of me, lying on top of me. He talks to me. I have a special purpose. I am God's lover."

254. content

255. An apophanous autochthonous idea springs fully formed in the patient's mind. A delusional perception is based on a real stimulus, personalized, and made significant.

256. Apophanous phenomena is a category of phenomena characterized by false or arbitrary ideas developed without adequate proof.

(Note: No one should be totally happy with this definition. We can better define the specific phenomena of apophanous mood and ideas (primary and secondary).

257.   Draw lines between appropriate items in the two columns:

Delusional mood   "I'm going to die tomorrow. Why else would my mail not arrive?"

Autochthonous delu-sional idea   Sudden fully-formed apophanous idea

Primary delusional idea   "I feel as if someone or something sinister is watching me."

Secondary delusional idea   "I'm going to die tomorrow, the voice told me."

258.   Next to each of the following descriptions, indicate which apophanous phenomena it best illustrates:

"Something is going on out there. They're up to something. I can feel it. They're watching me."   _____

"I know they are after me. The voices tell me."   _____

"I know they are after me. The blue shirt you are wearing is the sign."   _____

"I know they are after me. I was walking down the street and it just came to me. It was a revelation."   _____

"I know they are after me. It just makes sense; people looking at me, the lights not working at home. They've done something to my house. They bugged it."   _____

259.   Next to each of the following descriptions, indicate which apophanous phenomena it best illustrates:

"I feel so bad...as if I'm dead. I want to cry but I can't. It's horrible I'm all dried up. It's hopeless...I'm dead ...I'm a corpse."   _____

"There must be machines in the wall. They must have placed them there. I can feel them putting radioactive waves in my body. The waves make me weak and then force me to do things."   _____

"The President's in on it. I heard him speaking to my brother last night. He won't kill me, however, I know his plans now."   _____

"I know they're trying to take over... I just know."   _____

257. Delusional mood —————— "I'm going to die tomorrow. Why else would my mail not arrive?"

Autochthonous delusional idea ————— Sudden fully formed apophanous idea

Primary delusional idea ————— "I feel as if someone or something sinister is watching me."

Secondary delusional idea ————— "I'm going to die tomorrow, the voice told me."

258. "Something is going on out there. They're up to something. I can feel it. They're watching me."

Delusional mood _____

"I know they are after me. The voices tell me."

Secondary delusional idea _____

"I know they are after me. The blue shirt you are wearing is the sign."

Delusional perception _____

"I know they are after me. I was walking down the street and it just came to me. It was a revelation."

Autochthonous delusional idea (one form of primary delusional ideas)

"I know they are after me. It just makes sense: people looking at me, the lights not working at home. They've bugged it."

Primary delusional idea _____

259. "I feel so bad...as if I'm dead. I want to cry but I can't. It's horrible I'm all dried up. It's hopeless...I'm dead...I'm a corpse."

Secondary delusional idea _____ (to a mood)

"There must be machines in the wall. They must have placed them there. I can feel them putting radioactive waves in my body. The waves make me weak and then force me to do things.

Secondary delusional idea _____ (to the feeling of waves coming into the body)

"The President's in on it. I heard him speaking to my brother last night. He won't kill me, however, I know his plans now."

Secondary delusional idea _____ (to hallucinated voices)

"I know they're trying to take over...I just know."

Primary delusional idea _____

260.   Next to each of the following descriptions, indicate which apophanous phenomena it best illustrates:

"It's eerie ...as if someone were watching
me. People are acting funny. Something
is wrong. It's frightening."   _____

"I am the king of the world. I have so
much energy, so many ideas. It's wonderful. I'm ecstatic."   _____

"When the man in the subway yawned,
I knew the train would crash."   _____

"He's trying to poison me. The TV
keeps telling me over and over again."   _____

260. "It's eerie...as if someone were
watching me. People are acting
funny. Something is wrong.
It's frightening."   Delusional mood

"I am the king of the world. I
have power beyond your imagin-
ation. I have so much energy,
so many ideas. It's wonderful.   Secondary delusional idea
I'm ecstatic."   (to a mood)

"When the man in the subway
yawned, I knew the train would
crash."   Delusional perception

"He's trying to poison me. The
TV keeps telling me over and   Secondary delusional idea
over again."   (to voices from the TV)

PERCEPTION AND FIRST RANK SYMPTOMS

261.   You have now learned a good deal about the recognition of behaviors classified under the five mental status headings of:

_____ _____ ,
_____ , _____ , _____ , and
_____ . The next area of examination is perceptual
function. Perceptual disturbances are very common among psychiatric patients. As with other areas of behavior, the form not the
content of these disturbances is of diagnostic importance.

262.   Perception is the brain's interpretation of exogenous and endogenous stimuli. The stimulus modalities we are interested in are
generally the traditional sensory systems of the body: visual, auditory, olfactory, gustatory, tactile and visceral. Perception is one
major process by which we know the real world and our reality perception is a complex process, inadequately understood, but obviously influenced by multiple genetic, constitutional, social, environmental, and pathological factors. When these factors distort, limit, or
otherwise damage the process of perception, a person's reality perception can be said to be disordered. Thus, if a person sees something that is not there, he has had a perception without a stimulus
and his reality perception is _____ .

263.   A hallucination is a disordered perception because it occurs
when no _____ has occurred.

264.   A hallucination is an example of disordered _____
_____ .

265.   Reality testing refers to the individual's ability to recognize
what perceptions are real--that is, reflecting real stimuli--and what
perceptions are not real--that is, distorted interpretations of real
stimuli or perceptions which develop without stimulus. Perceptions
which develop without stimulus are termed _____ .

261. general appearance, motor behavior, affect, thought processes, apophany

262. disordered

263 stimulus

264. reality perception

265. hallucinations

266.   The distinction between reality perception and reality testing is clinically important because many psychiatric patients have disturbed reality perception but are aware they are misperceiving and thus have good reality _____. Psychotic patients usually have both disordered reality _____ and poor reality _____. As they first begin to respond to treatment, patients continue to misperceive but begin to become aware of their misperceptions. Their _____ _____ improves first.

267.   Your ability to differentiate reality testing from reality perception will give you an early clue to your patient's beginning response to treatment. Write a sentence defining the difference between reality testing and reality perception.

268.   Hallucinations can occur in all sensory modalities: visual, auditory, olfactory, gustatory, tactile, and visceral. Hallucinations or _____ that occur without sensory _____ can happen under a variety of non-pathological conditions such as fatigue, distractability, and normal pre- and post-sleep states. Nearly 50% of people without any mental disorder have hallucinated at some time in their lives (31 pp. 18-22).

269.   Pseudo, or false hallucination is a term that refers to vague, poorly formed hallucinations or hallucinations which are experienced as occurring in inner subjective space (an "inner voice"). Pseudo-hallucinations occur in many people without mental disorder. Unfortunately, the prefix "pseudo" is a poor one since these phenomena are indeed hallucinations. Their vagueness and lack of intensity has lead to their being separated by the term "pseudo" from clear, fully-formed and intense hallucinations (62,63). Write a sentence defining a hallucination.

270.   Not infrequently, pseudo-hallucinations occur near sleep-onset. They are called hypnagogic hallucinations. When they occur upon awakening they are called hypnopompic hallucinations. Although they are given different names, these phenomena are most likely manifestations of identical processes. _____ hallucinations occurring as one falls asleep and _____ hallucinations occurring as one wakes up, have significance only for the diagnosis of altered sleep states (65).

271.   Vague, poorly formed perceptions occurring without real stimuli are termed _____. When they occur as a person falls asleep they are termed _____.

272.   A vague, poorly formed hallucination occurring as one falls asleep is termed hypnagogic. A similar phenomena occurring as one awakes is termed _____.

273.   One of the most commonly hallucinated phenomena is termed incomplete auditory hallucinations (42). Incomplete auditory hallucinations are voices. They are muffled, whispered, often experienced as coming from inside the head and are usually limited to a few words or phrases. _____ _____ auditory hallucinations occur with great frequency in all psychoses.

266. testing, perception, testing, reality testing

267. Reality perception is your ability to accurately interpret exogenous and endogenous stimuli. Reality testing is your ability to determine the accuracy of your perceptions.

268. perceptions, stimuli

269. A hallucination is a perception without a stimulus.

270. hypnagogic, hypnopompic

271. pseudo hallucinations, hypnagogic

272. hypnopompic

273. incomplete

274.　　　Some patients experience unformed hallucinations such as flashes of light, unidentified noises, smells and tastes. These phenomena are termed elementary hallucinations (31,32,62,63). A muffled whispered voice termed an _____ is not an elementary hallucination because even though it is vague it has form, i.e., the patient identifies it as a voice.

275.　　　Although not necessarily a manifestation of pathology, unformed hallucinations occur in numerous morbid states (toxic, depressive, epileptic, schizophrenic). These unformed unidentified noises, smells, lights and tastes are termed _____.

276.　　　If a patient complains about a whispered voice that is bothering him at night, but he knows the voice is not real, his reality _____ is disordered, but his reality _____ remains intact.

277.　　　A hallucinated whispered voice is an example of an _____
_____ _____.

278.　　　Not infrequently, patients will hallucinate only immediately after ordinary stimulation in that particular sensory modality. For example, a patient heard voices only when the electric fan was on. This phenomenon is termed a functional hallucination and can occur in numerous morbid states (depressive, epileptic and schizophrenic) (32,63,64). Unformed hallucinations, termed _____ hallucinations, can also occur in these conditions.

279.　　　Occasionally, patients report hallucinations which occur outside the normal sensory field. They see people behind them or hear voices in another country. This phenomenon is termed an extracampine hallucination and, like hallucinations occurring immediately after ordinary stimulation (termed _____) and unformed hallucinations (termed _____), can occur in numerous morbid states (toxic, depressive, epileptic, and schizophrenic) (31).

280.　　　Draw lines between appropriate items in the two columns:

Elementary hallucination

Hypnagogic hallucination

Functional hallucination

Reality testing

A hallucination only after sensory stimulation

Unformed hallucinations

A pseudo-hallucination upon falling asleep

The ability to tell real from false perceptions

281.　　　Draw lines between appropriate items in the two columns:

Reality perception

Pseudo-hallucination

Incomplete auditory hallucination

Hypnopompic hallucination

A vague poorly formed hallucination

A brief, whispered voice

A pseudo-hallucination while awakening

Ability to accurately perceive sensory stimuli

274. incomplete auditory hallucination

275. elementary hallucinations

276. perception, testing

277. incomplete auditory hallucination

278. elementary

279. functional, elementary

280.

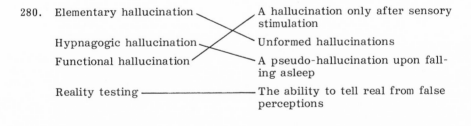

Elementary hallucination — A hallucination only after sensory stimulation

Hypnagogic hallucination — Unformed hallucinations

Functional hallucination — A pseudo-hallucination upon falling asleep

Reality testing ———————— The ability to tell real from false perceptions

281. Reality perception — A vague poorly formed hallucination.

Pseudo-hallucination — A brief, whispered voice

Incomplete auditory hallucination — A pseudo-hallucination while awakening

Hypnopompic hallucination — Ability to accurately perceive sensory stimuli

282. Draw lines between appropriate items in the two columns:

Extracampine hallucinations — Muffled, voices, vague music

Hypnagogic hallucination — Flashing lights

Incomplete auditory hallu-
cinations — Significant only in altered sleep
states

Elementary hallucination — A hallucination outside the normal sensory field

283. The particular sensory modality of a hallucination can provide
a clue to the nature of a patient's disorder. The modality of the
hallucination is part of its form. The hallucination's vividness
(clarity), perceived source (inside inner subjective space or outside the self) and duration are also part of its form. What the hallucination is about, or its _____, is rarely of diagnostic significance.

284. The most frequently observed perceptual disturbances among
psychiatric patients are visual and incomplete auditory hallucinations
(13,40-42,71,72). Although no hallucination is pathognomonic, some
are characteristic of specific psychiatric conditions. Visual hallucinations, for example, including functional and elementary hallucinations,
are most often manifestations of coarse brain disease, particularly
toxic states (31). Muffled voices, footsteps, groans, and voices of
short duration termed _____ _____ _____,
are most often associated with manias, depressions and schizophrenia
(13,33,40-42,58,65,71,72).

285. Tactile or somatosensory, haptic or visceral, olfactory and gustatory hallucinations are not uncommon among psychiatric patients
but unfortunately, many clinicians fail to inquire about the presence
of these phenomena. Although they can all occur in affective disorders (that is, mania and depressions), and in schizophrenia,
their presence should suggest _____ brain disease (13,33,
40-42,58,65,71,72).

286. A perception when no sensory stimulus has occurred is termed
a _____. A false or misperception of a real sensory stimulus
is termed an illusion.

287. Misperceptions of real sensory stimuli or _____ can occur
in normals as well as in most psychiatric conditions.

288. Misperceptions of real stimuli or _____, often occur because
of fatigue or an extremely intense mood.

289. A frightened person, misperceiving shadows as threatening people, demonstrates an example of an _____.

290. Write a sentence defining the difference between a hallucination
and an illusion.

282. Extracampine hallucinations   Muffled, voices, vague music

Hypnagogic hallucination   Flashing lights

Incomplete auditory hallu-cinations   Significant only in altered sleep states

Elementary hallucination   A hallucination outside the normal sensory field

283. content

284. incomplete auditory hallucinations

285. coarse

286. hallucinations

287. illusions

288. illusions

289. illusion

290. A hallucination is a perception without a stimulus; an illusion is a misperception of a real stimulus.

115

291.   Some perceptions take the form of distortion of the real stimulus. Objects can be visualized as smaller or larger than their real size; sounds are perceived as louder or softer than their true intensity or depth perception is suddenly lost. On the other hand, misinterpretations of a real stimulus are termed _____.

292.   Perceiving objects as becoming larger is termed macropsia. Perceiving objects as becoming smaller is termed micropsia. Macropsia and micropsia are examples of perceptual _____.

293.   Perceptual distortion can take the form of objects becoming larger _____opsia or smaller, _____opsia.

294.   Macropsia and micropsia are examples of perceptual distortion where objects are perceived as changing in _____. These phenomena come under the general heading of dysmegalopsia and are often experienced in epileptic states (15,23).

295.   Draw lines between appropriate items in the two columns:

Illusion   "I feel a snake crawling in my stomach"

Micropsia   "Everything suddenly becomes small & far away"

Elementary hallucination   "I was running home and as the trees moved, I thought I saw a giant"

Haptic hallucination   "I see flashes of light"

296.   Draw lines between appropriate items in the two columns:

Haptic hallucination   "I see objects becoming suddenly larger"

Macropsia   "I hear a voice only when the water is running from the faucet"

Functional hallucination   Whispered voices

Incomplete auditory   A visceral perception without a stimulus
hallucination

297.   As patients relate what has happened to them, many will inadvertently reveal experiences which are obviously hallucinations:

Example: "I saw a man with a knife standing at the foot of the bed. He disappeared when I turned on the light."

"I see a shining cross in the sky."

"God is talking to me now."

However, in the seriously ill, it is likely that they believe their hallucinations to be real. They have poor _____ _____ and poor _____ _____. In this situation, the examiner must be skilled in obtaining information about hallucinatory experiences.

291. illusions

292. distortion

293. macro, micro

294. size

295. Illusion 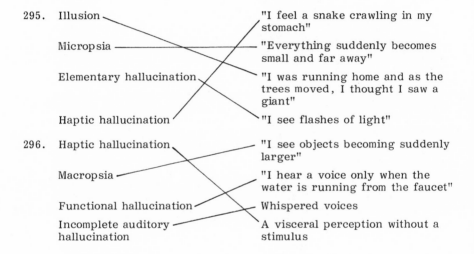 "I feel a snake crawling in my stomach"

Micropsia "Everything suddenly becomes small and far away"

Elementary hallucination "I was running home and as the trees moved, I thought I saw a giant"

Haptic hallucination "I see flashes of light"

296. Haptic hallucination "I see objects becoming suddenly larger"

Macropsia "I hear a voice only when the water is running from the faucet"

Functional hallucination Whispered voices

Incomplete auditory hallucination A visceral perception without a stimulus

297. reality perception, reality testing

298.   When examining a patient for apophany, we ask him about "trouble with neighbors, co-workers, or family members" which might reveal the patient's delusional ideas, or perceptions about these or other people. Hallucinatory experiences can, at times, be elicited in a similar manner. Questions such as: "Have any of the neighbors or any other people been bothering you or trying to harm you?"... "Have you seen any of them following you?"..."Can you hear them talking about you or saying bad things about you?"   This will often encourage a patient to describe voices, visions, and other perceptual phenomena. The development of good rapport with the patient is vital if you are to obtain adequate information about apophanous and perceptual phenomena. Patients will converse with you more readily if you can make them feel that you are concerned, interested in their experiences (as if they were real), and that you have heard about such things before. Frequently, a statement like the following is helpful: "I have spoken with other people with similar experiences (feelings, situations) to yours and they also..." You then simply give examples of apophany, hallucinations, or illusions and many patients will respond with "Yes, I've had that happen to me too." Details usually follow.

        Once this process has begun, the introduction of more obvious "crazy" experiences is less likely to be met with resistance. "Have any of these people (who are talking about you and trying to hurt you) tried to spy on you?...Bug your house with machines?...Do they use the TV or radio?...Do they try to control you?...I know a man who felt that some machine in the wall was controlling his thoughts. Did you ever experience something like that?"

        Throughout the conversational examination, the patient should feel that you know about such things and that you know people believe such things, and also that you are simply interested. Should the patient ask you directly, "Do you think I'm right?" the best reply is, "I understand what you're saying and I know you feel these (frightening) experiences to be true, but I wonder whether there isn't another explanation." If the patient says, "No, there isn't", go on to the next logical topic. If the patient insists on your opinion, offer the explanation that the experiences are signs and symptoms of an illness. After you've said your peace, don't argue. You're on the record; you've told the patient the truth without attacking him. Many patients will trust you even more for being truthful and disagreeing, than for appeasing them and treating them as if they're crazy, or for disregarding their feelings and fighting with them about the validity of their experiences. On rarer occasions, a fruitful question might be: "Have you recently had any frightening experiences or experiences that you couldn't explain?" You can then give the patient some examples of voices or visions. One in a hundred patients will respond positively to the questions, "Do you hallucinate? Do you hear voices?"

        It is not easy to examine for apophany and perceptual phenomena in the manner just described. It takes time, self-control and a bit of acting skill. If you master it even partially, however, it will serve you well.

298.   (No answer required. Just rest and think about it.)

299.   Popular literature, music, and art often express experiences
which we observe in patients. Label each pop music phrase with
the appropriate phenomenologic term:

"I hear singing and there's no
one there."

_____

"She dances overhead, on the
ceiling near my bed."

_____

"Lucy in the sky with diamonds

_____

300.   Label each description with the appropriate phenomenologic
term:

"It's frightening---suddenly
everything becomes very small
as if I were looking through the
wrong end of a telescope."

_____

"It happens many times during
the day. I suddenly smell burning rubber or rotting flesh. I
feel dizzy and then it's all right
again."

_____

"It's a frightening man. I can
see him walking behind me.
Sometimes I see him in another
city."

_____

"I can't make it out. It's
some sort of a noise or hum
but I hear it all over the
place."

_____

301.   Next to each of the following descriptions, indicate which perceptual disturbance it best illustrates:

"I can hear him talking all the
way from California: 1900 miles!"

_____

"It's horrible. Everything
becomes flat and then bigger
as if swollen. It makes me
sick to my stomach."

_____

"I woke up in the middle of the
night and saw this transparent
figure standing over my head."

_____

"It's like a buzzing noise. I
can just make it out."

_____

299. "I hear singing and there's no one there."

Incomplete auditory hallucination
(auditory hallucination)

"She dances overhead, on the ceiling near my bed."

Hypnagogic hallucination

"Lucy in the sky with diamonds."

Visual hallucination

300. "It's frightening---suddenly everything becomes very small as if I were looking through the wrong end of a telescope."

Micropsia (dysmegalopsia)

"It happens many times during the day. I suddenly smell burning rubber or rotting flesh. I feel dizzy and then it's all right again."

Olfactory hallucination

"It's a frightening man. I can see him walking behind me. Sometimes I see him in another city."

Extracampine visual hallucination

"I can't make it out. It's some sort of a noise or hum but I hear it all over the place."

Elementary auditory hallucination

301. "I can hear him talking all the way from California: 1900 miles!"

Extracampine hallucination

"It's horrible. Everything becomes flat and then bigger as if swollen. It makes me sick to my stomach."

Macropsia (dysmegalopsia)

"I woke up in the middle of the night and saw this transparent figure standing over my head."

Hypnopompic hallucination

"It's like a buzzing noise. I can just make it out."

Elementary hallucination

302. Next to each of the following descriptions, indicate which perceptual disturbance it best illustrates:

"I feel a hand moving in my stomach." _____

"I taste metal." _____

"I am sitting alone in my room and I suddenly smell burning rubber or rotting flesh." _____

"Everything is o.k. until the phone rings or the door bell goes off - then I hear this voice calling me names." _____

"Every time I heard a noise it sounded like a person moving around in the house. It was scary." _____

303. Next to each of the following descriptions, indicate which perceptual disturbance it best illustrates:

"I see light rays bouncing off things. It's like a glow...a haze of light." _____

"Just before I fell asleep I saw this animal jump about in the corner of the room." _____

"The room suddenly became small and far away. I felt dizzy." _____

"I hear this voice. It says my name or mumbles something to me." _____

"I feel these things, like worms, crawling about under my skin." _____

"The shadow looked like a gorilla." _____

304. Kurt Schneider was the first person to describe systematically the phenomena he labeled first rank symptoms (60). Schneider asserted that, in the absence of coarse brain disease, the presence of any one of these phenomena was decisive in the diagnosis of schizophrenia. Schneider's assertion was based on anecdotal clinical observations. He believed these phenomena to be "first rank" only in a clinical sense with no etiological significance. Even though his descriptions and definitions have generated great interest in the phenomenological study of schizophrenia, studies (1,19,52,70-72, 74) have demonstrated that although Schneiderian's first rank symptoms occur in 60 to 75 percent of rigorously defined schizophrenics, they are also experienced by individuals with affective disease, particularly during manic episodes. Although no longer "first rank" in the diagnostic sense, first rank symptoms are still useful in determining severe illness.

302.   "I feel a hand moving in my
      stomach."   Haptic (visceral) hallucination

      "I taste metal."   Gustatory (taste) hallucination

      "I am sitting alone in my room
      and I suddenly smell burning
      rubber or rotting flesh."   Olfactory (smell) hallucination

      "Everything is o.k. until the
      phone rings or the door bell
      goes off - then I hear this
      voice calling me names."   Functional hallucination

      "Every time I heard a noise it
      sounded like a person moving
      around in the house. It was
      scary."   Auditory illusion

303.   "I see light rays bouncing off
      things. It's like a glow...a
      haze of light."   Elementary hallucination

      "Just before I fell asleep I
      saw this animal jump about in
      the corner of the room."   Hypnagogic hallucination

      "The room suddenly became
      small and far away. I felt
      dizzy."   Micropsia (form of dysmegalopsia)

      "I hear this voice. It says
      my name or mumbles some-
      thing to me."   Incomplete auditory hallucination

      "I feel those things, like
      worms, crawling about under
      my skin."   Tactile (somatosensory) hallu-
                             cination

      "The shadow looked like a
      gorilla."   Visual illusion

304.   No answer required

305.   Although Schneider listed eleven _____ _____
symptoms, they can be conveniently categorized under five major
headings:

1) Thought broadcasting, 2) Experiences of alienation, 3) Experiences of influence, 4) Complete auditory hallucinations, 5) Delusional perceptions.

306.   According to Schneider, in thought broadcasting, the patient
experiences that as his thoughts occur, they escape from his head
aloud into the external world. Some clinicians assume thought ___
_____ to be a hallucinatory experience, but as Schneider
described it and as patients relate it, _____
_____ is the experience, the feeling of losing one's
thoughts to the outside world. Patients with both thought broadcasting and auditory hallucinations experience them as different phenomena.

307.   Patients will often have secondary delusional ideas involving
telepathy, electronic surveillance or power rays that explain the
phenomena that their thoughts escape aloud from their heads so that
others can hear them. This is termed _____
_____.

308.   Once a patient has told you about his apophanous ideas and you
have been asking detailed questions about "how he knows," it is a
natural sequence to ask about plots involving electronic surveillance,
or attempts at telepathy. From this progress to questions such as,
"Do you feel that people are reading your mind?...Can others really
(literally) hear your thoughts?...You mean it's like your thoughts
were coming out of your head, as loud as my voice?...Come on,
you're kidding me. You mean to say it's as if your head were like
a radio and everybody here can hear what you're thinking?" If a
patient responds positively to these questions, he is admitting to the
first rank symptom of _____.
Sometimes naive observers object to such a line of questioning. It
appears to them that you are "putting words in the mouths of patients." Don't let this attitude faze you. You must ascertain whether or not a patient has apophanous ideas in order to arrive at a diagnosis. The form of these ideas has diagnostic value. Your apparently "leading questions" are in response to statements your patient
has made. If the patient denies experiencing any of the phenomena
I have described, you obviously won't ask him if his head is "like a
radio."

309.   When a patient expresses the feeling that others can read his
mind or says that he believes that people know what he's thinking
by the expression on their faces, we can conclude that he has apophanous ideas. These are not sufficient statements, however, to
qualify for the experience of others hearing his thoughts coming a-
loud out of his head. When a patient was asked what he was planning to do that day, he laughed and then said testily, "You know
perfectly well what my plans are; everyone in this room does; you're
hearing them right now...All those machines in the floor are letting
everyone hear them." This is an example of _____
_____.

305. first rank

306. broadcasting, thought broadcasting

307. thought broadcasting

308. thought broadcasting

309. thought broadcasting (if you added secondary delusional idea you would also be correct).

310.   Many seriously ill patients describe the experience that their body sensations, feelings, impulses, thoughts and actions are imposed upon them by some external agency; that they are literally "being controlled," can literally "feel" the controlling force, and they must passively submit to the experience. Schneider termed this phenomenon experiences of influence. Patients often develop _____ _____ delusional ideas that explain the nature of their experiences of _____ .

311.   A frightened 19-year-old female student described her teacher as continually "emitting energy waves" which made her think homosexual thoughts, and which made her assume "certain sexual" body postures. The student "felt" the teacher "control" her body, "touching her genitals" and vibrating over her skin while she remained still, unable to move or resist. This student was experiencing the Schneiderian _____ _____ symptom of ____ _____ .

312.   In experiences of alienation the patient's feelings, impulses, thoughts or actions are felt not to be his own but to literally belong to someone else. Secondary delusional ideas explaining the nature of this external force are common.
    Experiences of alienation are the subjective disowning of one's feelings, thoughts, or movements, i.e., "it's not mine". In contrast, experiences of _____ are primary subjective feelings of being controlled by some outside force and of involuntary submission.

313.   If it's yours, but it's being controlled, it's an experience of _____ . If it's not yours, but somehow attached to your body, or in your mind, it's an experience of _____ .

314.   Some people refer to the feeling of loss of contact or empathy with family, friends or society as "alienation." The Schneiderian _____ _____ is quite different. The patient experiences his feelings, thoughts, or movements as "foreign," not part of the self, and as though they "do not belong" to him.

315.   Some patients with large parietal lobe lesions will deny any relationship to certain of their body parts (21). They will say: "That arm is not mine, I don't know what that thing is but it's not mine, mine is over there next to it." While this phenomenon is similar in many ways to the Schneiderian first rank symptom of _____ _____ , cerebral localization has never been demonstrated for any first rank symptom.

310. secondary, influence

311. first rank, influence

312. influence

313. influence, alienation

314. experience of alienation

315. alienation

316.   A 19-year-old patient complained of concentration difficulties resulting from unwanted thoughts which suddenly appeared in his stream of consciousness but which were "obviously" not his own. He insisted that: "someone keeps putting things in my head...and the pressure is too much." He spent hours cleaning the ward kitchen but insisted the cleaning activity was not part of him. He knew he was there while it happened, but the action was "disconnected" from his "self" like a "foreign body" and was attributed to the "actions of God." This young man's complaint is an example of an _____ _____. His belief that God was literally responsible for the actions people said were his is an example of a _____ delusional idea.

317.   The 19-year-old man in the previous item felt that God was putting thoughts in his head. This is often referred to as thought insertion because the inserted thought is experienced as a foreign body, this phenomenon is termed an experience of _____.

318.   Some patients describe the phenomena of suddenly losing all mental and motor activity, i.e., suddenly going blank as in petit mal epilepsy or as observed in the thought disorder termed_____ _____. Patients with these experiences will sometimes state that someone or something has taken their thoughts away. This experience is often referred to as thought withdrawal and is often literally experienced or felt as the result of some outside force (e.g., gamma rays, thought vacuum). In this form, it is an experience of _____.

319.   Schneider listed experiencing foreign thoughts being placed in one's head or thought _____, having one's thoughts taken away or _____, and blocking, as separate first rank symptoms. Since there is no evidence that their separation enhances the selection of more homogenous patient groups, they have been included under the terms experiences of _____ and of _____.

320.   In the presentation of perceptual disorders, you learned about whispered voices of short duration or _____ _____. Schneider described hallucinated voices which: occurred in clear consciousness, were clearly audible, were experienced as coming from outside the patient's head (inner subjective space) and were sustained in duration. He termed these voices phonemes or complete auditory hallucinations.

321.   Phonemes, or _____ auditory hallucinations are prolonged voices, continually commenting upon the patient's actions, discussing the patient among themselves or repeating the patient's thoughts.

322.   The auditory hallucination of a voice continually repeating a patient's thoughts is an example of a complete auditory hallucination or a _____.

316. experience of alienation, secondary

317. alienation

318. blocking, influence

319. insertion, withdrawal, alienation, influence

320. incomplete auditory hallucinations

321. complete

322. phoneme

323.   The phenomenon of a voice repeating the patient's thoughts is also termed thought echo. This should not be confused with the patient's experience of his thoughts escaping aloud from his head which is termed _____ . _____ .

324.   When a patient hears someone repeat his thoughts to him, it is termed thought echo or a _____ hallucination. When a patient literally feels his thought escaping aloud from his head, it is termed _____ _____ _____ .

325.   In the presentation of apophany, you have learned about primary delusional ideas that develop from real perceptions. Schneider termed these _____ _____ . This is the last form of first rank symptoms.

326.   A delusional perception is based upon the patient perceiving a real stimulus, making it significant ("that's important"), making it personal ("that's important to me"), and then reaching a conclusion for which you (the empathic examiner) cannot feel a meaningful connection between the real stimulus (the "proof") and the patient's conclusion (the delusion).

327.   A delusional perception has all of the following characteristics except:

a)   Based upon a real stimulus

b)   The real stimulus is given special meaning by the observer

c)   The content of the conclusion is always persecutory

d)   There is no meaningful connection between the real stimulus and the patient's conclusion as to its significance.

328.   A patient entered the examiner's office, frowned and said, "I see, you're in on it too!" When asked to explain, she reluctantly pointed to the coffee cup on the desk and said, "You see that, don't you? Well, isn't it obvious? You're in on it! It (the cup) is all the proof I need to show me you're with those bastards against me." This patient perceived a real stimulus, the _____ ; she personalized it: proof that you are against me"; she made the perception significant: "You're in on it," i.e., made a connection between the cup and the idea for which there is no understanding (meaningful connection) and she stated an apophanous phenomenon which is the Schneiderian first rank symptom of _____ _____ .

329.   Draw lines between matching items in the two columns:

Thought broadcasting   "I feel someone putting his thoughts in my head. I feel them in there now."

Phoneme (complete auditory hallucination)   "My thoughts came out of my head like a radio."

Experience of alienation   "Comes from outside my house and yells at me all day long."

323. thought broadcasting

324. complete auditory, thought broadcasting

325. delusional perceptions

326. no answer required

327. c)

328. cup, delusional perception

329. Thought broadcasting   "I feel someone putting his thoughts in my head. I feel them in there now."

Phoneme (complete auditory hallucination)   "My thoughts came out of my head like a radio."

Experience of alienation   "Comes from outside my house and yells at me all day long."

330.   Draw lines between matching items in the two columns:

Experience of influence | "Every time I have a thought that bastard says it back to me."

Delusional perception | "The machine makes me stand still."

Thought echo | "The yellow bus didn't come to-day. I am going to die."

331.   Label the description with all the appropriate phenomenologic terms:

"You know perfectly well what's happening to me! You and those machines! I know, you're in it with the rest of them. They're all trying to hurt me. I can feel that machine pull the thoughts right out of my head. Everyone hears them. What do you mean 'What are you thinking about?' You hear them too, you liar!"

332.   Draw lines between appropriate items in rows 1 and 2, and be-tween rows 2 and 3:

Thought insertion | The patient sud-denly becomes silent, immobile & unresponsive & after a few moments becomes animated again & begins speak-ing. | Thought withdrawal

Phoneme | Experiences of alienation | A clear, sustained hallucinated voice coming from outside one's head.

Blocking | A patient stated that a man's voice constantly talked to her and that it came from a spot on the wall. | A patient was very upset because someone else's leg seemed to be attached to her body.

132

330. Experience of influence   "Every time I have a thought, that bastard says it back to me."

Delusional perception   "The machine makes me stand still."

Thought echo   "The yellow bus didn't come to-day. I am going to die."

331. secondary delusional ideas
experiences of influence with an irritable mood
thought broadcasting

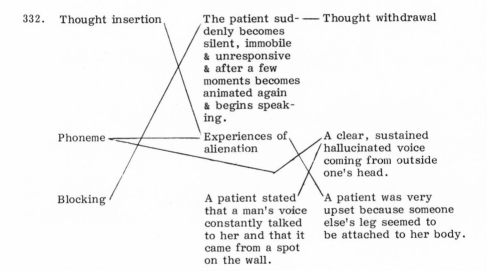

332. Thought insertion   The patient sud- —— Thought withdrawal
denly becomes
silent, immobile
& unresponsive
& after a few
moments becomes
animated again
& begins speak-
ing.

Phoneme   Experiences of   A clear, sustained
alienation   hallucinated voice
coming from outside
one's head.

Blocking   A patient stated   A patient was very
that a man's voice   upset because someone
constantly talked   else's leg seemed to
to her and that it   be attached to her body.
came from a spot
on the wall.

333.   Next to each of the following descriptions, indicate which Schneiderian first rank symptom it best illustrates:

"They're talking all the time, both of them. They yell at me, say vile things. Can't shut them up. I hear them now yelling from the other room."

_____

"The rays come from the television station. They go into the antenna on the roof, into the wires and then through the house and into me. They vibrate and tingle, Sometimes they make me weak and I can't move. They keep my arms at my side and I can't overcome it."

_____

"There are too many things in my head. I can't think. He keeps putting them in there and they move about. The thoughts he puts there jumble things up and I can't think my own thoughts."

_____

334.   Next to each of the following descriptions, indicate which Schneiderian first rank symptom it best illustrates:

"A green phone...a green phone! As soon as I saw that I knew what was happening. They've infiltrated the government."

_____

"Sure everyone can hear them. They come out of my head as if someone is sucking them out. Everytime I think I feel them being sucked out. Everyone hears my thoughts once they're outside my head."

_____

"I can't make a move without that bastard telling me what I'm doing. All day long he talks to me. I think he put a transmitter into a freckle on my back."

_____

333. "They're talking all the time, both of them. They yell at me, say vile things. Can't shut them up. I hear them now yelling from the other room."

Complete auditory hallucination / phoneme

"The rays come from the television station. They go into the antenna on the roof, into the wires and then through the house and into me. They vibrate and tingle. Sometimes they make me weak and I can't move. They keep my arms at my side and I can't overcome it."

Experience of influence (with secondary delusional ideas)

"There are too many things in my head. I can't think. He keeps putting them there and they move about. The thoughts he puts there jumble things up and I can't think my own thoughts."

Experience of alienation / Thought insertion (with a secondary delusional idea)

334. "A green phone...a green phone! As soon as I saw that I knew what was happening. They've infiltrated the government."

Delusional perception

"Sure everyone can hear them. They come out of my head as if someone is sucking them out. Everytime I think I feel them being sucked out. Everyone hears my thoughts once they're outside my head."

Thought broadcasting

"I can't make a move without that bastard telling me what I'm doing. All day long he talks to me. I think he put a transmitter into a freckle on my back."

Complete auditory hallucination / phoneme (with a secondary delusional idea of a transmitter in a freckle)

COGNITIVE FUNCTION

335. A complete mental status examination must include a thorough evaluation of cognitive function. Numerous investigators (11,57, 73,75,77) have demonstrated significant cognitive impairment in as many as 60 percent of severely ill psychiatric patients. Although an evaluation of cognitive functioning should be systematic, the examiner should maintain the flow of the interview by asking questions or eliciting tasks which clarify the patient's complaints or difficulties. Specific questions can be asked however, and the patient can be requested to perform structured tasks without fear of losing the rapport vital to proper examination.

336. In this part of the mental status examination, we are concerned with behaviors which reflect known cerebral cortical and subcortical functioning. It usually takes about 20 minutes to evaluate these behaviors properly. Once this task is completed, you will have obtained a reasonably reliable and valid profile of cerebral _____ function. Some understanding of cerebral anatomical landmarks and functional regions is essential if the profile of cerebral function is to be correlated with localization of lesions or area in dysfunction.

337. In the preceding sections of this text, we have followed a sequence of mental status areas which parallels the usual natural sequence of observations. Thus we begin with an evaluation of _____ _____ and then _____ _____ before we find out about affect and thought processes, i.e., we evaluate what we see in the patient before we evaluate what the patient says.

338. To simplify the material, this section will break with the natural sequence of evaluation and present the mental status of cognition organized by cerebral _____ regions or functional areas rather than by the conversational sequence of a good interview.

335. No answer required

336. cognitive

337. general appearance, motor behavior

338. cortical

339.   A patient's responses to tests of cognitive functioning must be interpreted in the context of his previous education, cultural background, motivation for doing his best on the tests, and the situation in which the examination is conducted. Tests of cognitive function are essentially evaluating cerebral _____ function.

340.   If a patient has only an elementary school education or comes from a socially deprived environment, responses to questions regarding fund of information and vocabulary must be interpreted with caution. Persons from other countries are also often handicapped when asked to perform certain "American" tests of cognition. Their responses must therefore be cautiously evaluated. Education, motivation, acculturation and native language are all important factors affecting the performance on tests of cognition. Circle the factors below which can affect performance on tests of cognition:

High school drop-out   Extremely tall   Lack of interest

Fluency in language   Literary   Divorced
of test

341.   Cerebral _____ impairment is frequently observed in psychiatric patients. Standard concepts use the terms "delirium" or "acute organic brain syndrome" to refer to conditions where the cognitive impairment is diffuse and reversible.

342.   A diffuse, coarse brain disorder which develops rapidly, is transient, and reversible is termed a _____ .

343.   In contrast to delirious states, dementias are diffuse, coarse brain disorders where the cognitive impairment develops slowly and is _____ .

344.   Since some patients with so-called acute onset diffuse, reversible conditions termed _____ become chronically ill and some patients with slow onset diffuse, irreversible conditions termed _____ recover in part, it is often best, when examining a patient, to cautiously use these terms and evaluate specific functions or cortical regions and whether each is impaired or intact.

339. cortical

340. (High school drop-out)   Extremely tall   (Lack of interest)
     (Fluency of language   (Literary)   Divorced
     of test

341. cognitive

342. delirium

343. irreversible

344. deliriums, dementias

139

345.   During the examination you will obtain a general impression of
the patient's cognitive ability from your informal observations of
the patient's vocabulary, fund of information and ability to accurately
relate details and sequence of personal events. Some examiners inquire whether the patient "remembers" or becomes "confused" about
such things as local politicians, current events, national politicians.
This line of discussion often leads to the questions:

"Who is the Mayor?"

"Who is the Governor?"

"What is the capital of this state?...the country?"

"Who is the President?...Before him?...and before him?...
What happened to him?...etc."

These questions and those about the population of the United States,
distances between the West and East coast and recent major news
events are all helpful, as is your general impression of the patient's
abilities. Nevertheless, they are crude and should not substitute
for methodological testing of specific functions of cerebral
_____ regions.

346.   During the past two decades, rapid, reliable and valid methods
have been developed for testing cognitive function. These tests,
in part, focus on the localization of certain cognitive functions in the
dominant cerebral hemisphere. Other functions are localized in the
non-_____ hemisphere.

347.   For more than 97 percent of individuals, the dominant cerebral
hemisphere is the left (29,44,45,61), the non-dominant cerebral hemisphere is usually the _____.

348.   Dominant function usually refers to symbolic cognition and language related processes (29,44,45,47,61,76). In about 97 percent
of individuals, these functions are performed by the _____
hemisphere.

349.   Non-dominant functioning usually refers to non-symbolic spatial/
perceptual cognition. In most individuals, these functions are performed by the _____ hemisphere (44,45,47,61).

350.   Dominant, non-dominant cerebral function is, in actuality, not
a single separation. For our purposes, however, we will assume
simplicity and learn to evaluate patient's cognition as if verbal cognition was clearly _____ functioning and non-verbal
spatial/perceptual cognition clearly _____ functioning.

345. cortical

346. dominant

347. right

348. left

349. right

350. dominant, non-dominant

351.   A gross test of cerebral dominance requires the patient to write his name (see below). The preferred hand held in a "hooked" position above the line of writing suggests the dominant hemisphere is on the same side as the preferred hand. The preferred hand held below the line of writing (most common) suggests the dominant hemisphere is on the opposite side to the preferred hand (46).

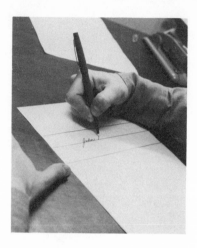
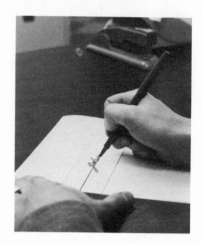

<table>
<tr><td align="center">Same Side
Dominant Hemisphere</td><td align="center">Opposite Side
Dominant Hemisphere</td></tr>
</table>

352.   When asked to write her name, a patient held her right hand below the line of writing. This suggests that her _____ hemisphere is dominant for language.

353.   Since about 97 percent of people have a dominant left hemisphere and most people also write with their contralateral (opposite) hand, the right one, most people must also write with their right hand _____ the line of writing.

354.   Specialized tests of cerebral dominance involve electroencephalographic monitoring and intracarotid injections of sedatives (76). For purposes of a mental status examination, the location of the preferred hand to the line of writing (above or below) can determine the _____ _____. In most individuals, it is the _____ hemisphere.

355.   In addition to hand position when writing, information about hand preference for different tasks can aid in determining the dominant hemisphere. If you were to test the entire population, how many would you find to be left cerebral dominant? _____

351. No answer required

352. left

353. below

354. dominant hemisphere, left

355. 97 percent

356. The examiner asked the following questions:

"Which hand do you throw a ball with?"

"Which hand do you write with?"

"Which hand do you pour liquids with?"

To each question the patient responded: "my right." In such a clear-cut situation (a pure right-hander), the odds are overwhelming that the patient's dominant cerebral hemisphere will be contralateral to the preferred right hand. If so, what is the writing hand position of such a person? _____

357. Between 5 and 10 percent of the population is left handed. Nevertheless, _____ of the population is left cerebral dominant. What can you conclude from these figures regarding the cerebral dominance and writing hand position of most left handers? Write down your conclusion.

358. Draw lines between matching items in the two columns:

Dominant hemisphere is ipsilateral (same side) to preferred hand	Writes with hand below the line of writing
Dominant hemisphere function	Writes with hand above the line of writing
Dominant hemisphere is contralateral (opposite) to preferred hand	Language function
Non-dominant hemisphere function	Non-verbal function

359. Following a stroke, a patient spoke with difficulty. The area of damage most likely was in the _____ hemisphere.

360. Following a stroke a patient spoke with difficulty and had trouble using his preferred hand, the left. An electroencephalogram showed abnormality in the left temporo-parietal area. This suggests that this person's dominant hemisphere for language was the _____ _____, but that unlike most individuals the preferred hand was _____, not contralateral to the dominant hemisphere.

361. From the information about the patient in item 360 you would predict that when writing he held his hand _____ the line of writing.

144

356. below the line

357. 97% - Many left handers are left cerebral dominant and write in the "hooked" position above the line of writing.

358. Dominant hemisphere is ipsilateral (same side to preferred hand)

Dominant hemisphere function

Dominant hemisphere is contralateral (opposite) to preferred hand

Non-dominant hemisphere function

Writes with hand below the line of writing

Writes with hand above the line of writing

Language function

Non-verbal function

359. left

360. left, ipsilateral

361. above

145

FRONTAL LOBE COGNITIVE DYSFUNCTION

362.   The frontal lobes rostral to (in front of) the motor areas have executive function over other areas of the cerebral _____ (47 pp. 187-225).

363.   Unlike other cortical regions, the differentiation of the frontal lobes into dominant and non-dominant functions is not clear-cut. Although language function is lateralized in the dominant, usually the _____ frontal lobe, other frontal lobe functions appear more diffuse (47 pp. 187-225).

364.   The frontal lobes focus attention (concentration), regulate (organize and program) motor behavior, synthesize information from all other cortical regions, monitor all behaviors and plan new ones (47 pp. 270-279). It is not unlike a futuristic computer that implements and monitors its old programs and develops its own new programs as needed. Unlike other cortical regions most frontal lobe functions cannot be _____ to the right or left lobe.

365.   In the mental status examination, we can evaluate the frontal lobe functions of:

1.   Global orientation in clear consciousness

2.   Concentration

3.   Regulation of motor behavior

4.   Language

5.   Active perception

6.   Judgment and abstract thinking

146

362. cortex

363. left

364. lateralized

365. No answer required

366.　　　All too frequently the inexperienced clinician assumes that "crazy" is a synonym for disoriented and following "Hello," blurts out, "What's today's date, and who is the President?"

　　　Not only is this approach not conversational, but it is not exactly the best way of establishing the rapport vitally needed for the examination. Better to wait for the appropriate moment in the conversation and then ask questions which will provide you with the necessary information regarding the patient's global orientation. Often this can be accomplished at the outset of the exam. "How long have you been in the hospital...Let's see, you said you came in on Friday, that means you've been here, uh...how many days?" Yes, a bit of acting is required, but certainly no more than the usual cocktail party or business luncheon dramatics.

　　　Often, in discussing the events of the present illness, a patient will say that he's confused, not sure of time-sequence, or that he can't remember. This provides an excellent opportunity to become "concerned" about the patient's memory and ability to remember dates, places and people. Frequently, helpful are statements such as: "When you say you have difficulty remembering things, do you mean dates? Do you mean where you are?...For example, is your memory problem such that you don't remember today's date...the name of the place we're in...my name?" Once the patient begins to respond to these questions, it appears more natural to ask for more details "just to clarify the difficulty in my own mind." "The day of the week," "the year," "what kind of building are we in?," all become less jarring to your relationship with the patient.

367.　　　Global orientation refers to one's precise awareness of place, person and _____ .

368.　　　If a patient doesn't remember your name but knows your job function, he's oriented to person. If it's a Tuesday and he thinks it's a Friday, he's _____ . If he's in a hospital and he thinks he's home, he is _____ _____ to _____ .

369.　　　As part of your concerned questioning about all the patient's "difficulties" and possible "confusion" you should acquire information about the patient's awareness of:

　　　The date
　　　Day of the week
　　　Month
　　　Year
　　　Season
　　　Building location and name
　　　Town or county
　　　State

this information reflects _____ to _____ and _____ .

370.　　　Concentration or the ability to attend to a task must always be evaluated prior to testing or properly interpreting information about other cognitive function (47 pp. 270-279). If a patient cannot attend to a task, he will be unable to perform well on other tests of _____ .

366.   No answer required

367.   time

368.   disoriented to time, disoriented to place

369.   global orientation, place and time

370.   cognition (cortical function)

371.   Before beginning any formal testing, the patient should be asked about his subjective feelings, regarding his memory and concentrating capacities. If he is satisfied, begin with a simple, "Well, I'm glad to hear that, so I'd just like to ask you a few questions to help me to better understand your situation." If he is not satisfied, begin with "That must be troublesome (or upsetting). I'd like to find out more about your memory (difficulties)." What would you say to introduce the topic of global orientation? Write down your statements.

372.   When a patient's anxiety or fatigue is marked, it may interfere with his ability to attend to a task. An altered mood (depression or euphoria), intrusive thoughts or perceptions can also interfere with _____ .

373.   A series of numbers stated by the examiner and repeated backwards by the patient is a test of concentration and not of memory (47 pp. 270-279,66,67,79). The patient's ability to accurately repeat in sequence five numbers backward should be considered a normal response. Directions for this task should be clear and the patient's actual trial preceded by an example: "I'm going to say several numbers and I'd like you to repeat them for me...If I say: 1, 2, 3, I'd like you to say 1, 2, 3." After the patient's actual trial with numbers forward, you should say: "I'm now going to say several numbers, and this time I'd like you to repeat them for me backwards ...If I say: 1, 2, 3, what will you say?" You can proceed only after (sometimes with several examples) the patient responds, "3, 2, 1." A poor performance of this test of concentration could reflect many things. Circle those examples below which could account for concentration problems:

Depression   Hallucinations   Anxiety

Stupor   Euphoria   Intrusive thoughts

374.   The subtraction of serial sevens or serial threes beginning at 100 is a test of attention to a task, not memory (66). Another test of attention to a task is _____ .

375.   In testing with serial sevens, directions should, as always, be explicitly stated and an example of two given, using another number. You should, for example, do it first serially, subtracting twos, and then ask the patient to do the same thing with sevens. No errors and completion close to zero in 90 seconds or less is considered a normal response. An abnormal performance of serial sevens suggests a deficit in _____ .

376.   Some patients who have difficulty with numbers will be unable to perform serial sevens properly or repeat numbers backward. These tests of _____ can be supplemented by asking the patient to spell simple words (world, money, truck) and then spell them backwards. If the patient has no spelling difficulties, spelling a simple word backwards is also a test of _____ .

377.   The frontal lobes regulate motor behavior (47 pp. 182-185, pp. 250-255). When we observe and categorize a patient's motor behavior, we are evaluating the functioning of the _____ .

371. How long have you been in the hospital? You've been here how many days? Today is.....? You came here when?

     OR

     When you say you have difficulty remembering things, do you mean dates? For example, do you remember today's date?

372. concentration

373. (Depression)   (Hallucinations)   (Anxiety)
     (Stupor)   (Euphoria)   (Intrusive thoughts)

374. numbers backwards

375. concentration

376. concentration
     concentration

377. frontal lobe

378.   Frontal lobe function is reflected in part by an extreme increase in motor activities or _____ or its opposite, very few motor activities or _____ .

379.   The removal of the frontal lobes of animals can cause them to show stereotypes, posturing and echopraxias (47 pp. 89-90). Thus an evaluation of the _____ syndrome also partially tests frontal lobe function.

380.   Echophenomena are also suggestive of frontal lobe dysfunction. A patient repeating your questions rather than answering them, termed _____, or a patient reflecting your movements despite your commands to the contrary, termed _____ , may have serious frontal lobe dysfunction.

381.   Equal resistance to an examiner's attempts to move a limb, termed _____ , is a catatonic feature and also a sign of dysfunction or dysregulation of motor behavior of the _____ lobe.

382.   Tests of cognitive function include the copying of shapes. These tests require the patient to make his copy of approximately the same size, in the middle of a blank sheet of paper and without taking his pencil off the paper. Patients with frontal lobe dysfunction can copy the shape reasonably well, but are unable to keep from repeating their effort until multiple lines distort the shape (motor perseveration). In the drawing below, for example, the patient was asked to copy a circle (47 pp. 182-185).

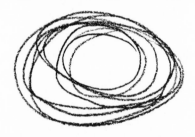

383.   Patients also can be asked to copy changing visual patterns such as Ɛ or ⌐\/\/\/W . Errors in which the patient is unable to keep from making extra shapes, e.g., § ⌐\/\/\/\/\/\/V indicates the dysfunction termed motor _____. This is an example of _____ lobe dysfunction.

384.   Frontal lobe motor regulation can also be tested by asking the patient to rapidly tap with his index finger while the heel of his hand is resting upon a flat surface (47 pp. 182-185, pp. 250-255). Standardized methods for evaluation of finger tapping require several trials but in general dysrhythmic and uncoordinated tapping or less than 35 taps in 10 seconds suggests frontal lobe dysfunction.

378. hyperactivity, hypoactivity

379. catatonic

380. echolalia, echopraxia

381. gegenhalten, frontal

382. No answer required

383. perseveration, frontal

384. No answer required

385.　　　Unlike other frontal lobe functions, fine motor control is later-alized. Thus, the finger tapping of the right hand tests functions in the contralateral or _____ frontal lobe whereas the fin-ger tapping of the left hand tests functions in the contralateral or _____ frontal lobe.

386.　　　Draw lines between matching items in the two columns. The frontal lobe functions in the left hand column can be used more than once.

Concentration	Knows the year, but not the date
Motor regulation	Hyperactivity
Orientation	Hospitalized patient doesn't know hospital's name or location
	Echopraxia
	Cannot perform serial 7's

387.　　　Circle the words or phrases related to frontal lobe function:

Aware of place, person, and time	Accurately perceives tactile stim-ulation
Able to attend to a task	Able to spell
Able to read	Able to regulate fine hand movements

388.　　　Orientation, concentration, motor regulation, are all frontal lobe functions. Next to each item below, indicate to which frontal lobe function it relates by placing an O next to orientation items; a C next to concentration items; and a M next to motor regulation items.

1. Knows the day of the week ____

2. Finger tapping dysrhythmic and slow ___

3. Echopraxia, gegenhalten ____

4. Hypoactivity or hyperactivity ___

5. To the command copy this: the patient responds: ___

6. Can do serial sevens well ___

7. "Where am I?" ____

8. Spells world "WORLD" but spells it backwards "ALOW" ___

9. To the command "Draw a circle" ___

389.　　　We have evaluated the frontal lobe functions of _____, _____, and _____. The frontal lobe also actively synthesizes perceptions (active per-ception) (47 pp. 240-244) and engages in abstract thinking (47 pp. 323-340,48).

385. left, right

386. Concentration — Knows the year, but not the date
Motor regulation — Hyperactivity
Orientation — Hospitalized patient doesn't know hospital's name or location
Echopraxia
Cannot perform serial 7's

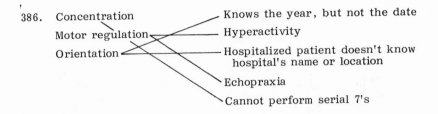

387. Aware of (place, person, and time) — Accurately perceives tactile stimulation
Able to (attend to a task) — Able to spell
Able to read — Able to (regulate the fine hand movements)

388. 1. Knows the day of the week O
2. Finger tapping dysrhythmic and slow M
3. Echopraxia, gegenhalten M
4. Hypoactivity or hyperactivity M
5. To the command copy this: the patient responds: M
6. Can do serial sevens well C
7. "Where am I?" O
8. Spells world "WORLD" but spells it backwards "ALOW" C
9. To the command "Draw a circle" M

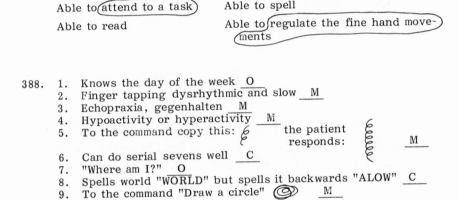

389. global orientation, concentration, regulation of motor behavior

390.   If your patient has no difficulty in naming objects, show him a picture of a simple object upside down. Active perception requires the reversing of the perception to its proper orientation. If the patient is unable to identify the object (such as a hat, candle stick, cup and saucer) turn the picture right-side up. Proper identification then signifies loss of _____ _____ and frontal lobe dysfunction.

391.   Abstract thinking is the final _____ _____ function to be evaluated in this section. (Language will be evaluated later on.) Begin by telling the patient:

"I'd like to ask you about some things and I'd like you to tell me what they have in common or how they are most alike. For example, a cat and a dog are most similar in that they are animals."

You can proceed only if the patient understands what your expectations are. If so, then:

Q. "What is the similarity between an orange and an apple?"

A. _____

Q. "What is the similarity between an airplane and a bicycle?"

A. _____

Q. "What is the similarity between a fly and a tree?"

A. _____

Proper answers to the first two questions suggest normal abstraction. Proper answers to all three questions suggest above average abstraction.

392.   Abstract thinking can also be tested by asking the patient to solve problems. If you have determined that the patient can do simple math you can then ask the following:

a) "If you had four apples and I had three more than you, how many would I have?"

b) "If you had 18 books and you wanted to put them on two different book shelves so that one shelf had twice as many books as the other, how many would be on each shelf?"

c) "If you had a candle 15 inches long and it casts a shadow four times its length, how long is the shadow?"

The mathematics in the above problems are not difficult. The real task is to determine the principle involved. This is abstract thinking and a major function of the _____ lobe.

393.   If a fully alert patient cannot problem solve or abstract he most likely has dysfunction in what brain area? _____

394.   Draw lines between matching items in the two columns:

Concentration   Finger tapping

Global orientation   Place, time, person

Motor regulation   Serial 7's

156

390. active perception

391. frontal lobe
    A. Both are fruit
    A. Both are means of transportation
    A. Both are alive

392. frontal

393. frontal

394. Concentration ⟍   ⟋ Finger tapping
     Global orientation ─╳─ Place, time, person
     Motor regulation ⟋   ⟍ Serial 7's

157

395.   Draw lines between matching items in the two columns:

Active perception	Motor perseveration
Motor regulation	Similarities
Abstract thinking	Recognizing upside down figures

396.   Judgment refers to the ability to evaluate various situations and information and reach an effective conclusion. Unfortunately, the evaluation of judgment is too greatly affected by the examiner's personal and cultural biases, and is rarely of diagnostic importance. Although psychiatrists are called to assess people's judgmental capacities for legal purposes, the subtleties of the area of "judgment" in the legal sense is beyond the scope of this book (if not of the profession). Tradition suggests that the evaluation of a patient's judgment can be achieved by asking the following questions:

A. "What would you do if you found a stamped, addressed and sealed envelope on the street?"

B. "What would you do if you were in a crowded theater and were the first person there to discover a fire?"

C. "What would you do if you were lost in the woods?"

After being subjected to such responses as:

A. "Open it up and look for money..." or "I don't pick up things off the street!"

B. "Run like hell"...

C. "Are you kidding? I never even go to the park!"

I decided there must be a better way. There is! Decisions concerning the patient's life situations and reality problems offer the best chance to evaluate judgment, e.g., "What are you going to tell your boss about this?...What are your plans when you leave the hospital? ...What advice would you give your daughter about her problem?"

395. Active perception   Motor perseveration
     Motor regulation   Similarities
     Abstract thinking   Recognizing upside down figures

396. No answer required

397.   Below are examples of responses to tasks evaluating frontal lobe function. Indicate with an x if the response is abnormal and in each case write where indicated, the function being tested.

"93...86...79...72...65...58
...51...44...37...30...23...
16...9...2."

_____

"A flower has a green stem and so does grass."

_____

"Oh, a cup. I didn't recognize it when you held it upside down."

_____

"Copy ⌐W W W⌐"

Response ⌐VVVVVV

_____

Finger taps (less than 35 taps with index finger in 10 seconds)

_____

Despite instructions to the contrary, patient repeats (copies) examiner's movements.

_____

"T H E A R"

_____

"It's July 1, 1959"

_____

"If I had 4 and you had 3 more than me, you'd have 7."

_____

"A plane and a bicycle both have wheels."

_____

160

397. "93...86...79...72...65
...58...51...44...37...
30...23...16...9...2."   Concentration

"A flower has a green stem
and so does grass."   X   Abstract thinking

"Oh, a cup. I didn't recognize it when you held it

upside down."   X   Active perception

"Copy ⌐\/\/⌐\/⌐\/\⌐"

Response ⌐\/\/\/\/\/   X   Motor regulation

Finger taps (less than 35
taps with index finger in
10 seconds)   X   Motor regulation

Despite instructions to the
contrary, patient repeats
(copies) examiner's move-
ments.   X   Motor regulation

"T H E A R"   X   Concentration

"It's July 1,1959."   X   Orientation

"If I had 4 and you had 3
more than me, you'd have
7."   Abstract thinking

"A plane and a bicycle
both have wheels."   Abstract thinking

161

VERBAL MEMORY

398.　　　Formal memory testing is part of the mental status examination. Information concerning past historical events, family history and recent personal events including those of the day of the interview can obviously provide information concerning a patient's memory capacity (7). A patient who is unable to accurately relate these details or sequence of events in his personal life should be suspect for having a memory deficit. List some of the life events which would be helpful indicators for evaluating a patient's memory.

399.　　　Memory, however, is not a holistic brain function (7,47, p.297, 67,78). Long-term memory (months to years), recent memory (hours to weeks), short-term memory (minutes) and immediate recall can all be selectively affected in mental illness. Draw lines between appropriate items in the two columns:

Immediate recall	Recalling events years back
Long-term memory	What happened last week
Recent memory	What happened 10 seconds ago

400.　　　Except in severe bilateral hippocampal dysfunction or an altered state of consciousness, immediate recall is rarely, if ever, impaired. Short-term memory (minutes) is often disturbed in psychiatric patients, particularly those suffering from psychomotor states (recurrent paroxysms of behavior often associated with temporal lobe dysfunction), intoxications and other acute coarse brain processes. Recent memory (hours to weeks) is frequently disturbed in more chronic coarse brain processes while the most established memory patterns or _____ _____ is often the last to be disturbed by illness.

401.　　　Draw lines between matching lines in the two columns:

Short-term memory	Memories of years past
Long-term memory	Memories of the last 30 seconds
Recent memory	Memories of this morning
Immediate recall	Memories of the past few minutes

162

398. Birth and marriage dates; numbers and ages of children; job sequences, duration and inclusive years; sequence of events and duration of present complaints; dates, duration and sequence of past
illnesses.

399. Immediate recall   Recalling events years back
     Long-term memory   What happened last week
     Recent-term memory   What happened 10 seconds ago

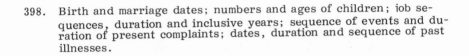

400. long-term memory

401. Short-term memory   Memories of years past
     Long-term memory   Memories of the last 30 seconds
     Recent memory   Memories of this morning
     Immediate recall   Memories of the past few minutes

402. Once you have established to your satisfaction that a patient is able to concentrate, i.e., attend to a task, you can then proceed with formal memory testing. Memory can be tested utilizing words or drawings (e.g., the Wechsler memory scale) (49,78). The patient is asked to remember several words or word pairs; the words or pairs are stated and the patient asked to repeat immediately the words. This tests immediate assimilation and immediate _____. Repetition after ten minutes tests _____ _____ memory. Reproduction of standard figures can be similarly utilized.

403. Immediate repetition of a series of words, letters, or numbers tests the memory function of immediate recall. The repetition of a series of words, letters, or numbers backwards tests _____.

404. Long-term memory is best tested by questions concerning past personal and family history. Questions concerning recent personal events, particularly those of the previous day, is the best clinical test of _____ memory.

405. One reasonable short-term memory test is to ask the patient to remember the following words: blue, chair, swim, glove. Five minutes later, ask him to recall the words in any order. Be careful, don't give hints such as: "Do you remember the four words I asked you?" Three or more words recalled correctly should be considered a normal response. A ten-word test, if time permits, is more reliable and valid.
      One word of caution: Write the words down or you're sure to forget them! List all the memory functions we have discussed. This is a test of your _____ - _____ memory.

406. Inability to repeat words, letters or numbers backwards termed poor _____ is different from poor memory. Amnesia refers to the inability to recall past events. (The only time I've seen global amnesia in a "psychiatric patient" has been at the movies.)

407. Decreased memory capacity can take several forms. The inability to recall past events or _____ can be retrograde (inability to recall events preceding the injury or illness onset) or anterograde (inability to recall events following the injury or illness onset).

408. The inability to recall events prior to a psychological or physical traumatic event is _____ amnesia, and except for the moment or two immediately prior to the trauma, it is rarely permanent.

409. When a person, hit upon the head, cannot remember the events immediately preceding the blow, he is said to suffer from a mild traumatic _____ amnesia.

410. Anterograde amnesia refers to the inability to recall events following the traumatic incident. Inability to recall events preceding the traumatic incident is termed _____.

411. When a person, hit upon the head, cannot remember the events immediately following the blow, he is said to suffer from a mild traumatic _____ amnesia.

402. recall, short-term

403. concentration

404. recent

405. short-term memory: immediate recall, short-term memory,
                            recent memory, long-term memory

406. concentration

407. amnesia

408. retrograde

409. retrograde

410. retrograde amnesia

411. anterograde

412.   The inability to recall events following a traumatic incident is
called _____ amnesia. It results from the faulty registration
of new material because of a continuing altered consciousness and
acute cerebral dysfunction. Anterograde amnesia is almost always
permanent though almost always self-limiting in duration (i.e., events during the period of amnesia are not recalled, even after the
amnesic processes resolve). The longer the period of _____
amnesia, the more severe the dysfunction.

413.   Persons suffering head injury often appear dazed, perplexed,
or "out-of-sorts" for several hours or even days following the injury. Suddenly, they seem to become their "usual selves" again
but insist that they cannot remember clearly what happened since
the injury. Such people have had an episode of _____
amnesia.

414.   Periods of memory dysfunction often occur in association with
an altered consciousness. An apparent perplexity, dazed appearance or "fuzziness" in response to questions often signals such an
alteration of consciousness. When an altered consciousness follows
a traumatic event and the person upon recovery cannot remember
post-traumatic events, we can say that he had _____
amnesia.

415.   Not infrequently, psychiatric patients appear perplexed, dazed,
or fuzzy in their responses, but without any evidence of coarse
brain dysfunction. They may appear to have "spotty" recall of
events prior to the onset of their illness termed _____ and
difficulty recalling events following the onset of their illness termed
_____ but their responses are not as consistent as those
observed in patients with coarse brain disease. Upon recovery (the
usual course) from this perplexed condition, patients will describe
themselves as having been in a clouded, dream-like state. The term
for this is oneroid state.

416.   Clouded, dream-like conditions termed _____ states,
occur frequently in acute psychoses. When there is no evidence of
head trauma, such a state prognosticates a good recovery (51,72).

417.   Patients suffering from acute and chronic anxiety syndromes
will often describe periods of detachment in which everything feels
fuzzy around the edges, and in which they feel themselves, as if
in a dream, watching themselves "go through the motions." This
condition is termed depersonalization and should not be confused
with an altered sensorium or a clouded, dream-like _____
state.

418.   A person suffering from anterograde amnesia almost always exhibits an altered _____; a person in an _____
state appears clouded and perplexed but has no traumatic history;
a person in a _____ or detached feeling state has a clear
sensorium.

419.   The inability to remember events prior to and following a traumatic event are termed _____ and _____ amnesia. Some
patients, however, can recall "memories", but these memories turn
out to be false.

412. anterograde, anterograde

413. anterograde

414. anterograde

415. retrograde amnesia, anterograde amnesia

416. oneroid

417. oneroid

418. consciousness, oneroid, depersonalized

419. retrograde, anterograde

420.   Some false memories are the result of coarse brain disease (retrospective falsification); others are associated with apophanous psychosis. False memories associated with delusional ideas are called pseudomemories. These pseudomemories seem to support the patient's apophanous notions with "historical" evidence. Only careful history taking, validation from family and friends and your own common sense can determine what are real and what are false or _____ memories.

421.   Confabulation (making things up) is another form of false _____. It is falsified memory in response to the questions or statements of others. Example: A manic patient with grandoise ideas claims that he has had "a telephone conversation with the President of the United States". When he is questioned about that, he adds: "Actually, he calls me all the time. He and I are old buddies. He always asks my advice on how to deal with the Russians."

422.   Confabulated memory can be elicited by suggesting false events to the patient who may agree and elaborate. A "Good morning, Mr. Jones. How did you like that party last night?...And how about the steak we had for breakfast?" can often lead you and the patient down the garden path of confabulation. Confabulation, then, is a most dramatic example of false or _____.

423.   Confabulated memory is most frequently observed in Korsakoff's encephalopathy. Fantastic confabulations in which patients relate trips to other planets, flying sans plane across the country, etc., is similar to obviously false tall tales and is associated with cortical atrophy in the frontal lobe (69), but can occur in mania, sociopathy, and normal children. I assume the last from anecdotal observation, and conclude that confabulation is either normal in children or that my younger son, age six at this writing, is a chronic alcoholic.
Write a sentence describing confabulated memory.

424.   There is a common form of falsification of memory in which an individual feels he has experienced an event before. This is given the French term deja vu (already seen). Jamais vu (never seen) is another French term for the rarer experience of not recognizing a familiar situation. When pathological, deja vu and jamais vu are often related to psychomotor states (15,23). They can also be observed in toxic states and some sociopaths (65). What is the term for each of the following experiences?

A patient stated that she returned home from work to find that she was "unfamiliar" with her apartment, furniture and personal belongings. "I knew it was crazy but I felt as if I had never been there before."   _____

A patient said that during the past few weeks, several times each day she would experience the overwhelming sensation that what was happening at that moment had happened before.   _____

420. pseudo

421. memory

422. pseudomemories

423. Confabulation is the falsification of memory in response to the questions of others.

424. A patient stated that she returned home from work to find that she was "unfamiliar" with her apartment, furniture and personal belongings. "I knew it was crazy, but I felt as if I had never been there before."   Jamais vu

A patient said that during the past few weeks, several times each day she would experience the overwhelming sensation that what was happening at that moment had happened before.   Deja vu

425.   Draw lines between matching items in the two columns

Oneroid state   Amnesia for events following a trauma

Anterograde amnesia   Clouded, dream-like state

Depersonalization   Clear sensorium but detached from
                                self

426.   Draw lines between matching items in the two columns:

Pseudomemory   Amnesia for events prior to trauma

Retrograde amnesia   False memories associated with apo-
                                phanous ideas

Confabulation   Falsification of memories, often fan-
                                tastic which can be stimulated by
                                examiner's questions

427.   Draw lines between matching items in the two columns:

Deja vu   Permanent though circumscribed
                                memory loss

Jamais vu   Unfamiliar events experienced as
                                familiar

Anterograde amnesia   Amnesia for events prior to trauma

Retrograde amnesia   Familiar events experienced as un-
                                familiar

428.   Label each clinical item with the appropriate phenomenologic
term. Indicate with an X which items or patient responses you feel
are not normal or reflect illness.

When asked to repeat 5 1 0 9, a young
woman said, "6 9 5 1." When asked
__ to subtract sevens from 100 (after a   Testing for:
demonstrated twos from 100), she
said: "100, 93, 89, 87, 65, 58." Be-   _____
cause of this response, the examiner
did not test _____.

__ The patient complained of feeling
"funny," as if in a dream-like state,
as if surrounded by a fog or haze.   _____

429.   Label each item with the appropriate phenomenologic term. Indicate with an X which items or patient responses you feel are not
normal or reflect illness.

When asked to repeat 6 1 0 9 8, a   Testing:
young man said "6 1 0 9 8." He
— completed serial sevens in 45   _____
seconds.   Testing:

                                         _____

He was next asked to remember:
Blue, chair, swim, glove, and as   Testing:
__ instructed, repeated them to the
examiner. Five minutes later, when   _____
asked to repeat the words, he said,   Testing:
"Blue, glove, chair, swim."
                                         _____

170

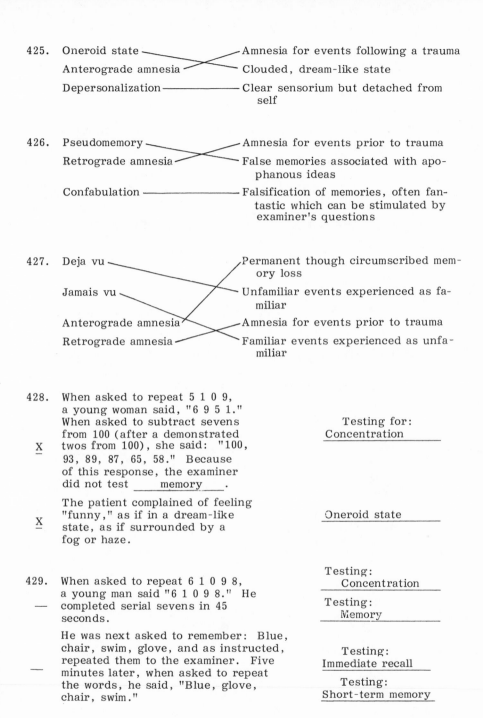

425. Oneroid state ———— Amnesia for events following a trauma

Anterograde amnesia ———— Clouded, dream-like state

Depersonalization ———————— Clear sensorium but detached from self

426. Pseudomemory ———— Amnesia for events prior to trauma

Retrograde amnesia ———— False memories associated with apophanous ideas

Confabulation ———————— Falsification of memories, often fantastic which can be stimulated by examiner's questions

427. Deja vu ———— Permanent though circumscribed memory loss

Jamais vu ———— Unfamiliar events experienced as familiar

Anterograde amnesia ———— Amnesia for events prior to trauma

Retrograde amnesia ———— Familiar events experienced as unfamiliar

428. When asked to repeat 5 1 0 9, a young woman said, "6 9 5 1." When asked to subtract sevens from 100 (after a demonstrated

X   twos from 100), she said: "100, 93, 89, 87, 65, 58." Because of this response, the examiner did not test ____memory____ .

Testing for:
Concentration

The patient complained of feeling "funny," as if in a dream-like

X   state, as if surrounded by a fog or haze.

Oneroid state

429. When asked to repeat 6 1 0 9 8, a young man said "6 1 0 9 8." He

— completed serial sevens in 45 seconds.

Testing:
Concentration

Testing:
Memory

He was next asked to remember: Blue, chair, swim, glove, and as instructed, repeated them to the examiner. Five

— minutes later, when asked to repeat the words, he said, "Blue, glove, chair, swim."

Testing:
Immediate recall

Testing:
Short-term memory

430.　　　Label each item with the appropriate phenomenologic term. To a patient who has been hospitalized for a week:

Dr.: "Good morning, Mr. Caldwell. You look like you're feeling a little better this morning."

Pt.: "I'm just great, Doc."

Dr.: "It must have been that party last night. Did you like the punch?"

Pt.: "Ha, you ain't kiddin', it was really good...But I only took a sip, Doc. I don't drink much you know."

Dr.: "I understand. By the way, did they give you the steak for breakfast?"

Pt.: "Sure did...lot of other stuff, too. They're treatin' me real nice here."

A man with a bandage on his forehead said: "What happened? You say today's Friday? The last thing I remember it was Monday and I was in the car."

431.　　　Label each item with the appropriate phenomenologic term:

"I can't explain it. I know it's impossible. But I can't get away from the feeling that things that are happening to me have all happened before. It's all familiar." _____

"I remember the accident and falling. But I don't remember what happened just before the accident. I know I was talking, but I don't remember anything else, not even who I was talking to." _____

"I've been everywhere. Why the other day I took a space-ship to Venus. It was extremely hot there. Then I came back here and began building a new skyscraper in the city. Actually I've built most of the big buildings in the city." _____

430. confabulation
anterograde amnesia (since he doesn't remember the accident, he
also has retrograde amnesia)

431. deja vu
retrograde amnesia
fantastic confabulation

PARIETAL LOBE FUNCTION

432.   In most individuals, the dominant parietal lobe is on the
_____.

433.   In general, the left or _____ parietal lobe controls verbal
or symbolic abilities related to spatial orientation and categorization
while the right or _____ parietal lobe controls non-verbal
motor-perceptual abilities (21,47 pp. 147-168).

434.   A person who has severe difficulties with verbal or symbolic
abilities related to spatial orientation or categorization may have
dysfunction in the _____ _____
_____.

435.   A person who has severe difficulties with non-verbal motor perceptual tasks may have dysfunction in the _____
_____ _____.

436.   Many psychiatric patients, although oriented to place, are disoriented to right and left, and/or their body parts (11). A complete mental status examination will include questioning about this
cortical function. Any good history will include questions about
the patients' general health and "somatic" complaints. Ask the patient about weakness, particularly in the arms and legs. The statements "Hold out your right arm," "Show me your left hand" become
natural. They maintain the doctor-patient relationship while testing
for right-left _____.

437.   Disorientation to time, place and _____ grossly suggests
frontal lobe dysfunction. Right-left _____ suggests brain
dysfunction in the dominant parietal lobe (21,26,34,54).

438.   The patient should also be asked to place his hand to the opposite ear or elbow. Several trials should be required involving different contralateral body parts. This is a test of _____
disorientation and thus dominant _____ lobe function.

174

432. left

433. dominant, non-dominant

434. left (dominant) parietal lobe

435. right (non-dominant) parietal lobe

436. orientation

437. person, disorientation

438. right-left, parietal

439.   When told "Place your left hand on your right ear" a patient hesitated, looked at both his hands, turned them over several times, and then with great hesitation placed his left hand on his right ear. This is a mild form of _____ disorientation suggestive of _____ _____ lobe dysfunction.

440.   Following testing of orientation to body parts and right-left orientation a patient should be asked to name each finger of each hand. Failure to accomplish this like right-left disorientation suggests _____ _____ lobe dysfunction.

441.   Inability to properly identify one's fingers is called finger agnosia and suggests dysfunction in the dominant _____ _____ (21,26,38,54,68). Psychotic patients often (11) have difficulties in naming their fingers.

442.   In testing the inability to recognize and name one's fingers, termed _____ _____ the examiner should first point to each finger and require the patient to name each. This can be followed by holding up your hand and asking the patient to show you your index finger, ring finger, etc. If there is any doubt about the patient's responses, the fingers should be numbered, the patient instructed as to the number of each finger and the tests repeated with the correct number for each finger being the required response.

443.   An examiner pointed to a patient's fingers one at a time and asked: "What do you call this one?" Beginning with the right thumb the patient responded:

"Thumb...straight finger...middle systems finger...index and outer or end finger."

This is an example of finger _____ and suggests dysfunction in the dominant _____ _____ .

444.   Circle those words or phrases suggestive of dominant parietal lobe dysfunction.

Unable to do serial 7's

Difficulty in identifying one's fingers

Difficulty in identifying upside-down objects

Difficulty with symbolic categorization

Difficulty with non-verbal motor-perceptual abilities

Difficulty in knowing right from left

445.   When asked to identify the fingers on his right hand, a patient said "thumb...finger next to thumb...large finger...index finger ...smaller index finger." If this patient has a localized brain lesion, is he likely to do well on tests of right-left orientation? _____ Is he likely to do well on tests of symbolic or language categorization? _____ Is he likely to do well on tests of non-verbal motor-perceptual? _____ Where is this patient's lesion likely to be? _____

439. right-left, dominant parietal

440. dominant parietal

441. parietal lobe

442. finger agnosia

443. agnosia, parietal lobe

444. Unable to do serial 7's
Difficulty in identifying one's fingers
Difficulty in identifying upside-down objects
Difficulty with symbolic categorization
Difficulty with non-verbal motor-perceptual abilities
Difficulty in knowing right from left

445. no, no, yes, dominant parietal lobe

177

446.   Patients with significant brain dysfunction often have difficulty performing simple motor behaviors even though they have no sensory loss, paralysis or muscle weakness. These difficulties are called apraxias. Some apraxias suggest dysfunction in the dominant parietal lobe (16,21,24,25,27,28). What other cognitive difficulties suggest dysfunction in the dominant parietal lobe?

447.   If persons cannot perform simple motor tasks even though they have no sensory loss, paralysis or muscle weakness, they are said to have _____ .

448.   If a person cannot identify his fingers he is said to have

_____ _____ .

449.   Non-recognition (or inability to identify) is an _____ . Non-performance without motor sensory deficit is an _____ .

450.   Some patients without sensory or motor deficits cannot demonstrate (without props) the use of simple objects (a hammer, a key, flipping a coin, using a straw, blowing out a candle). This inability is a special form of _____ .

451.   The inability to demonstrate the use of simple objects such as a key or a hammer is termed an ideomotor apraxia. Many patients with ideomotor apraxia have dominant parietal lobe dysfunction. What other cognitive deficits can be observed in patients with dysfunction in this cortical region?

452.   When asked: "Show me how you would: throw a ball; hammer a nail; flip a coin; use a key;" a patient without sensory deficit or motor weakness was unable to follow the commands although she understood them. This inability to demonstrate the use of simple objects is _____ .

453.   In most instances when a patient has difficulty demonstrating the use of objects with both hands and there is no sensory/motor loss the dysfunction is in the dominant _____ (16,21,24, 25). Bilateral (right and left hand) ideomotor apraxia can also result from lesions in fibers running between the dominant temporoparietal area and the frontal lobe (28,30).

454.   When asked to demonstrate the use of a key, a patient could only do so by extending his index finger as if it were the key. This is called body-part as object and is a manifestation of _____ apraxia.

455.   When asked to demonstrate the use of a key, a hammer, and how to flip a coin, a patient was able to do so only when first saying what he was going to do, i.e. "I take the key like this and put it into the lock. Then I turn it this way." Despite instructions to the contrary, the patient could not demonstrate the use of simple objects without describing what he was going to do. This is called "verbal overflow" and, as "body part as object", is a manifestation of _____ apraxia.

446. finger agnosia, right/left disorientation, difficulty with symbolic or language categorization

447. apraxia

448. finger agnosia

449. agnosia, apraxia

450. apraxia

451. finger agnosia, right/left disorientation
difficulty with symbolic or language categorization

452. ideomotor apraxia

453. parietal lobe

454. ideomotor

455. ideomotor

456.   When asked to demonstrate the flipping of a coin, a patient without sensory or motor deficit mimicked a movement with open palm,
his hand going up and down without flipping his thumb against his
index finger. Even when asked to do so, he was unable to flip his
thumb against his index finger. This dysfunction suggests a lesion
in the _____ hemisphere usually the parietal lobe but
also among the fibers running between the parietal and frontal lobes.

457.   When asked to demonstrate the hammering of a nail, a patient
without sensory or motor deficit did so by raising and lowering his
arm without any wrist movement. When asked to demonstrate the
use of a key he did so by sticking out his index finger as the key.
This latter performance termed _____ _____ and the lack
of wrist movement while demonstrating the use of a hammer, are
examples of _____ _____.

458.   Write a sentence or two defining or describing the following:

Verbal overflow:
Body part as object:
Ideomotor apraxia:

459.   Some patients will have ideomotor apraxia of only one hand, usually the left. Often, this is associated with a type of language disorder we will learn about later in the program. This unilateral ideomotor apraxia of the left hand is due to a lesion or dysfunction in
the left frontal lobe (30) which prevents the information required
to perform the task with the left hand from crossing over into the
right hemisphere which regulates movement on the left side.

460.   Ideomotor apraxia of only the left hand suggests a lesion in the
_____ _____ _____ because a lesion
here would prevent information required to perform a motor task
from crossing over into the other hemisphere.

461.   Ideomotor apraxia of both hands (bilateral) can be due to a lesion in the fibers connecting the dominant temporo-parietal region
to the dominant frontal lobe or, more commonly due to a lesion in
the _____ _____ _____.

456. dominant (left)

457. body part as object
     ideomotor apraxia

458. Verbal overflow: The inability to demonstrate the use of simple ob-
                      jects without describing the movements. A form
                      of ideomotor apraxia.

     Body part as object: The use of a body part, such as a finger, as
                          the object to be demonstrated. A form of
                          ideomotor apraxia.

     Ideomotor apraxia: The inability to demonstrate the use of simple
                        objects despite no sensory or motor deficit.

459. No answer required

460. dominant (left) frontal lobe

461. dominant (left) parietal lobe

462.   Identify the site of the lesion:

The patient demonstrates finger
agnosia, body part as object, verbal
overflow, right/left disorientation   _____

The patient demonstrates body part
as object in the left hand only,
verbal overflow with the left hand
only, flips an imaginary coin with an
open palm with the left hand only,
uses an imaginary hammer without
moving his wrist, left hand only   _____

The patient demonstrates good
right/left orientation, good
finger recognition, bilateral
ideomotor apraxia   _____

463.   Draw lines between matching items in the two columns:

Unable to demonstrate the use   Right dominant hemisphere
of simple objects despite normal
motor strength

Unable to name own fingers   Ideomotor apraxia

Writes name with right hand   Finger agnosia
above line of writing

Writes name with right hand   Left dominant hemisphere
below line of writing

464.   Patients with parietal lobe dysfunction (particularly in the posterior area), may have trouble copying the examiner's movements (25,
47 pp. 147-168). They cannot regulate their body parts in space.
Ask your patient to do what you do.

1. Right arm extended; 2. then bend arm, hand open, arm raised;
3. then hand closed in a fist. Repeat with left arm (see below).

Inability to copy these simple movements despite normal sensory and
motor function indicates parietal lobe dysfunction opposite (contralateral) to the arm-hand having difficulty and is a form of _____ .

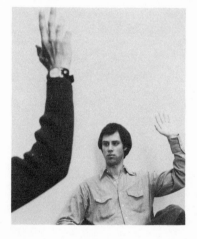
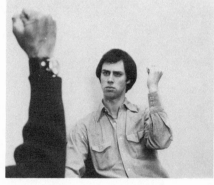

462. dominant (left) parietal lobe
dominant (left) frontal lobe
fibers between dominant temporo-parietal region and frontal lobe

463. Unable to demonstrate the
use of simple objects despite
normal motor strength

Right dominant hemisphere

Unable to name own fingers

Ideomotor apraxia

Writes name with right hand
above the line of writing

Finger agnosia

Writes name with right hand
below line of writing

Left dominant hemisphere

464. apraxia

465.   Inability to demonstrate without props the use of simple objects despite normal sensory and motor function is termed _____ . The inability to copy simple movements despite normal sensory and motor function is termed a movement or kinesthetic apraxia.

466.   Identify the site of the dysfunction:

Cannot copy examiner's hand
and arm movements with right
hand, poor verbal categorization,
right/left disorientation   _____

Kinesthetic apraxia of right hand,
ideomotor apraxia of both hands,
finger agnosia of both hands,
right/left disorientation   _____

Bilateral ideomotor apraxia,
good finger identification,
no kinesthetic apraxia, good
right/left orientation   _____

Left hand ideomotor apraxia,
no kinesthetic apraxia, good
right/left orientation, good
finger identification   _____

467.   Psychiatric patients often have difficulties copying the outline of simple figures, even though they have no motor weakness and understand the task (73,75). This is called a construction apraxia. When a patient cannot demonstrate the use of a simple object even though he has no motor weakness, this is called an _____ apraxia.

468.   Ideomotor apraxia is a sign of _____ _____ . Construction apraxia is a dysfunction in non-verbal motor-perceptual organization and is therefore a sign of dysfunction in the ___ _____ (10,21,47 pp. 147-168).

469.   Inability to copy the outline of simple figures, termed _____ _____ can be tested by asking the patient to copy simple figures such as a square, a cross and a triangle (73,75). When you ask a patient to copy one of the figures say, "I'm going to ask you to copy something. This is not a drawing test, but I'd like you to try your best. Just draw the outline of the picture and once you start, don't take your pencil off the paper. Make your copy a bit bigger than the picture and place it in the middle of the paper." Use a different piece of paper for each drawing.

465. ideomotor apraxia

466. left parietal lobe
      left parietal lobe
      fibers between dominant (temporo-parietal region and dominant fron-
        tal lobe)
      dominant frontal lobe

467. ideomotor

468. dominant parietal lobe dysfunction (occasionally frontal and fiber
      tracts between lobes), non-dominant parietal lobe

469. construction apraxia

470.   When asked to copy the square, cross and triangle pictured on the left, a patient draws figures depicted on the right.

These are examples of marked _____ _____ and indicate dysfunction in the _____ _____ lobe.

471.   Place an F for frontal, D-P for dominant parietal and N-P for non-dominant parietal, next to the appropriate items:

Construction apraxia   ____

Right/left disorientation   ____

Finger agnosia   ____

Ideomotor apraxia   ____

Echopraxia   ____

472.   Identify the example of cortical dysfunction and give localization:

Unable to copy a cross   _____

Unable to recognize and name fingers   _____

Unable to copy examiner's hand and arm movements   _____

Unable to keep from copying examiner's arm movements   _____

Unable to demonstrate the use of a key with either hand   _____

186

471. Construction apraxia   N-P
     Right/left disorientation D-P
     Finger agnosia   D-P
     Ideomotor apraxia   D-P
     Echopraxia   F

472. Unable to copy a cross   Construction apraxia, non-dominant
                                       parietal lobe

     Unable to recognize and   Finger agnosia, dominant parietal lobe
     name fingers

     Unable to copy examiner's   Apraxia, contralateral parietal lobe
     hand and arm movements

     Unable to keep from copying   Echopraxia, frontal lobe
     examiner's arm movements

     Unable to demonstrate the   Ideomotor apraxia, dominant parietal
     use of a key with either   lobe
     hand

473.   A person's awareness of right and left and the ability to recognize and name his body parts is located in the _____
_____. This brain area is also the locale for the ability to calculate (21,26,47 pp. 147-168,54).

474.   Inability to do simple math (to calculate) is called acalculia and results from dysfunction in the _____ _____
_____.

475.   In testing for inability to do simple math, termed _____, first ask the patient to write a series of numbers like: 7, 9, 3, 5, 7, next ask the patient "How much is": 3 x 3; 5 x 4; 7 - 4; 8 - 5; 3 + 4; 6 + 7; or similar problems. Inability to do this task is indicative of _____.

476.   Many patients are able to do very simple math problems but are unable to do problems requiring "carrying" or "borrowing" numbers. To test for this ask the patient to: add 27 + 8; 44 + 57; subtract 31 - 7; 41 - 14; or problems of similar complexity. Inability to do these problems while solving simpler ones like 3 x 3, 7 - 4, indicated dyscalculia. Dyscalculia or the more severe acalculia is a dysfunction of the _____ _____ _____.

477.   Place a check in the box which best matches the dysfunction with the related brain region:

Dysfunction	Frontal lobe	Dominant Parietal	Non-Dominant Parietal
Acalculia			
Ideomotor apraxia			
Finger agnosia			
Echopraxia			
Poor concentration			
Construction apraxia			
Global disorientation			

473. dominant parietal lobe

474. dominant parietal lobe

475. acalculia, acalculia

476. dominant parietal lobe

477.

Dysfunction	Frontal Lobe	Dominant Parietal	Non-Dominant Parietal
Acalculia		√	
Ideomotor apraxia	√(left hand only)	√Bilateral	
Finger agnosia		√	
Echopraxia	√		
Poor concen- tration	√		
Construction apraxia			√
Global disorienta- tion	√		

478.   Place a check in the box which best matches the dysfunction with the related brain region:

Dysfunction	Frontal lobe	Dominant Parietal	Non-Dominant Parietal
Poor abstract thinking			
Can't copy a cross			
Can't do serial 7's			
Can't demonstrate use of simple objects			
Can't do simple math			
Can't keep from mimicking examiner's movements			
Can't name fingers			
Doesn't know right from left			

479.   The dominant parietal lobe is the way station between visual perception and language; thus reading and writing as well as mathematical abilities are located in this brain region (21,28,47 pp. 147-168). List all of the functions you have learned including those mentioned above, associated with the dominant parietal lobe.

480.   Inability to write or difficulty writing is termed agraphia or dysgraphia (the less severe form). Inability to calculate or difficulty calculating is termed _____ or _____ .

481.   Inability to read or difficulty reading is termed alexia or dyslexia (the less severe form). Inability to write is termed _____ or _____ .

482.   When you test for reading difficulties termed _____ or _____ ask the patient to read aloud simple sentences and then do what it says. For example, "Put this paper in your pocket." Any error should be considered pathological and warrants further evaluation. Proper testing of reading and comprehension requires more elaborate standardized tests.

478.

Dysfunction	Frontal Lobe	Dominant Parietal	Non-Dominant Parietal
Poor abstract thinking	√		
Can't copy a cross			√
Can't do serial 7's	√		
Can't do simple math		√	
Can't keep from mimicking examiner's movements	√		
Can't name fingers		√	
Doesn't know right from left		√	
Can't demonstrate use of simple objects	√ (left hand only)	√ Bilateral	

479. calculations, writing, reading, recognizing and naming body parts, right/left orientation, regulation of contralateral body parts in space, kinesthetic practic function, motor programs for using simple objects (ideomotor practic function)

480. acalculia, dyscalculia

481. agraphia, dysgraphia

482. alexia, dyslexia

483.   When you test for writing difficulties termed _____
ask the patient to copy a simple sentence such as "John went to the
store for a loaf of bread." Inability to write words or to write in
script (loss of that ability) should be considered pathological and
warrants further evaluation.

484.   The final dominant parietal lobe function we will consider in this
section is recognition and naming of relationships, or categorization
(47 pp. 147-168). Ask the patient to identify the following individuals:

    "Your father's brother"
    "Your brother's father"

Try it yourself! Inability to properly recognize the relationships
suggests dysfunction in the dominant parietal lobe.

485.   Place a check in the box which best matches the dysfunction
with the related brain region:

Dysfunction	Frontal Lobe	Dominant Parietal	Non-Dominant Parietal
Acalculia			
Poor concentration			
Construction apraxia			
Agraphia			
Ideomotor apraxia			
Echopraxia			
Can't do similar-ities			
Finger agnosia			
Can't define rela-tionships			
Dyslexia			
Can't identify upside-down objects			
Can't copy exa-miner's hand positions, both hands			
Can't do serial 7's			

483. agraphia, or dysgraphia

484. my uncle, my father

485.

Dysfunction	Frontal Lobe	Dominant Parietal	Non-Dominant Parietal
Acalculia		√	
Poor concentration	√		
Construction apraxia			√
Agraphia		√	
Ideomotor apraxia	√(left hand only)	√(Bilateral)	
Echopraxia	√		
Can't do similarities	√		
Finger agnosia		√	
Can't define relationships		√	
Dyslexia		√	
Can't identify upside-down objects	√		
Can't copy examiner's hand positions, both hands		√	√
Can't do serial 7's	√		

LANGUAGE DISORDER

486.   Since thought process is inferred from a person's speech, when we describe "thought disorder" we are really describing language and/or speech disorder. There are numerous schema for classifying language disorder and the following brief integration with "thought disorder" will utilize the classification described by Jason Brown (17).

487.   You have previously learned that many psychiatric terms have their neurological equivalent. Thus, the psychiatric term drivelling speech, where the syntax is intact but the meaning is lost, is called by the neurologist _____ _____ and stereotyped, repetitive speech is called _____ by the psychiatrist and _____ by the neurologist.

488.   Schema of language disorder are based upon the functional type of the disorder and/or its "localizing" value. Whatever system is used, it is rare for a patient to have a pure form. In psychiatric patients with major mental illness, complex forms of language dysfunction indicating widespread cerebral dysfunction is the rule rather than the exception. Thus, the use of new words termed _____ is often observed with the use of substitute words termed _____ _____. Both are forms of paraphasic speech.

489.   The language schema we will use separates language into posterior (temporo-parietal) and anterior (frontal) systems. As both deal with symbolic function, the language system is in the _____ hemisphere, usually the _____ .

490.   The _____ hemisphere is dominant in better than _____ percent of the general population.

491.   The organization of language in the left hemisphere can be separated into _____ and _____ systems.

194

486. No answer required

487. jargon agrammatism, verbigeration, palilalia

488. neologisms, word approximations

489. dominant, left

490. left, 97

491. posterior, anterior

492.   The posterior language system relates to the left temporo-parietal brain region. The _____ language system relates to the left frontal lobe.

493.   The posterior language system is localized in the posterior temporoparietal brain regions of the _____ cerebral hemisphere. In most individuals, this is located on the _____.

494.   The posterior language system relates to the _____ brain regions. This system is functionally separated into semantic, nominal and phonemic language functions.

495.   The left temporo-parietal brain region includes an area termed Wernicke's area. Language disorders from this region are sometimes termed Wernicke's language disorder or more properly Wernicke's aphasia. Wernicke's aphasia indicates dysfunction in the _____ _____ language system.

496.   Wernicke's language disorder or Wernicke's _____ suggests dysfunction in the posterior language system. This relates to the _____ brain regions in the _____ hemisphere.

497.   The posterior language system involves disorder described as semantic, nominal and phonemic. This type of language disorder is localized in the _____ brain regions of the _____ hemisphere.

498.   The posterior language system involves disorder described as _____, _____, and _____.

499.   Semantic disorder refers to dysfunction of the meaning of speech. It includes jargon agrammatism or the psychiatric term _____, nonsequitive speech, semantic paraphasia (word substitution) or _____ _____ and speech where associations suddenly skip to a new and often paralleled topic. This last form is given the psychiatric term _____.

500.   Match the words or phrases in the two columns:
Drivelling speech   Semantic paraphasis (word substitution)
Derailment   Meaning of speech is broken followed by a new train of thought
Word approximation   Responses unrelated to questions
Non-sequitur   Syntax is retained but meaning of speech is lost.

501.   Drivelling speech, word approximations, derailment, non-sequitive speech, are all examples of _____ language disorder and suggests dysfunction in the _____ brain regions of the _____ hemisphere.

502.   Nominal disorder refers to a deficit in naming objects (nominal aphasia) and a deficit in the use of nouns so that speech is often "empty" and "circumlocutory." In contrast, when the meaning of speech is lost we use the term _____ disorder.

196

492. anterior

493. dominant, left

494. temporo-parietal

495. posterior

496. aphasia, temporo-parietal, left (dominant)

497. temporo-parietal, left (dominant)

498. semantic, normal, phonemic

499. drivelling, word approximations, derailment

500. Drivelling speech   Semantic paraphasia (word substitution)
Derailment ——— Meaning of speech is broken followed by a new train of thought
Word approximation Responses unrelated to questions
Non-sequitur Syntax is retained but meaning of speech is lost.

501. semantic
temporo-parietal
left (dominant)

502. semantic

197

503.   "Empty" and "circumlocutory" speech with a deficit in the use of nouns suggests _____ language disorder.

504.   Word approximations less severe than the semantic type, as well as inability to name objects, is observed in _____ language disorder.

505.   Inability to name objects is termed anomia. It is a form of __ _____ language disorder.

506.   Place an S next to the word or phrase suggestive of semantic language disorder and an N next to the word or phrase suggestive of nominal language disorder.

Drivelling speech ___   Derailment ___

Anomia ___   Jargon agrammatism ___

Circumlocutory speech ___   Non-sequitive speech ___

507.   Anomia and "empty" speech suggest _____ language disorder. Drivelling and derailment suggest _____ language disorder.

508.   Phomenic language disorder along with nominal and semantic language disorder functionally represent the _____ language system located in the _____ brain regions of the _____ hemisphere.

509.   Phonemic language disorder refers to a deficit in the use of sounds to make spoken language. Associations by sound rather than meaning, termed _____ _____ and new words, termed _____, produced because the sounds have been altered are observed in this form of language disorder.

510.   Match the words or phrases in the two columns:

Semantic aphasis   Neologisms, clang associations

Nominal aphasia   Drivelling, derailment, non-sequitive speech

Phonemic aphasia   Anomia, loss of use of nouns

511.   Wernicke's aphasia, also termed fluent/receptive/sensory aphasia, is for our purpose equivalent to posterior aphasia which includes: _____, _____, _____ types.

512.   Fluent, receptive or sensory aphasia are terms equivalent to Wernicke's aphasia and suggest dysfunction in the _____ brain region.

513.   If a man is unable to speak with meaning, uses "circumlocutory, empty" speech and an occasional new word, he most likely has dysfunction in his _____ _____ brain region. The terms for this group of aphasias are Wernicke's aphasia, _____, _____, and _____.

503. nominal

504. nominal

505. nominal

506. Drivelling speech S   Derailment S
     Anomia N   Jargon agrammatism S
     Circumlocutory speech N   Non-sequitur speech S

507. nominal, semantic

508. posterior, temporo-parietal, left

509. clang associations, neologisms

510. Semantic aphasia   Neologisms, clang associations

     Nominal aphasia   Drivelling, derailment, non-sequitive
                               speech

     Phonemic aphasia   Anomia, loss of use of nouns

511. semantic, nominal, phonemic

512. temporo-parietal

513. dominant temporo-parietal, fluent, receptive, sensory

514.   Which of the following statements about posterior language disorder is incorrect?

   a. Posterior language disorder correlates with dysfunction in the dominant temporo-parietal brain regions.

   b. Posterior language disorder incompasses the terms: Wernicke's aphasia, receptive aphasia, sensory aphasia, fluent aphasia.

   c. Posterior language disorder includes the subtypes semantic, nominal, phonemic.

   d. Phonemic disorder refers to the meaning of speech whereas nominal disorder refers to the use of proper nouns.

515.   Paraphasias: word approximations, neologisms, jargon agrammatisms (drivelling speech) are characteristic of _____
aphasia, a term equivalent to _____ language disorder.

516.   Sensory aphasia or _____ aphasia results from dysfunction in the _____ _____ areas.

517.   The best clinical "test" of language ability requires careful listening to how the patient is speaking. Once again, you must focus upon _____ not _____ .

518.   If a patient refers to a pen as "a writer," a key as "a lock or opener" a watch as "a timer," a comb as "you know, to fix your hair with," he is using word _____ . The presence of these paraphasias indicates dysfunction in _____ brain areas and dysfunction of the posterior language system. Which of the subtypes of the posterior system does the above example best fit?

_____

519.   Word approximations, neologisms, tangential speech (talking past the point), drivelling (jargon agrammatisms) are all observed in patients with demonstrable lesions in the dominant posterior temporo-parietal brain area. Encompassing terms for these disorders are _____ , _____ , _____ , or _____
aphasia.

520.   As part of a language evaluation, ask each patient to name simple objects such as a pen, a watch, a key, a comb and then the smaller parts of these objects (e.g., penpoint, watchband). Inability to name objects or parts of objects is termed _____ .

521.   Anomia is associated with Wernicke's aphasia and thus indicates dysfunction in the _____ _____ _____ .
Another term for this _____ language dysfunction is _____ aphasia.

522.   Inability to understand spoken words, termed word deafness, as is the inability to name simple objects, termed _____ ,
are indications of _____ aphasia and suggest dysfunction in the _____ _____ brain region.

523.   A test of posterior language function is also a partial test of function in the _____ _____ brain region.

514.   d. Phonemic disorder refers to the sound of speech.

515.   Wernicke's, posterior

516.   Wernicke's (receptive, fluent), dominant temporal/temporo-parietal

517.   form, content

518.   approximations, dominant temporo-parietal, nominal

519.   Wernicke's, fluent, receptive, sensory

520.   anomia

521.   dominant temporo-parietal brain regions, posterior, nominal

522.   anomia, nominal, dominant temporo-parietal

523.   dominant temporo-parietal

524.   The terms Wernicke's, fluent, sensory or receptive aphasia refer to posterior language disorder which can be further divided into _____, _____, and _____. Anterior language disorder which relates to dysfunction in the dominant frontal lobe can also be separated into subtypes.

525.   An individual who exhibits jargon speech, anomia or neologisms, has dysfunction in the _____. Anterior language disorder suggests dysfunction in the _____ _____.

526.   Patients with anterior language disorder often have difficulty in articulation. Their speech is slow, labored and distorted in rhythm and pronunciation. A patient with this speech pattern may have dysfunction in the _____ _____ _____.

527.   Patients with anterior language disorder often speak in a "telegraphic" pattern in which small words and word endings are eliminated from the flow of speech. Patients with anterior language difficulties will have trouble with the fluency of their speech and in repeating spoken speech. What are some other characteristic speech patterns of patients with dominant frontal lobe dysfunction?

528.   During an examination, a patient was unable to speak fluently. Her speech was dysrhythmic and slow and she had great difficulty in "getting words out." When she did speak, her speech was "telegraphic." This speech pattern is characteristic of _____ language disorder and suggests a lesion in the _____. The term for this pattern is Broca's aphasia.

529.   Anterior language disorder frequently results in a reduction in the amount of fluency of speech. This non-fluent aphasia, also termed _____ aphasia, can take the form of uncontrolled automatic repetition of syllables in the middle of and at the end of words or phrases. The psychiatric term for this anterior language disorder is _____. Its equivalent neurologic term is _____.

530.   Circle the words or phrases which best describe Broca's aphasia.

Speech is fluent   Speech is non-fluent

Poor articulation of words   Word approximations

Neologisms   Labored speech

Small words and word   Jargon agrammatism
endings missing

524.   semantic, nominal, phonemic

525.   dominant temporo-parietal region, dominant frontal lobe

526.   dominant frontal lobe

527.   slow, labored speech, difficulty in articulation, distortion in rhythm
        and pronunciation.

528.   anterior, dominant frontal lobe

529.   Broca's, verbigeration, palilalia

530.   Speech is fluent   Speech is non-fluent
          Poor articulation of words Word approximations
          Neologisms   Labored speech
          Small words and word   Jargon agrammatism
          endings missing

531.   Often, motor aphasia is a term used interchangably with Broca's aphasia. Is motor aphasia fluent or non-fluent? _____

532.   Broca's aphasia, also termed motor aphasia, results from dysfunction in the _____ _____ _____ .

533.   Broca's aphasia, also termed motor aphasia, is language disorder in the _____ language system.

534.   Broca's area is located in the posterior, inferior region of the outside surface (lateral) of the dominant frontal lobe (16,17). Describe the speech pattern of this aphasia.

535.   Psychiatric patients rarely have classical Broca's aphasia; however, patients with intoxications or chronic brain syndromes will often exhibit motor speech dysfunction (9,16). This can be tested by asking the patient to repeat phrases such as: "No ifs, ands or buts," "Methodist Episcopal," "Massachusetts Avenue." Patients with anterior language dysfunction will have difficulty with the above phrases often leaving out a word or two: "No ifs or buts," or the endings of words: "No if an buts," or adding syllables that don't belong: "Methodist Episcacapal." Difficulties in repetition such as the above, suggest dysfunction in the inferior, posterior area of the _____ _____ _____ .

536.   Non-fluent aphasia can present with poverty of speech to the point of mutism. General motor behavior can also be reduced in frequency. This speech "arrest" disorder, as Broca's aphasia, is a form of anterior language disorder and thus can result from dysfunction in the _____ _____ _____ .

537.   The combination of paucity of speech with Broca's type responses can also be observed in patients with bilateral frontal lobe dysfunction. This presentation has been termed transcortical motor aphasia and, as Broca's aphasia, is a form of _____ _____ _____ (9,16,17).

538.   Place an A next to those words and phrases indicative of anterior language disorder and a P next to those words and phrases indicative of posterior language disorder.

Motor aphasia ___   Sensory aphasia ___

Receptive aphasia ___   Fluent aphasia ___

Non-fluent aphasia ___   Transcortical motor aphasia ___

Wernicke's aphasia ___   Broca's aphasia ___

Nominal aphasia ___   Speech arrest ___

Phonemic aphasia ___   Semantic aphasia ___

531. non-fluent

532. dominant frontal lobe

533. anterior

534. slow, labored, poor articulation, loss of small words and word endings, telegraphic, non-fluent

535. dominant frontal lobe

536. dominant frontal lobe

537. anterior language disorder

538. Motor aphasia A   Sensory aphasia P
Receptive aphasia P   Fluent aphasia P
Non-fluent aphasia A   Transcortical motor aphasia A
Wernicke's aphasia P   Broca's aphasia A
Nominal aphasia P   Speech arrest A
Phonemic aphasia P   Semantic aphasia P

539.   In the space provided, write all the terms that describe each example of language disorder.

"I couldn't rerubish it"   _____

"Not happy...not content ...not satisfied here... home"   _____

"It could always be, but I'm not the indicator that one would need to require it."   _____

"1......1......"   _____

"It's episodada...da ...da...cal"   _____

"It's a door-turner, a twister, a door mover-on."   _____

540.   In the space provided, write all the terms that describe each example of language disorder:

"Open door...in open door ...street."   _____

"....Harold go....car...."   _____

"The rotarator tribbled its output."   _____

"I can't find the cover-upper to the pot."   _____

541.   The relationships between the dominant frontal, temporal, and parietal lobes in the organization of verbal or symbolic function are extremely complex. Disconnections between areas and combination lesions can lead to a variety of syndromes (28,30). This material is beyond the scope of this text.

539. "I couldn't rerubish it"   Neologism, phonemic language disorder.
Wernicke's aphasia, posterior language
disorder, fluent aphasia, sensory aphasia,
receptive aphasia

"Not happy...not   Broca's aphasia, motor aphasia, anterior
content...not satis-   language disorder, non-fluent aphasia
fied here...home"

"It could always be,   Drivelling, jargon agrammatism, semantic
but I'm not the indi-   language disorder, Wernicke's aphasia,
cator that one would   posterior language disorder, fluent apha-
need to require it"   sia, sensory aphasia, receptive aphasia

"1......1......"   Paucity of thought, speech arrest, anterior language disorder, motor aphasia,
non-fluent aphasia

"It's espsodada...   Verbigeration, palilalia, anterior language
da...da...cal"   disorder, motor aphasia, non-fluent aphasia

"It's a door-turner,   Word approximations, nominal language
a twister, a door   disorder, Wernicke's aphasia, posterior
mover-on."   language disorder, fluent aphasia, sensory aphasia, receptive aphasia

540. "Open door...in open   Broca's aphasia, motor aphasia, anterior
door...street."   aphasia, non-fluent aphasia

"...Harold go...car..."   Transcortical aphasia (speech arrest,
Broca's combination), motor aphasia, an-
terior aphasia, non-fluent aphasia

"The rotarator tribbled   Neologisms, phonemic language disorder,
its output."   Wernicke's aphasia, receptive aphasia,
sensory aphasia, fluent aphasia, posterior
aphasia

"I can't find the   Word approximation (for "lid"), nominal
cover-upper to the pot."   aphasia, posterior aphasia, Wernicke's
aphasia, receptive aphasia, sensory apha-
sia, fluent aphasia

541. No answer required

542.   Draw lines between matching items in the two columns:

Anomia   "How much is 85 - 27 ?"

Spelling apraxia   "What is the name of this object?"

Alexia   "Spell cross"

Acalculia   "Read this"

543.   Draw lines between matching items in the two columns:

Apraxia   Unable to recognize objects

Agnosia   Unable to read

Alexia   Unable to do math

Acalculia   Unable to perform simple motor tasks
                          despite normal motor and sensory
                          function

544.   Fill in the blanks with the appropriate terms:

The inability to name objects is _____.

The inability to read is _____.

The inability to compute simple numbers is _____.

The inability to write words is _____.

545.   Fill in the blanks with the appropriate terms:

The inability to recognize objects is _____.

This function can be specifically sublabeled: the inability to recognize letters is letter _____; the inability to recognize numbers is number _____.

546.   Circle the terms indicating dominant hemisphere dysfunction:

Construction apraxia   Anomia

Spelling apraxia   Alexia

Ideomotor apraxia   Agraphia

Acalculia   Letter agnosia

547.   When you are testing for dominant and non-dominant dysfunction, give directions clearly and precisely. Don't give hints such as "What is the name of this geometric figure?" Simply say "What is the name of this shape" or "Please copy this shape."

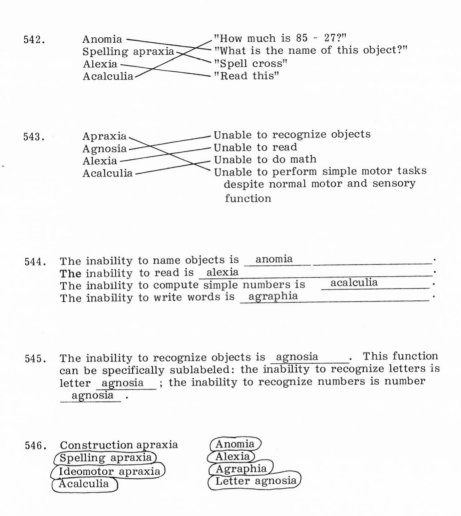

542.   Anomia ———————— "How much is 85 - 27?"
        Spelling apraxia ————— "What is the name of this object?"
        Alexia ———————— "Spell cross"
        Acalculia ———————— "Read this"

543.   Apraxia ———————— Unable to recognize objects
        Agnosia ———————— Unable to read
        Alexia ———————— Unable to do math
        Acalculia ———————— Unable to perform simple motor tasks
                            despite normal motor and sensory
                            function

544.   The inability to name objects is   anomia   .
        The inability to read is   alexia   .
        The inability to compute simple numbers is   acalculia   .
        The inability to write words is   agraphia   .

545.   The inability to recognize objects is   agnosia   . This function
        can be specifically sublabeled: the inability to recognize letters is
        letter   agnosia   ; the inability to recognize numbers is number
        agnosia .

546.   Construction apraxia   (Anomia)
        (Spelling apraxia)   (Alexia)
        (Ideomotor apraxia)   (Agraphia)
        (Acalculia)   (Letter agnosia)

547.   No answer required

209

548. Review the following tasks and responses. Which hemisphere(s) is(are) affected in this patient?

TASKS

a. Name these shapes (square, cross, triangle)

b. Copy the shapes (cross, square, triangle)

c. Write the name of each shape

RESPONSES

a. *Box, Cross, Triangle*

b. (drawn cross) (drawn square) (drawn triangle)

c. *Criso, Scare, Srangl*

549. Review the following tasks and responses. Which hemisphere(s) is(are) affected in this patient?

TASKS

a. Name these shapes (square, cross, triangle)

b. Read this. "He is a friendly animal, a famous winner of dog shows."

c. Calculate 85 - 27 =

RESPONSES

a. Box, cross, pyramid

b. "He is a famous animal, a friendly winner of dog shows."

c.
$$\begin{array}{r} 85 \\ -27 \\ \hline 78 \end{array}$$

550. Review the following tasks and responses. Which hemisphere(s) is(are) affected in this patient?

TASKS

a. Name these (square, clock)

b. To calculate 85 - 27.

c. To place the left hand on the right ear.

d. "Show me how you hammer a nail."

RESPONSES

a. "Box", "Time"

b.
$$\begin{array}{r} 85 \\ -27 \\ \hline 28 \end{array}$$

c. Left hand placed on left ear, even when told it was incorrect.

d. Unable to perform

210

548. both

549. dominant

550. left (dominant)

551.   Check the appropriate box that best matches each behavior with its most likely cortical functional region:

Behavior	Frontal	Dominant Parietal	Non-Dominant Parietal	Dominant Temporal
Loss of recent memory				
Can't copy simple shapes				
Can't do serial 7's				
Global dis-orientations				
Can't do simple math				
Jargon agram-matism				
Telegraphic speech				
Can't remember four items, concentration intact				
Can't concentrate				
Can't demonstrate the use of simple objects				
Copies examiner's movements, despite instructions to the contrary				
Disoriented to left-right				
Uses multiple overlapping lines when copying a circle				
Can't name simple objects				

212

551.

Behavior	Frontal	Dominant Parietal	Non-Dominant Parietal	Dominant Temporal
Loss of recent memory				√
Can't copy simple shapes			√	
Can't do serial 7's	√			
Global dis-orientations	√			-
Can't do sim-ple math		√		
Jargon agram-matism				√
Telegraphic speech	√			
Can't remem-ber four items, concentration intact				√
Can't concen-trate	√			
Can't demon-strate the use of simple objects		√		
Copies examiner's movements, des-pite instructions to the contrary	√			
Disoriented to left-right		√		
Uses multiple over-lapping lines when copying a circle	√			
Can't name simple objects				√

552.   Place the number of the appropriate item on the proper brain region:

Left Hemisphere   Right Hemisphere

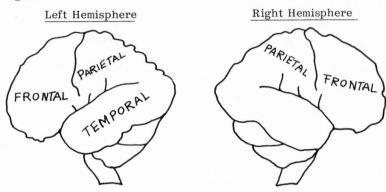

1. Active perception (identification of upside-down objects)

2. Wernicke's area

3. Broca's area

4. Ability to copy (reconstruct) objects

5. Ability to orient oneself to right/left

6. Ability to do simple math

7. Ability to concentrate

8. Abstract thinking

9. Reading and writing

10. Memory

11. Recognition and categorization of symbolic relationships

12. "Methodist Episcopal"

13. Naming simple objects

14. Regulating motor behavior (no perseveration)

15. Regulating motor behavior (no echopraxia)

16. Ability to demonstrate use of objects

17. Ability to recognize and name body parts (i.e. - fingers)

18. Global orientation

19. Usually the dominant hemisphere

553.   You noticed that in the last item there were no tasks or behaviors for the right _____ _____ _____ or for both _____ lobes. These areas are difficult to test without special equipment.

Left Hemisphere   Right Hemisphere

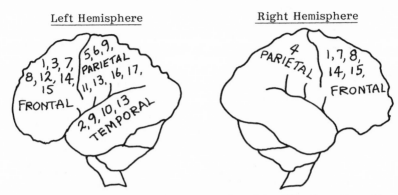

LEFT FRONTAL: 1. Active perception (identification of upside-
down objects)
   3. Broca's area
   7. Ability to concentrate
   8. Abstract thinking
  12. "Methodist Episcopal"
  14. Regulating motor behavior (no perseveration)
  15. Regulating motor behavior (no echopraxia)

RIGHT FRONTAL: 1. Active perception (identification of upside-
down objects)
   7. Ability to concentrate
   8. Abstract thinking
  14. Regulating motor behavior (no perseveration)
  15. Regulating motor behavior (no echopraxia)

LEFT PARIETAL: 5. Ability to orient oneself to right/left
   6. Ability to do simple math
   9. Reading and writing
  11. Recognition and categorization of symbolic
relationships
  13. Naming simple objects
  16. Ability to demonstrate use of objects
  17. Ability to recognize and name body parts
i.e. - fingers)

RIGHT PARIETAL: 4. Ability to copy (reconstruct) objects

LEFT TEMPORAL: 2. Wernicke's area
   9. Reading and writing (accepted)
  10. Memory
  13. Naming simple objects

Left hemisphere usually the dominant hemisphere.

553. non-dominant temporal lobe, occipital

554.   Even though the right (non-dominant temporal lobe) and both occipital lobes are difficult to test and are sometimes referred to as the "silent area," patients can be asked to perform several tasks which will at least screen for dysfunction. What functions of the dominant temporal lobe have you learned?

555.   Occipital lobe function can be tested by evaluating visual acuity in all quadrants of the visual fields. This is part of every complete physical examination, but it tests only the primary visual cortex and not the visual associational areas also located in the occipital lobe. Once you have established that a patient's visual acuity is intact (with or without corrective lenses) show him a card similar to the following (you can make up your own or purchase standard cards). Ask the patient to "choose the best match for the missing part in the pattern." (The correct answer is the third pattern, in the top row on the right.) (47 pp. 107-127)

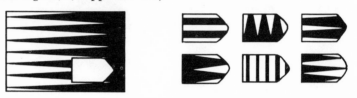

Another method involves the use of camouflaged figures such as this one. Ask the patient to tell you "what he sees in the picture."

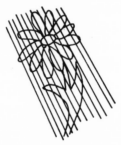

An individual with intact visual perception should be able to extract the figure from the camouflage. Once extracted, the inability to name the figure is an example of _____ and suggests dysfunction in the _____ _____ _____ (47 pp. 107-127).

554. posterior language, verbal memory

555. anomia, dominant temporal-parietal region

556.   The non-dominant temporal lobe, usually on the _____
side of the brain, perceives rhythm and music (47 pp. 128-146).

557.   To test for non-dominant temporal lobe function, ask the patient
to sing simple songs or repeat your singing of songs (e.g., "Happy
Birthday"). Another test of non-dominant temporal function is to
ask the patient the following:

"I am going to tap on the desk, I want you to tell me how many taps
I make."

Then proceed: --, ---, ----. If the patient responds accurately,
say: "I am going to tap on the desk; I want you to tap on the desk
exactly the way I do."

Then proceed. The dots represent short or soft sounds, the
bars represent longer or louder sounds.

‾‾ , ‾‾ , ‾‾ , ‾‾ ,

..‾ , ..‾ , ..‾ , ..‾ ,

‾. , ‾. , ‾. , ‾. ,

‾‾... , ‾‾... , ‾‾... , ‾‾... ,

...‾‾ , ...‾‾ , ...‾‾ , ...‾‾ ,

Inability to repeat the rhythm or numbers of your taps or to "sing
along" suggest dysfunction in the _____ _____ _____.
How would you test for occipital lobe function?

558.   Verbal memory and language functions are located in the ____
_____: perception of music and rhy-
thm are located in the _____ _____

_____.

559.   Inability to identify camouflaged figures suggests _____
_____ dysfunction; inability to identify rhythm suggests
_____ _____ lobe dysfunction.

556. right

557. non-dominant temporal lobe, test patient for visual acuity, ability to identify patterns and perceive camouflaged objects.

558. dominant temporal lobe, non-dominant temporal lobe

559. occipital lobe, non-dominant temporal

560.   Place the number of the appropriate item on the proper brain region:

Left Hemisphere   Right Hemisphere

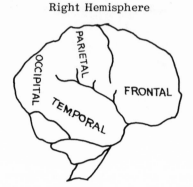

1. Global orientation

2. Calculations

3. Name 4 objects

4. Identify hidden objects

5. Copy cross

6. Repeat rhythm and musical tones

7. Draw circle

8. Finger identification

9. Serial 7's

10. Identification of upside-down objects

11. Right-left orientation

12. Echophenomena

13. Demonstrate use of simple objects

14. "Methodist Episcopal"

15. Writing

16. Recognition and categorization of relationships

17. Verbal memory

18. Wernicke's area

19. Broca's area

20. Abstract thinking

560.

Left Hemisphere　　　　　　　　　　Right Hemisphere

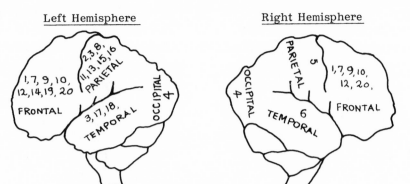

LEFT FRONTAL:　　1.　Global orientation
　　　　　　　　　　7.　Draw circle
　　　　　　　　　　9.　Serial 7's
　　　　　　　　　10.　Identification of upside down objects
　　　　　　　　　12.　Echophenomena
　　　　　　　　　14.　"Methodist Episcopal"
　　　　　　　　　19.　Broca's area
　　　　　　　　　20.　Abstract thinking

LEFT PARIETAL:　　2.　Calculations
　　　　　　　　　　3.　Name 4 objects
　　　　　　　　　　8.　Finger identification
　　　　　　　　　11.　Right-left orientation
　　　　　　　　　13.　Demonstrate use of simple objects
　　　　　　　　　15.　Writing
　　　　　　　　　16.　Recognition and categorization or relationships

LEFT TEMPORAL:　3.　Name 4 objects
　　　　　　　　　17.　Verbal memory
　　　　　　　　　18.　Wernicke's area

LEFT OCCIPITAL:　4.　Identify hidden objects

RIGHT FRONTAL:　1.　Global orientation
　　　　　　　　　　7.　Draw circle
　　　　　　　　　　9.　Serial 7's
　　　　　　　　　10.　Identification of upside down objects
　　　　　　　　　12.　Echophenomena
　　　　　　　　　20.　Abstract thinking

RIGHT PARIETAL: 5.　Copy cross

RIGHT TEMPORAL: 6.　Repeat rhythms and musical tones

RIGHT OCCIPITAL: 4.　Identify camouflaged objects

561.   Check the appropriate box that best matches each behavior with its most likely cortical functional region:

Behavior	Frontal	Dominant Temporal	Dominant Parietal	Non-Dominant Temporal	Non-Dominant Parietal	Occipital
Motor perseveration						
Poor short-term memory						
Finger agnosia						
Construction apraxia						
Cannot identify camouflaged objects						
Cannot do similarities						
Poor serial 7's						
Cannot repeat rhythms & songs						
Acalculia						
Ideomotor apraxia (both hands)						
Right/left disorientation						
Cannot recognize or categorize relationships						
Anomia						
Agraphia						
Echopraxia						
Dyslexia						
Word approximations						

561.

Behavior	Frontal	Dominant Temporal	Dominant Parietal	Non-Dominant Temporal	Non-Dominant Parietal	Occipital
Motor perseveration	√					
Poor short-term memory		√				
Finger agnosia			√			
Construction apraxia					√	
Cannot identify camouflaged objects						√
Cannot do similarities	√					
Poor serial 7's	√					
Cannot repeat rhythms & songs				√		
Acalculia			√			
Ideomotor apraxia (both hands)			√			
Right/left disorientation			√			
Cannot recognize or categorize relationships			√			
Anomia		√	√			
Agraphia			√			
Echopraxia	√					
Dyslexia			√			
Word approximations		√	√			

REVIEW SECTION

562.   The phenomenological mental status examination utilizes three
basic principles of clinical method. In addition to separating form
from content, they are _____ _____ and _____
_____ _____.

563.   Place a check mark in the appropriate box to indicate which mental status heading each clinical item best fits:

	General Appearance	General Motor Behavior	Catatonia	Affect	Thought Disorder
Clang associations					
Hyperactivity					
Posturing					
Flight-of-ideas					
Verbigeration					
Intense affect					
Lability of mood					
Euphoria					
Tangential speech					
Irritability					
Sadness					
Unkempt clothes					

562. objective observation, precise terminology

563.	General Appearance	General Motor Behavior	Catatonia	Affect	Thought Disorder
Clang Associations					✓
Hyperactivity		✓			
Posturing			✓		
Flight-of-ideas					✓
Verbigeration			✓		✓
Intense affect				✓	
Lability of mood				✓	
Euphoria				✓	
Tangential speech					✓
Irritability				✓	
Sadness				✓	
Unkempt clothes	✓				

564.   Place a check mark in the appropriate box to indicate which mental status heading each item fits. More than one check per item is possible.

	Mania	Catatonia	Schizophrenia	Coarse Brain Disease
Apophany				
Violence				
Inappropriate mood				
Thought disorder				
Poor personal hygiene				
Tardive dyskinesia				
Agitation				
Loose associations				
Illusions				
Hallucinations				
Persecutory delusions				
Catalepsy				

564.	Mania	Catatonia	Schizophrenia	Coarse Brain Disease
Apophany	√	√	√	√
Violence	√	√	√	√
Inappropriate mood	√	√	√	√
Thought disorder	√	√	√	√
Poor personal hygiene	√	√	√	√
Tardive dyskinesia	√	√	√	√
Agitation	√	√	√	√
Loose associations	√	√	√	√
Illusions	√	√	√	√
Hallucinations	√	√	√	√
Persecutory delusions	√	√	√	√
Catalepsy	√	√	√	√

There are no pathognomonic signs of the major psychoses.

227

565.   Place a check mark in the appropriate box to indicate which mental status heading each clinical item best fits. More than one check mark per item is possible.

	General Appearance	Motor Behavior	Affect	Thought Process	Apophany	Perceptual Dysfunc.	1st Rank Symptom
Delusional perception							
Delusional mood							
Hyperactivity							
Incomplete auditory hallucination							
Flight-of-ideas							
Irritability							
Autochthonous delusional ideas							
Clang associations							
Euphoria							
Depression							
Posturing							

565.

	General Appearance	Motor Behavior	Affect	Thought Process	Apophany	Perceptual Dysfunc.	1st Rank Symptom
Delusional perception					√		√
Delusional mood					√		
Hyperactivity		√					
Incomplete auditory hallucination						√	
Flight-of-ideas				√			
Irritability			√				
Autochthonous delusional ideas					√		
Clang associations				√			
Euphoria			√				
Depression			√				
Posturing	√						

566.   Place a check mark in the appropriate box to indicate which mental status heading each clinical item best fits.

	General Appearance	General Motor Behavior	Catatonia	Affect	Thought Disorder
Thin					
Agitated					
Echolalia					
Grimacing					
Dishevelled					
Labile affect					
Anxiety					
Rambling speech					
Non-sequiturs					
Irritability					
Clouded consciousness					
Perseveration of association (stock words)					

567.   Circle all the thought disorder terms best associated with schizophrenia:

Non-sequiturs   Flight-of-ideas

Circumstantial speech   Paraphasia

Blocking   Tangential speech

566.

	General Appearance	General Motor Behavior	Catatonia	Affect	Thought Disorder
Thin	√				
Agitated		√			
Echolalia			√		
Grimacing			√		
Dishevelled	√				
Labile affect				√	
Anxiety				√	
Rambling speech					√
Non-sequiturs					√
Irritability				√	
Clouded consciousness	√				
Perseveration of association (stock words)					√

567. (Non-sequiturs)   Flight-of-ideas

   Circumstantial speech   (Paraphasia)

   (Blocking)   (Tangential speech)

568.   Label with the appropriate terms the following behaviors:

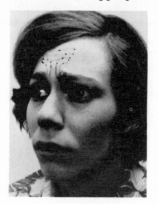 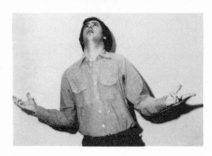

569.   Label with the appropriate term(s) the following behaviors:

A. "Why are you in the hospital?"
"What's the trouble? It's been a long time...I can tell you that, trouble, trouble, the whole world is troubled not just me, so why should I complain? Think of all those other people."

B. "What's a nice girl like you doing in an address like this?"

C. "Doctor, I'm dead. I don't care what they (staff) say---even if I can move and talk, I know I'm dead, it has to be so, I just know it."

570.   Label with the appropriate terms the following behavior:

"My husband is trying to poison me, he is unfaithful; the radio keeps reporting his activities to me."   _____

"Hello, Doc---How am I today? Today?---I'm fine, I feel great, g-great, g-great, ate, ate, ate, ate."   _____

568. Picture A: Omega Sign, veraguth folds, a sad facial expression

Picture B: Posturing, a cataleptic state - catatonia

569. A. Tangential speech with perseveration: talks past the point,
does not answer the question and perseverates the stock word
"trouble."

B. Word approximation ("address" for "place").

C. Primary delusional idea

570. Secondary delusional idea, verbigeration/palilalia

571.   Label each description with the appropriate phenomenologic term(s):

"It's frightening---suddenly everything becomes very small as if I
were looking through the wrong
end of a telescope."   _____

"It happens many times during
the day. I suddenly smell burning rubber or rotting flesh. I
feel dizzy and then it's all
right again."   _____

"They're all in on it. They're
trying to kill me, then they're
going to wipe out the country.
It's all over, I can tell. The
radio and TV say it; the ma-
chines in my room say it."   _____

572.   Label each description with the appropriate phenomenologic term(s):

"Doctor, you've got to do something. She spends all day standing in the middle of the room,
looking at the ceiling. She won't
answer me..."   _____

"...Then, suddenly, she'll start
to clean the house, sew clothes,
go shopping. It's as if she's do-
ing everything at once."   _____

"...When I try to talk to her, she
becomes angry, yells, curses,
threatens me. Then, almost in
the next second, she laughs, and
then cries."   _____

573.   Label each description with the appropriate phenomenologic term:

"It's a frightening man. I can see
him walking behind me. Some-
times I see him in another city."   _____

"I can't make it out. It's some
sort of a noise or hum but I hear
it all over the place."   _____

"Well, if the place pictures like a
next moment I can't be written
in sections."   _____

"Yeah. I know...a kid could
do something like that...I'm
tired, my mouth is dry...What
time is it...Did you read in the
papers..."   _____

234

571. Micropsia, olfactory hallucination, secondary delusional idea

572. Catalepsy and posturing, hyperactivity, lability of affect

573. extracampine hallucination; elementary auditory hallucination; drivelling; rambling speech

574.   Label each item with the appropriate phenomenologic term:

"I don't know. I just feel funny. Detached...nervous, sort of... like I'm going through the motions, watching myself."

_____

"It's horrible. Everything becomes large, then small. People's faces become large and distorted."

_____

"I can't stand it. Every time the phone rings or the door bell rings, that son of a bitch turns on the machine and the voice screams at me."

_____

"You know. You hear it too. Everyone must. They're talk-ing all the time...(Shouting at the ceiling). Stop it, stop it! They never stop. They talk about me all the time...Of course, as loud as your voice, you idiot. They're talking so loud it drives me crazy."

_____

575.   Place a P next to the items suggesting perceptual dysfunction, an O next to the items suggesting memory dysfunction, and a Y next to the items suggesting an abnormality of motor behavior.

1. Mitmachen ___   7. Deja vu ___

2. Illusion ___   8. Extracampine hallucination ___

3. Anterograde amnesia ___   9. Catalepsy ___

4. Haptic hallucination ___   10. Hypnagogic/hypnopompic ___

5. Functional hallucination ___ 11. Confabulation ___

6. Echopraxia ___   12. Waxy flexibility ___

576.   Beside each heading, place the numbers of the appropriate items below:

Memory _____   Affect_____

Thought process_____   Apophany _____

1. Euphoria   9. Paraphasia
2. Retrograde amnesia   10. Appropriate mood
3. Delusional perception   11. Jamais vu
4. Derailment   12. Non-sequiturs
5. Expansive mood   13. Delusional mood
6. Confabulation   14. Verbigeration
7. Perseveration   15. Pseudomemory
8. Autochthonous idea   16. Relatedness

574. depersonalization; macropsia and micropsia (dysmegalopsia); functional auditory hallucination; phoneme or complete auditory hallucination

575. Mitmachen Y

   Illusion P

   Anterograde amnesia O

   Haptic hallucination P

   Functional hallucination P

   Echopraxia Y

   Deja vu O

   Extracampine hallucination P

   Catalepsy Y

   Hypnagogic/hypnopompic P

   Confabulation O

   Waxy flexibility Y

576. Memory 2, 6, 11, 15   Affect 1, 5, 10, 16

   Thought process 4, 7, 9, 12, 14 Apophany 3, 8, 13

577.   Draw lines between matching items in the 2 columns (items on the right can be used more than once).

Unable to name own fingers

Unable to demonstrate use of key, hammer or flipping a coin with both hands

Dominant Parietal Lobe

Unable to copy the outline of a key

Non-Dominant Parietal Lobe

Unable to perform a non-verbal spatial task

Unable to read

578.   Draw lines between matching items in the two columns:

Apraxia   Unable to recognize previously known objects

Agnosia   Unable to write a sentence to dictation but able to copy a sentence

Acalculia   Unable to do simple math

Agraphia   Unable to perform simple motor tasks despite normal muscle strength

579.   Check off the tests of dominant parietal lobe function:

"Show me how you thread a needle."   _____

"What finger is this?"   _____

"Copy the outline of this object."   _____

"How do you use a key?"   _____

"Subtract 29 from 66."   _____

"Spell earth backwards."   _____

"Hold out your right hand...Put your right hand on your left ear."   _____

577. Unable to name own fingers

Unable to demonstrate use of key, hammer or flipping a coin with both hands

Unable to copy the outline of a key

Unable to perform a non-verbal spatial task

Unable to read

Dominant Parietal Lobe

Non-Dominant Parietal Lobe

578. Apraxia

Agnosia

Acalculia

Agraphia

Unable to recognize previously known objects

Unable to write a sentence to dictation but able to copy a sentence

Unable to do simple math

Unable to perform simple motor tasks despite normal muscle strength

579. "Show me how you thread a needle." √

"What finger is this?" √

"Copy the outline of this object." _____

"How do you use a key?" √

"Subtract 29 from 66." √

"Spell earth backwards." _____

"Hold out your right hand... put your right hand on your left ear." √

CLINICAL EVALUATIONS

Excerpts from clinical cases will be presented in the final section
of Part I. As each patient is described, you will be asked to identify
behaviors and make clinical comments.

CASE I

A 43-year-old white, medium-built man,
dressed in a leather suit is brought into
the emergency room by the police. He has
been running through the street waving a
large knife and attacking buildings.

When you first observe him, the handcuffed
patient is being held in a chair as he shouts
unintelligible phrases, makes comments to
the emergency room staff, and occasionally
bursts into intense satanic laughter.

This patient's general motor
behavior is characterized
by _____.
The most severe form of this
motor state is termed
_____ and
can lead to cardiovascular
collapse and death.

When released from his handcuffs, the
patient rapidly paces around the examining
room, commenting on every item, yelling to
any staff member who passes by the open
door.

Throughout the interview, the patient's
manner is exalted, agressive, and on
occasion, suspicious. He appears alert.
He frequently laughs loudly, expresses
great joy, expounds on the feeling of great
power and "superhuman" strength but, upon
questioning, becomes suddenly irritable and
angry. His speech is rapid. He speaks
constantly and can be interrupted only with
difficulty.

This patient's affective
_____ is expanded.
His affected intensity is
_____. His moods
of _____ and _____
are _____
to the examination situation
and their sudden appearance
and disappearance suggest
a _____ of
affect. His speech is both
rapid and _____.

240

This patient's general motor behavior is characterized by hyperactivity. The most severe form of this motor state is termed   excitement   and can lead to cardiovascular collapse and death.

This patient's affective   range   is expanded. His affective intensity is   increased   . His moods of   euphoria   and   anger   are   inappropriate   to the examination situation and their sudden appearance and disappearance suggest a   lability   of affect. His speech is both rapid and   pressured .

You are unable to keep him on the topic;
he is constantly jumping from subject to
subject. To the question, "What do you
mean by 'great power'?", he replies:
"Power is as power does; I am the resur-
rection, ha, I want an erection... rejection.
Did you know my girlfriend wanted to be a
psychiatrist?... She works for a law firm...
Those bastards... They keep the price of
everything up... No-fault insurance would
be the best. The best, the best, the
best, est, est, est!

An example of _____ .

An example of _____
associations.

An example of _____ .

The patient also says: "God speaks to me,
He tells me what to do. I hear him all the
time; I feel his power."

Possible delusional _____ .
Possible first rank symptom of
experience of _____ .

Your responses to the patient's last statement should be (list all the
questions to determine form):

CASE II

A 30-year-old, thin woman is hospitalized
because she has thrown herself in front of
a subway train in a suicide attempt. She
has sustained only superficial injuries.
Admission physical and all laboratory findings
are within normal limits.

When you first see her, the woman rushes
to you, grabs you by your white coat and
begins to moan, whine and plead: "Help
me, help me...What am I to do? I can't go
on like this."

The descriptions would be
placed under the mental
status heading of _____
_____ .

Once in your office, the patient continues
to pace back and forth, wringing her hands,
patting her breasts, shaking her head and
trembling. When you ask her to sit down,
she complies for a few minutes but soon
becomes restless, constantly moving her
hands, rocking back and forth, and finally
rising and again beginning her pacing.

This patient has moderate
to severe motor _____ .

Her photograph is on the previous page.
Observe it carefully. How would you
describe her?

Her expression is characteristic of _____ with
obvious _____
and _____ folds.

She is somewhat unkempt. Throughout the
interview she continues to whine; tries on
numerous occasions to cry without success;
looks and says she is in great distress; that
life is hopeless; that she is going to die;
that she is a bad person; that she is very
fearful and sad.

Her range of affect is
_____ but her
intensity is _____ .
The quality of her mood is
_____ .

242

An example of ___flight-of-ideas___ .

An example of ___clang___ associations.

An example of ___verbigeration___ .

Possible delusional ___idea___ .

Possible first rank symptom of experience of ___influence.___ .

"Do you mean you hear God's voice?... As loudly as you hear mine?...
Where does the voice come from?... Does he speak to you all the time?
Does anyone else talk to you like that? Is it like an energy wave? Does
it make you do things even when you don't want to?...You mean you actually feel the wave on your body?"

CASE II

These past descriptions would be placed under the mental status heading
of ___general appearance___ .

This patient has moderate to severe motor ___agitation___ .

Her expression is characteristic of ___depression___ with obvious
___omega___ ___sign___ and ___veraguth___ folds.

Her range of affect is ___constricted___ but her intensity is___increased.___
The quality of her mood is ___sad and anxious.___

She can offer no explanation for her fears or feelings of hopelessness (going to die) and guilt (bad person). She just feels it to be so.

She says she is convinced that people are suffering for her sins, even people whom she had never met. She feels this to be true because she feels so disgusting that her "badness" must affect others.

She had delusional ideas, which develop from her mood, therefore, they are _____.

She says she still feels like killing herself and would do so if we left her alone. She says that she feels worse in the morning, particularly at 2 or 3 a.m., and that she hears strange noises in her room. The noises sound like footsteps, breathing, or creaks and groans; but they are muffled and sometimes just noises. They frighten her, and fortunately, she does not hear them during the day. She denies hearing them during the interview.*

She is describing vague hallucinations also termed
_____
hallucinations.

*NOTE: Since she does not experience the noise phenomena during the examination, this information should not be written in the mental status evaluation but rather in the history under the heading Present Illness.

Secondary delusional ideas (secondary to her mood).

She is describing vague hallucinations also termed pseudo and elementary
hallucinations.

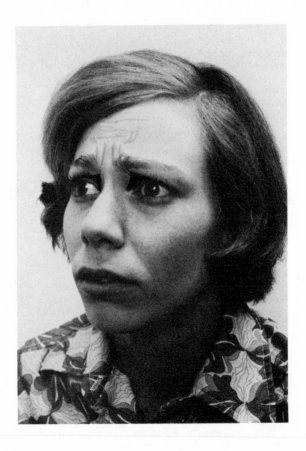

CASE III

A 24-year-old man is brought to the emergency room by his mother because of his increasing seclusiveness and "odd" behavior.

Throughout his admission interview, he sits quietly staring straight ahead, but when spoken to, he does look at the examiner and responds.

Although not conclusive, this does suggest that his consciousness is _____.

His movements are slow and somewhat awkward. His facial expression remains unchanged throughout the examination and generally gives no hint of emotion.

His general motor behavior can be characterized as moderately _____.

The patient speaks in a soft, monotonous voice which remains unchanged throughout the interview.

This suggests a _____ range of affect with _____ intensity.

On several occasions, he suddenly stops speaking, stops moving, and simply stares off into space. He seems unaware of these periods which last only a few seconds. On several occasions, these episodes are followed by a different train of thought.

A classical example of _____ and _____.

When he is asked about the events that led to his mother's bringing him to the hospital, he keeps repeating that the problem was his school where he had too many eight o'clock groups. When you realize that the patient means eight o'clock "classes" and you bring this to his attention, the patient becomes mildly irritated and says, "Well, you don't have to be so fickled about it!"

An example of _____. The word "fickled" is a _____. These errors in speech suggest _____ language dysfunction.

He says that his reason for secluding himself in his room is that his mother and father are surrounded by a green foul-smelling gas that makes him sick to his stomach. When you open the door so that the patient can see his mother in the waiting area, he says that he can still see and smell the gas. You tell him that you cannot see or smell the gas, that it certainly is an unusual situation; and you ask the patient whether he has any idea about what is happening, why it happens, and who or what is behind it all. The patient gives you a shallow smile (the only time during the interview) and says that you know perfectly well what he thinks since you can hear his thoughts. You deny this, question the patient more closely and learn that he is experiencing his thoughts coming out of his head so that everyone can hear them.

The patient is describing both _____ and _____. His reality _____ is also poor.

The patient is experiencing _____.

CASE III

Although not conclusive, this does suggest that his consciousness is
___clear___.

    His general motor behavior can be characterized as moderately
    __hypoactive__.

    This suggests a __constricted__ range of affect with
    __decreased__ intensity.

    A classical example of __blocking__ and __derailment__.

An example of word approximation (a paraphasia).

The word "fickled" is a neologism. These errors in speech suggest posterior language dysfunction.

The patient is describing olfactory and visual hallucinations. His reality testing is also poor.

The patient is experiencing thought broadcasting.

247

The patient also says that it is obvious that machines in the wall are generating a force and that the gas surrounding his parents is connected in some fashion to the machines.

These are _____ delusional ideas.

During cognitive testing, the patient remembers 5 numbers forward and 4 backwards. He remembers 3 of 4 words asked of him and subtracts sevens from 100 without error in 63 seconds.

Are any of these test responses abnormal?_____ What function are they testing?_____ What cortical region are they testing?_____

His fund of information is good and when asked: "What do an orange and an apple have in common?", he says: "They're both fruit."

Is this a good response?____

When asked: "What do a car and a boat have in common?", he says: "They're both means of transpalation."

While this response suggests adequate abstract thinking, the word "transpalation" suggests _____ and dysfunction in the _____
_____   _____

When you ask him to copy a cross and spell it, he does the following:

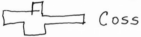 Coss

When you ask him to copy a triangle and spell it, he does this:

$\bigcup$ tringle

These test responses suggest cerebral dysfunction: (circle one): Non-dominant, dominant, bilateral

He calculates 85 - 27 this way:

85
-27
82 87

CASE IV

A 35-year-old white man is transferred from an outlying health facility to the general hospital's psychiatric unit because of an episode of "violent" behavior and for "catatonic schizophrenia".

These are <u>secondary</u> delusional ideas.

Are any of these test responses abnormal? <u>no</u>
What function are they testing? <u>concentration</u>
What cortical region are they testing? <u>frontal lobes</u>

Is this a good response? <u>yes</u>

While this response suggests adequate abstract thinking, the word "trans-palation" suggests <u>phonemic language disorder</u> and dysfunction in the <u>dominant temporo-parietal region.</u>

These test responses suggest: Non-dominant, Dominant, Bilateral

<u>CASE IV</u>

The patient had been working up to the day
of his hospitalization. Always a quiet and
shy person, he had become increasingly
aloof at work, speaking in a mumbled
almost unrecognizable English and moving
in an "odd manner". He was seen by a
local practitioner, given a neuroleptic drug
(chlorpromazine), and returned to work.
That same day he suddenly tried to rape
a passer-by: he was restrained and transferred for hospitalization.

Admission mental status examination reveals a six-foot, well-built, neat white
male, looking somewhat older than his
stated age. The patient appears anergic
(tired and without energy to initiate
activity), occasionally perplexed but at·
other times alert.

He walks to the examining room in a slow,
stilted fashion, often hesitates, holding
one foot several inches off the ground
before he takes a step. His gait is slightly
broad-based and, as he walks, he holds
his arms stiffly at his sides with his hand
and fingers hyperextended.

Is this gait normal?

His hand and arm positions become normal
when he stops, but occasionally his hand
suddenly supinates (turns palm upward)
in a short, rapid movement which, when
he notices it, he then extends into a
seemingly voluntary act.

This is an example of "chorea".
Can you find any examples to
justify the admission diagnosis
of "catatonia"? If so, underline. Are these signs of
agitation? Is he hypoactive
or hyperactive?_____ _____

The patient speaks slowly in a monotone
voice as thought his mouth were filled with
marbles. There is no hint of anger. When
questioned, he smiles in an automatic, prolonged, and exaggerated nonhumorous
fashion.

This facial expression is an
example of a _____.

His mood seems mildly sad, at other times
apathetic, but with little emotional expression. His emotional tone never varies
from this description.

This description illustrates
a _____ range of
affect and a _____
intensity of affect.

Is this gait normal? <u>No</u> His odd hand positions as he walks is also not normal motor behavior

Can you find any examples to justify the admission diagnosis of "catatonia"? <u>No</u> Are these signs of agitation? <u>No</u> Is he hypoactive or hyperactive? <u>Hypoactive</u>

An example of a <u>grimace</u>.

This description illustrates a <u>constricted</u> range of affect and a <u>decreased</u> intensity of affect.

When questioned, the patient takes several moments before answering and often his thoughts simply trail off unfinished. When this is pointed out, he picks up the same train of thought. When asked about the rape attempt, he replies, "I was working there for two years." When asked about the medicine he has been given he says, "My family comes from Alabama." His sentences are always short. He never volunteers information and never speaks unless spoken to.

Is this an example of derailment?_____

What type of thought disorder is this?

_____

The patient is able to repeat four numbers forward and three backwards. His responses to a serial 7's task is, "93, 97... 97...". His response to a serial 3's task is, "97, 93, 87, 80, 70..."

Are these responses within normal range?_____

Here the patient has responded to tests of

_____.

He is unable to give details about his family or of the past year of his life.

Some of his responses to cognitive test items are:

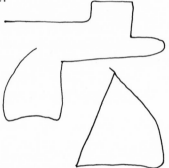

He reads "John went to the store to get a loaf of bread" as "John when to get a bread". He cannot name "key." He cannot demonstrate how to use a key.

Is his dysfunction: (circle one):

dominant, non-dominant, both

252

Is this an example of derailment? <u>No</u> It does suggest possible anterior
language dysfunction in his paucity of thinking. More data are needed.

These are examples of <u>non-sequiturs,</u> a form of formal thought disorder.
This also suggests possible posterior language disorder.

Is this within the normal range? <u>No</u> (5 forward and 4 backward and
correct subtraction in 90 seconds are considered normal)

Here the patient has responded to tests of <u>concentration.</u>

Is his dysfunction (circle one): dominant, non-dominant, (both)

A 45-year-old man is brought to a psychiatric clinic by his wife because of his "strange behavior" which developed suddenly during the past two days.

The patient had been a heavy drinker for most of his adult life but suddenly stopped drinking a year prior to this episode. He has no previous psychiatric history except that throughout his married life, he has had well-circumscribed periods in which he came home from work, hårdly spoke with his family, ate supper, and then either went immediately to sleep (often sleeping until the next morning) or simply sat in his chair staring at the newspaper, apparently without reading it. These episodes of one to two weeks' duration would suddenly lift, and he would be again his usual outgoing, energetic, infectiously happy-go-lucky self.

Two days prior to his clinic visit, while apparently sleeping, he suddenly sat up in bed, pointed to the window (second floor) and began shouting that there was someone watching him. He woke his wife and two children and accused them of plotting to harm him, and of being unfaithful and evil.

These are most likely apophanous or _____ ideas. Is there enough information to be sure of this? Explain your answer.

He spent the remainder of the night pacing all over the house, speaking rapidly to himself.

He slept throughout the following day, but that night he again became "agitated... confused" and frightened the family. They brought him to the clinic the next morning.

On examination, the patient is a middle-aged endomorphic (thick-boned, stocky, obese) neatly dressed man.

He moves slowly, stares ahead, making little eye contact with the examiner. His face is expressionless. His speech is slow and he rarely speaks unless spoken to. He says he is going to die... that they are out to get him for his past sins... that he is a "worthless person" and deserves his fate. You hospitalize him.

At home, he was agitated or hyperactive; now he's _____. Slowed motor behavior, speech and a paucity of thoughts is often referred to as psychomotor retardation.

These are most likely apophanous or delusional ideas. Is there enough information to be sure of this? No, because he must first be asked: "How do you know these things to be true?" and then the form of the primary or secondary nature of the phenomena must be established.

At home, he was agitated or hyperactive; now he is hypoactive. Slowed motor behavior, speech, and a paucity of thoughts is often referred to as psychomotor retardation.

Several hours after admission, the patient is found in bed, unresponsive to all but the most painful stimuli. He appears anesthetized although he has received no medication. After much prodding, he finally opens his eyes and in a thick-tongued voice says: "Get thee from me, Satan." He then falls back and does not respond for hours. His vital signs are stable and except for his general analgesia, physical exam is normal.

This extreme _____ active state is also termed _____. General analgesia is not an uncommon associated finding.

Later in the day, the patient suddenly wakes up and begins to sing. He follows this with some good-natured joking with the staff. He smiles, laughs, tries to teach them how to dance, and tries to help them do their work.

At this time, his affective intensity was _____, his mood _____.

He races from patient to patient, staff member to staff member, location to location, in an effort to carry out what he feels to be important tasks. Before he can finish any one of them, he is off on another "mission." His speech is rapid. He speaks to everyone, interrupts private conversations, cannot be stopped or interrupted, and only laughs and laughs when harshly spoken to by irritated patients and staff. He sings, whistles, dances, clowns for hours, finally collapsing on his bed once again in an uncommunicative analgesic state.

This extreme form of _____ activity is also termed _____.

In addition to the rapidity of his speech, his speech is also _____. Rapid pressured speech is a cardinal sign of _____. His intense _____ and euphoric mood is another cardinal sign of _____.

The following day, the patient becomes irritable. He begins shouting and shaking his fist in a threatening manner at both patients and staff. When placed in a seclusion room, he stands in one spot, staring out the window and speaking in a continuous flow. He can easily be approached, but he keeps on staring out the window even when he responds to questions. He says that there are machines in the ceiling that are constantly shouting to him.

This auditory phenomenon is called a _____ or a _____ _____.

The machines are loud and speak about events taking place in the hospital. He also says that there are other machines "out there" which are emitting gamma rays that spray his body and that this is the reason he is standing in one spot. The rays are doing "something" to his muscles "forcing" them to remain "stiff."

It is a Schneiderian _____ _____.

This phenomenon is termed an _____.

This extreme hypoactive state is also termed stupor. General analgesia is not an uncommon associated finding.

At this time, his affective intensity was increased; his mood euphoric.

This extreme form of hyper activity is also termed excitement.

In addition to the rapidity of his speech, his speech is also pressured. Rapid pressured speech is a cardinal sign of mania. His intense affect and euphoric mood is another cardinal sign of mania.

This phenomenon is called a phoneme or a complete auditory hallucination.

It is a Schneiderian First Rank Symptom.

This phenomenon is termed an experience of influence.

When not specifically questioned, he says
the following as he stares out the window:
"I see the sun. It's shining. It's shining.
All those trees green...grass...yellow
light; it's bright, it's bright but not
night. I see the sun. Cars are fast.
They are coming for me. They are coming
for me, me, me, me, me, me, me! Watch
out! Watch out! Slow down! You can't
go that fast...stop it, stop it. Is he dead?
No, there he is. I see him...The sun is on
his car... It's not too far, far, far, far
away, far away." Then he laughs.

Associations by sound are
called _____ associ-
ations.

This automatic repetition of
words is termed_____.

The overall speech form of
multiple interwining themes
and jumping from topic to
topic is termed _____

_____ _____.

CASE VI

A 45-year-old white man, formerly a university professor of statistical mathematics,
is brought to the hospital by his family
following air evacuation from England where
he had gone because he believed that he had
a professorship at Oxford. The British
authorities sent him back to the United
States because there was no record of him
at Oxford and because they observed some
of his psychopathology.

Throughout the mental status examination the
patient's facial expression remains unblinking
and without reflection of any mood. He
denies missing any friends or relatives and
says: "They're o.k.... they're on their
own." When asked about his feelings
about being hospitalized, he says blandly:
"I suppose I have to get it over with." His
plan for the future is to "apply for a position."

His overall affective re-
sponses suggest emotional
_____.

When you ask about the events in England
and during his trip back to the U.S...
he is vague in his answers and cannot
give details of events during the past
three weeks. He says he applied for many
positions, received replies and "has
positions."

A defect of _____
_____.

When asked "how come" he was hospitalized
in England and then sent back to the U.S.
he says: "It's just that I came to the
position and applied for the position".

These responses are talking
past the point or

_____ _____.

When pressed about the reason he is hospitalized he becomes mildly irritated and says:
"I've written many papers, positions, and
that's just the way it is."

The word "position" is a
stock word and is thus an
example of a _____.

Associations by sound are called clang associations.

This automatic repetition of words is termed verbigeration or palilalia.

The overall speech form of multiple intertwining themes and jumping from topic to topic is termed flight of ideas.

CASE VI

These behaviors suggest emotional blunting.

A defect of recent memory.

These responses are talking past the point or tangential speech. The word "position" is a stock word and is thus an example of a perseveration.

When asked about events which took place several years back, he is unable to give his birth date, his wedding date, or the age of his relatives. He says he is "38 or 39" and he denies any memory difficulty.

A deficit in _____ _____ _____

You inquire further about the patient's age. Then you ask math questions. The patient cannot subtract or add numbers that involve borrowing or carrying. He is unable to do serial 7's. Despite having a Ph.D. in mathematics, he is not troubled by his failure and says: "I did other mathematics in my position."

.An example of _____ and _____ _____ dysfunction.

Poor concentration suggests _____ _____ dysfunction.

Then you ask him about physical weakness, which he denies. (Previous physical examination has revealed no weakness).

Despite your repeated instructions to touch his nose when you touch your chest, the patient touches his chest.

Demonstrating _____ and dysfunction in the _____ _____ which regulate motor behavior.

When you question the patient about his fingers and ask him to name them, the patient says (from thumb outward) "Thumb, I don't know...straight finger?...index finger...I don't know...end finger."

An example of _____ _____ and _____ _____ dysfunction.

He calls a pen "a pencil," despite being told it is incorrect. He calls a watch "a clock" and cannot be more specific. He calls a key "a you know..." (and demonstrates its use with a poking, non-turning gesture).

Examples of _____ _____ and dysfunction in _____ _____ . These are examples of _____ language disorder of the _____ subtype.

The patient copies a cross in the following manner:

Is this abnormal? If so, what is the dysfunction called and where is it located?

A deficit in long-term memory.

An example of dyscalculia (or acalculia) and dominant parietal lobe dysfunction

Poor concentration suggests frontal lobe dysfunction.

Demonstrating echopraxia and dysfunction in the frontal lobes which regulate motor behavior.

An example of finger agnosia and dominant parietal lobe dysfunction.

Examples of word approximations and dysfunction in the dominant temporo-parietal region. These are examples of posterior language disorder of the semantic subtype.

Is this abnormal? yes
If so, what is the dysfunction called and where is it located? Construction apraxia, non-dominant parietal lobe.

Shade in the areas of probable dysfunction in this patient. List them.

Left Hemisphere   Right Hemisphere

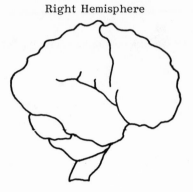

Left Hemisphere

Right Hemisphere

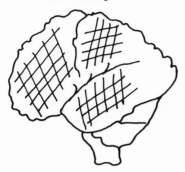
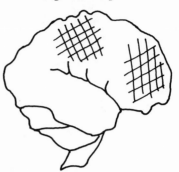

Dominant and non-dominant frontal
Dominant and non-dominant parietal
Dominant temporal

PHENOMENOLOGIC MENTAL STATUS OUTLINE

I. General Appearance

Age, race, sex, body type
State of consciousness, manner,
General health, hygiene, grooming

II. Motor Behavior

Gait
Rate, rhythm, activity,
Catatonic features

III. Affect

Range, intensity, stability
Quality of mood, appropriateness of mood, relatedness

IV. Thought Processes

Rate, rhythm and pressure of speech
Word use
Tightness and form of associational linkage
Thought content

V. Apophany

Delusional mood
Delusional ideas (primary, secondary)
Autochthonous ideas
Delusional perceptions

VI. Perceptual Disturbances

Illusions
Pseudo hallucinations
Elementary, functional, extracampine hallucinations
True hallucinations
Dysmegalopsia

VII. First Rank Symptoms

Thought broadcasting
Complete auditory hallucinations (Phonemes)
Delusional perceptions
Experiences of influence
Experiences of alienation

VIII. Cognitive Function

Global orientation
Judgment
Fund of information
Abstract thinking
Practic functions
Gnostic functions
Mnestic functions
Other

COGNITIVE FUNCTION EVALUATION OUTLINE

Cortical Region	Task	Dysfunction
A. Frontal Lobes	1. Global orientation	Disorientation
	2. Draw circle	Motor perseveration
	3. Serial 7's	Poor concentration
	4. Similarities	Poor abstract thinking
	5. Identification of upside down objects	Disability in active perception
	6. Echophenomena	Echopraxia
	7. "No ifs, ands or buts" "Methodist Episcopal"	Broca's aphasia (dominant lobe only)
	8. Repeat word series	Immediate recall
B. Dominant Parietal Lobe	1. Calculations	Acalculia
	2. Finger identification	Finger agnosia
	3. Right-left orientation	Right-left disorientation
	4. Reading	Alexia (dyslexia)
	5. Writing	Agraphia (dysgraphia)
	6. Demonstrate use of simple objects	Ideomotor apraxia
C. Non-dominant Parietal Lobe	1. Copy outline of simple shapes	Construction apraxia
D. Dominant Temporal Lobe		
Lateral Temporo-parietal region	1. Name simple objects	Anomia
	2. Speech	Wernicke's aphasia
Deep	1. Recall word series	Short-term memory
	2. Relate recent events	Recent memory
	3. Recall past events	Long-term memory (all verbal memory)
E. Non-Dominant Temporal Lobe	1. Repeat rhythms	Poor rhythm perception
	2. Repeat and recognize musical tones	Amusia
F. Occipital Lobes	1. Identification of camouflaged objects	Poor visual perception

REFERENCES

1. Abrams, R., Taylor, M.A.: First Rank Symptoms, Severity of Illness and Treatment Response in Schizophrenia. Compr. Psychiat. 14:353-355, 1973.
2. Abrams, R., Taylor, M.A.: Catatonia: A Prospective Clinical Study. Arch. Gen. Psychiat. 33:579-581, 1976.
3. Abrams, R., Taylor, M.A.: A Rating Scale for Emotional Blunting. Am. J. Psychiat. 135:226-229, 1978.
4. Abrams, R., Taylor, M.A.: Psychopathology and EEG. Biol. Psychiat. in press.
5. Andreasen, N.C.: Reliability and Validity of Proverb Interpretation to Assess Mental Status. Compr. Psychiat. 18:465-472, 1977.
6. Asnis, G.M., Leopold, M.A., Duvoisin, R.D., et al.: A Survey of Tardive Dyskinesia in Psychiatric Outpatients. Am. J. Psychiat. 134:1367-1370, 1977.
7. Barbizet, J.: Human Memory and its Pathology. Jardine, D.K. (Translator), San Francisco, W.H. Freeman & Co., 1970.
8. Bear, D.M., Fedio, P.: Quantitative Analysis of Interectal Behavior in Temporal Lobe Epilepsy. Arch. Neurol. 34:454-467, 1977.
9. Benson, D.F. Disorders of Verbal Expression, in Benson, D.F., Blumer, D., (Eds.) Psychiatric Aspects of Neurological Disease, New York, Grune & Stratton, 1975.
10. Benson, D.F., Barton, M.: Disturbance in Constructional Ability. Cortex 6:19-46, 1970.
11. Birkett, D.P.: Gerstmann's Syndrome. Brit. J. Psychiat. 113:801, 1967.
12. Bleuler, E.: Dementia Praecox. J. Ment. Pathol. 3:113-120, 1902-1903.
13. Bleuler, E.: Dementia Praecox on the Group of Schizophrenics, Zinkin, J. (Translator) New York, International Universities Press, 1950.
14. Bleuler, M.: Acute Mental Concomitants of Physical Diseases, in Benson, D.F., Blumer, D. (Eds.) Psychiatric Aspects of Neurological Disease, New York, Grune & Stratton, 1975, pp. 37-61.
15. Blumer, D. Temporal Lobe Epilepsy, in Benson, D.F., Blumer, D. (Eds.) Psychiatric Aspects of Neurological Disease, New York, Grune & Stratton, 1975, pp. 171-198.
16. Brown, J.W.: Aphasia, Apraxia and Agnosia: Clinical and Theoretical Aspects, Springfield, Charles C. Thomas, 1972.
17. Brown, J.: Mind, Brain and Consciousness: The Neuropsychology of Cognition. New York, Academic Press, 1977.
18. Carlson, G.A., Goodwin, F.K.: The Stages of Mania. Arch. Gen Psychiat. 28:221-228, 1973.
19. Carpenter, W.T., Jr., Strauss, J.S., Bartko, J.J.: An Approach to the Diagnosis and Understanding of Schizophrenia I. Use of Signs and Symptoms for the Identification of Schizophrenic Patients. Schizophrenia Bulletin, Issue 11, 37-49, 1974.
20. Crane, G.E.: Persistant Dyskinesia. Brit. J. Psychiat. 122:395-405, 1973.
21. Critchley, M.: The Parietal Lobes. New York, Hafner Press, 1953.
22. Critchley, M.: The Neurology of Psychotic Speech. Brit. J. Psychiat. 110:353-364, 1964.
23. Davidson, K., Bagley, C.R.: Schizophrenic-like Psychoses Associated with Organic Disorders, in Herrington, R.N. (Ed.) Current Problems in Neuropsychiatry: Schizophrenia, Epilepsy, the Temporal Lobe. Brit. J. Psychiatry Special Publication #4, Ashford, Kent, Headley Bros., Ltd. 1969, pp. 113-184.
24. DeAjuriagurerra, J., Hecaen, H., Angelerques, R.: Les Apraxies: Varretes Cliniques et Lateralisation Lesionnelle. Rev. Neurol. 102:566-1960.

25.	Denny-Brown, D.: The Nature of Apraxia. J. Nerv. Ment. Dis. 126: 9-32, 1958.

26.	Gerstmann, J.: Some Notes on the Gerstmann-Syndrome. Neurology 7:866-869, 1957.

27.	Geschwind, N.: The Apraxias: Neural Mechanisms of Disorders of Learned Movement. Am. Sci. 63:188-195, 1975.

28.	Geschwind, N.: Disconnection Syndromes in Animals and Man. Part II. Brain 88:585-644, 1965.

29.	Geschwind, N.: The Anatomical Basis of Hemisphere Differentiation, in Dimond, S. & Beaumont, J. (Eds.) Hemisphere Function in the Human Brain, New York, Halstead Press, 1977, p. 7-24.

30.	Geschwind, N., Kaplan, E.: A Human Cerebral Disconnection Syndrome. Neurology 12:675-685, 1962.

31.	Hamilton, M. (Ed.): Fish's Clinical Psychopathology, Signs and Symptoms in Psychiatry. Revised reprints, Bristol, John Wright & Sons, Ltd., 1974.

32.	Hamilton, M. (Ed.): Fish's Outline of Psychiatry, 3rd Edition, Bristol, John Wright & Sons, Ltd., 1978.

33.	Hamilton, M., White, J.M.: Factors Related to the Outcome of Depression Treated with ECT. J. Ment. Sci. 106:1031-1041, 1960.

34.	Hecaen, H., DeAjuriaguerra, J.: Meconnaissauces et Hallucinations Corporelles, Paris, Masson et cie, 1952.

35.	Hinsie, L.E., Campbell, R.J.: Psychiatric Dictionary, 3rd Edition, New Yor, Oxford University Press, 1960.

36.	Hinton, J., Withers, E.: The Usefulness of Clinical Tests of the Sensorium. Brit. J. Psychiat. 119:9-18, 1971.

37.	Kahlbaum, K.L.: Catatonia. Baltimore, The Johns Hopkins University Press, 1973.

38.	Kinsbourne, M., Warrington, E.: A Study of Finger Agnosia. Brain 85:47-66, 1962.

39.	Klonoff, H., Fibiger, C.H., Hutton, G.H.: Neuropsychological Patterns in Chronic Schizophrenia. J. Nerv. Ment. Dis. 150:291-300, 1970.

40.	Kraepelin, E.: Manic-Depressive Insanity and Paranoia. New York, Arno Press, 1976.

41.	Kraepelin, E.: Lectures on Clinical Psychiatry. Johnstone, T. (Ed.), London, Bailliere, Tindull and Cox, 1904.

42.	Lehmann, H.E.: Schizophrenia: Clinical Features, in Freedman, A.M., Kaplan, H.I., Sadock, B.J. (Eds.) Comprehensive Textbook of Psychiatry, 2nd Edition, Volume 1, pp. 892-3, 1967.

43.	Levin, N., Switzer, M.: Voice and Speech Disorders: Medical Aspects. Springfield, Charles C. Thomas, 1962.

44.	Levy, J.: The Origin of Lateral Asymmetry, in Harnad, S., Doty, R. & Goldstein, L. et al.(Eds.) Lateralization in the Nervous System, New York, Academic Press, 1977, pp. 195-209.

45.	Levy, J.: Psychobiological Implications of Bilateral Asymmetry, in Dimond, S.J., Beaumont, J.G. (Eds.) Hemisphere Function in the Human Brian, Halsted Press, New York, 1974, pp. 121-183.

46.	Levy, J., Reid, M.: Variations in Writing Posture and Cerebral Organization. Science 194:337-339, 1976.

47.	Luria, A.R.: The Working Brain, An Introduction to Neuropsychology, Haugh, B. (Translator), New York, Basic Books, 1973.

48.	Magoun, H.: The Waking Brain. Springfield, Charles C. Thomas, 1963.

49.	Matarazzo, J.D.: Wechsler's Measurement & Appraisal of Adult Intelligence. 5th Edition, New York, Oxford University Press, 1972.

50.	McHugh, P.R., Folstein, M.F.: Psychiatric Syndromes of Huntington's Chorea. A Clinical & Phenomenological Study, in Benson, D.F., Blumer, D. (Eds.) Psychiatric Aspects of Neurologic Disease, New York, Grune & Stratton, 1975.

51.	Meduna, L.J.: Oneirophrenia, Urbana, University of Illinois Press, 1950.

52.	Mellor, C.S.: First Rank Symptoms of Schizophrenia I. The Frequency in Schizophrenics on Admission to Hospital; II. Differences Between Individual First Rank Symptoms. Brit. J. Psychiat. 117:15-23, 1970.
53.	Morrison, J.R.: Catatonia: Retarded and Excited Types. Arch. Gen. Psychiat. 28:39-41, 1973.
54.	Nielsen, J.: Gerstmann's Syndrome: Finger Agnosia, Agraphia, Comparison of Right and Left and Acalculia. Arch. Neurol. Psychiat. 39:536-560, 1938.
55.	Pilleri, G.: The Kluver-Bucy Syndrome in Man. Psychiat. Neurol. 152:65-103, 1966.
56.	Reed, J.L.: The Proverbs Test in Schizophrenia. Brit. J. Psychiat. 114:317-321, 1968.
57.	Rochford, J., Detre, T., Tucker, G.J., et al. Neuropsychological Impairments in Functional Psychiatric Disease. Arch. Gen. Psychiat. 22:114-119, 1970.
58.	Roth, M.: The Phenomenology of Depressive States. Can. Psychiat. Assoc. J. 4:532-553, 1959.
59.	Rubens, A.B.: Anatomical Asymmetries of Human Cerebral Cortex, in Harnad, S., Doty, R. & Goldstein, L. et al. (Eds.) Lateralization in the Nervous System, New York, Academic Press, 1977, pp. 503-516.
60.	Schneider, K.: Clinical Psychopathology, Hamilton, M.W. (Translator) New York, Grune & Stratton, 1959.
61.	Seamon, J.G.: Coding and Retrieval Processes and the Hemispheres of the Brain, in Dimond, S. & Beaumont, J. (Eds.) Hemisphere Function in the Human Brain, New York, Halsted Press, 1977, p. 184-203.
62.	Sedman, G.: A Comparative Study of Pseudo-hallucinations, Imagery & True Hallucinations. Brit. J. Psychiat. 112:9-17, 1966.
63.	Sedman, G.: A Phenomenological Study of Pseudo-hallucinations and Related Experiences. Acta. Psychiat. Scand. 42:35-70, 1966.
64.	Segarra, J.M.: Cerebral Vascular Disease & Behavior. Arch. Neurol. 22:408-418, 1970.
65.	Slater, E., Roth, M.: Mayer-Gross Clinical Psychiatry, 3rd Edition. Baltimore, The Williams & Wilkins Co., 1969.
66.	Spear, F.G., Green, R.: Inability to Concentrate. Brit. J. Psychiat. 112:913-915, 1966.
67.	Strub, R.L., Black, F.W.: The Mental Status Examination in Neurology. Philadelphia, F.A. Davis Co.,
68.	Strub, R., Geschwind, N.: Gerstmann Syndrome Without Aphasia. Cortex 10:378-387, 1974.
69.	Stuss, D.T., Alexander, M.P., Lieberman, A., Levine, H.: An Extraordinary Form of Confabulation. Neurology 28:1166-1172, 1978.
70.	Taylor, M.A.: Schneiderian First Rank Symptoms & Clinical Prognostic Features in Schizophrenia. Arch. Gen. Psychiat. 26:64-67, 1972.
71.	Taylor, M.A., Abrams, R.: The Phenomenology of Mania: A New Look at Some Old Patients. Arch. Gen. Psychiat. 29:520-522, 1973.
72.	Taylor, M.A., Abrams, R.: Manic-Depressive Illness & Good Prognosis Schizophrenia. Am. J. Psychiat. 132:741-742, 1975.
73.	Taylor, M.A., Abrams, R., Gaztanaga, P.: Manic-Depressive Illness and Schizophrenia: A Partial Validation of Research Diagnostic Criteria Utilizing Neuropsychological Testing. Compr. Psychiat. 16:91-96, 1975.
74.	Taylor, M.A., Abrams, R.: The Prevalence & Importance of Catatonia in the Manic Phase of Manic-Depressive Illness. Arch. Gen. Psychiat. 34:1223-1225, 1977.
75.	Taylor, M.A., Greenspan, B., Abrams, R.: Lateralized Neuropsychological Dysfunction in Affective Disorders and Schizophrenia. Am. J. Psychiat. 136:1031-1034, 1979.
76.	Wada, J., Rasmussen, T.: Intra-Carotid Injection of Sodium Amytal for the Lateralization of Cerebral Speech Dominance. J. Neurosurg. 17:266-282, 1960.

77.   Watson, C.G., Thomas, R.W., Anderson, D., Filling, J.: Differentiation of Organics from Schizophrenics at Two Chronicity Levels by Use of the Reitan-Halstead Organic Test Battery. J. Consult. Clin. Psychol. 32:679-684, 1960.

78.   Wechsler, D.: A Standardized Memory Scale for Clinical Use. J. Psychol. 19:87-95, 1945.

79.   Withers, E., Hinton, J.: Three Forms of the Clinical Tests of the Sensorium and Their Reliability. Brit. J. Psychiat. 119:1-8, 1971.

Part II

INTRODUCTION

In Part I, we concentrated on the Mental Status Examination, that aspect of the diagnostic process which is perhaps the most difficult because its success depends upon your ability to observe and define the behaviors of patients.

Part II of the text takes you through the rest of the diagnostic process, with emphasis on the differential diagnosis, a process of refinement which is achieved by synthesizing the information you derive from your observation of the patient and from the patient's history. The ability to rule out and categorize a variety of subtle signs will lead you to the best possible diagnosis. In psychiatry, there are no pathognomonic signs; your ability to arrive at an intelligent diagnosis is therefore dependent upon a multiplicity of information. The more precise the information you gather, the more accurate your diagnosis.

Much of Part II requires a thorough understanding of Part I. You will be reminded, at strategic points in the text, to review areas in Part I about which you might feel uncertain. Part II makes increasingly greater demands on your diagnostic skills as your proficiency and confidence grow.

The DSM-III term "organic mental disorder" will not be used in this text as it implies the existence of "inorganic" or metaphysical brain syndromes, a notion which is contrary to basic biology and the generally accepted idea that the brain is the organ of behavior and that all behavior—pathological, deviant and normal—reflects brain function. As a substitute for the DSM-III term, I will use "coarse brain disease" to label clinical conditions which have demonstrable etiology or pathophysiology. These brain disorders are "coarse" in that their pathology is measurable with present technology. They contrast with other mental disorders in which the pathology is not yet measurable and in which the etiology or pathophysiology is unknown.

273

DIAGNOSIS

1.   In phenomenology, the fundamentals in the diagnostic process are
objective _____, precise _____, and the separation of
_____ from _____.

2.   The key to clinical diagnosis is the process of changing probabilities. Each bit of historical and mental status information continually
and gradually alters the probability of the patient having particular
conditions. Each datum decreases the likelihood of some disorders and
increases the likelihood of others. At the end of the process, the most
likely diagnosis is selected. Since there are no pathognomonic signs
in psychiatry, nor conclusive laboratory tests for mental illness, the
process of data collection: objective observation, precise terminology,
content separated from form, becomes extremely important. You have
learned about this process in Part I; to know it and use it you must
practice it. Part II will provide much of the data needed to determine
the probabilities of several major diagnostic conditions.

3.   Objective observation cannot be overemphasized. Even the small-
est mannerism, physical characteristic, word usage or other behavior
can be an essential diagnostic clue. For example: A patient was referred to a psychiatrist because of his deteriorating productivity at work
and because he spent increasing amounts of time in bed, complaining
of loss of interest. During the initial phases of the examination, the
man demonstrated no abnormalities. However, when he described his
work (as a clerk-typist), he said, "Well, I had some trouble...you
know..." and then made typing movements. Further testing of language functioning revealed other deficits in word finding, naming of
objects, reading and taking dictation. The patient had a localized
treatable lesion involving the _____ _____
_____. The lesion might have gone undetected if the examiner
had not noticed the small clue of the patient's typing movements. Pay
attention to details---they can help you in your diagnostic choices and
decrease the morbidity and mortality of your patients.

274

1.   observation, terminology, form, content

2.   No answer required

3.   dominant cerebral hemisphere or dominant temporo-parietal region

4.   Psychiatric diagnostic systems generally separate five major groups of disorders: the so-called functional psychoses: major affective disorder and schizophrenia, the organic brain syndromes (coarse brain disease), the neuroses, the personality and behavior disorders, and the psychophysiological disorders. The latest classification system of the American Psychiatric Association (DSM-III) (13), has reorganized this traditional nosology, scattering the neuroses among the other categories, adding new categories and renaming psychophysiological disorders: "Psychological factors affecting physical illness." As nosologies change with the rapidity and logic of hemline height, I will confine Part II to a description and characterization of traditional disorders, making reference only to their DSM-III counter term. In the first half of the text, I discussed the more dramatic mental conditions indirectly, and we will begin with them again here. Keep in mind, however, that most people seeking counsel or treatment for mental symptoms do not have major mental disease.

Major Affective Disorder

5.   Many investigations have demonstrated that people suffering from depressive and/or manic episodes can be separated phenomenologically into several disease groups. We will limit our focus to two broad groups: bipolar (two poles) and unipolar (one pole) affective disease (92,178).

6.   Bipolar and _____ affective diseases are characterized by a primary disturbance in mood. They are both periodic in course, and episodes usually end in remission. Most patients return to their premorbid level of function (88,177).

7.   When a person suffers from recurrent depressions, i.e., only one mood pole, he is said to have unipolar affective disease. When a person suffers from recurrent depressive and manic episodes, i.e., both mood poles, he is said to have _____ _____

_____.

8.   Some patients have only recurrent manic episodes. Even though they suffer from only one mood pole disorder, i.e., mania, they are nevertheless said to have _____ affective disease.

9.   Recent research (8,9) suggests that individuals with recurrent manic episodes and no depressions have a variant of bipolar disorder. Individuals who have only depressive episodes are said to have

_____ _____.

10.   The major affective disorders can be separated into _____ and _____ disorders. These are common conditions and women are affected more frequently than men by almost two to one (54,78,141,177).

11.   Bipolar patients suffer from both _____ and _____ episodes. Unipolar patients suffer from only recurrent _____ episodes.

4.   No answer required

5.   No answer required

6.   unipolar

7.   bipolar affective disease

8.   bipolar

9.   unipolar disorder.

10. bipolar and unipolar

11. manic, depressive, depressive

12. The major affective diseases, i.e., _____ and _____ diseases, are more common among _____ than among _____ .

13. The sex ratio difference for major affective disorder for females to males is _____ .

14. When all reported figures are averaged, approximately 2 percent of the general population is at risk (chances of getting disorder) for major affective disorder (unipolar and bipolar combined) (141 pp. 76-78, 151). Thus, during their lifetime, two out of every _____ people you know should theoretically develop affective disorder. It is very common.

15. Several studies suggest that among individuals with affective disorder 85 percent have the unipolar form and 15 percent have the bipolar form (10,178). In both instances, the sex most frequently affected is_____ .

16. Of 100 patients with affective disorder, how many should have the bipolar form and how many should have the unipolar form?

17. Of 85 unipolar and 15 bipolar patients, approximately how many of each group will be male and how many female?

18. Rank the following four patient categories by placing a number from 1 to 4 next to each, indicating its relative frequency of occurrence, e.g., 1 = the most common; 4 = the least common.

    Bipolar Males _____   Unipolar Males_____
    Bipolar Females _____   Unipolar Females _____

19. In Part I, item #122, you commented upon the observations of a patient who suffered from a severe depression. She has returned again and is first seen sitting quietly outside your office. Even though you say hello and ask her to come in, she remains seated, staring ahead until you repeat your introduction upon which she slowly gets up and moves to a chair next to your desk. There are deep furrows between her eyebrows. Her eyes have a sunken appearance, and the inner angle of the upper lid appears to rise. Throughout the interview, the patient remains seated, head bowed. Her only movements are the constant rubbing together of her hands. She speaks in a monotonous, slow, plodding fashion, is often close to tears and, despite an attempt at humor on your part, cannot even manage a smile. She says she feels like crying, but cannot. She says she feels she is a bad person, and that somehow her present condition is deserved and that people would be better off if she were dead. You find yourself feeling sad for her, and concerned about her pained expression. Later, in writing your report, you state that she exhibited _____ motor behavior. Because of her hand rubbing, you feel she showed mild motor _____ . Her facial expression, marked by an _____ sign, and _____ folds, was sad. In describing her affect, you state that her affective range was _____ , she showed _____ _____ lability and the intensity of her mood was one of constant _____ , but _____ to what was being discussed. Because of your emotional response to her, you felt her affect was _____ .

12. bipolar, unipolar, women, men

13. 2 to 1

14. 100

15. female

16. 85 unipolar, 15 bipolar

17. Using the 2:1 ratio, of 85 unipolar, 57 will be women and 28 males. Of the 15 bipolars, 10 will be female and 5 male.

18. Bipolar Males 4   Unipolar Males 2
    Bipolar Females 3   Unipolar Females 1

19. hypoactive, agitation, Omega, Veraguth, constricted, no increased, sadness, appropriate, related

    If you had difficulty with this question, you should review Part I again. You must be able to identify psychopathology before you can master the diagnostic process.

20. The characteristic aspects of major depression are a constricted range of _____ with a _____ mood. Anxiety is another mood associated with depression.

21. Since depressed people often are intensely sad and/or anxious, it is not surprising that their intense mood is sometimes expressed in increased frequency of motor behavior termed _____.

22. A marked decrease in activities and a slowing of movements or _____ is also characteristic of depressed individuals.

23. Circle the behaviors characteristic of a major depression:

Omega sign	Singing	Constricted affect
Anxiety	Hyperactivity	Agitation
Hypoactivity	Veraguth's folds	Flight-of-ideas

24. A severely depressed patient can sometimes stay motionless for hours, staring fixedly or following the examiner about the room with his eyes, unresponsive even to severe pain stimulation (general analgesia). This extreme hypoactivity is termed _____.

25. Thought content is helpful in reaching a diagnosis when the content reflects an intense mood. Once you have established the _____ of a patient's speech or how he is speaking, you should determine whether the thought _____ is helpful in the diagnostic process.

26. Feelings of hopelessness, worthlessness, helplessness, guilt and thoughts of suicide are often expressed in thought content. They reflect the presence of a sad mood. During the mental status examination, you must determine whether these feelings are present. Below write several of the questions you might ask to determine these feelings:

27. Depressed people are often suicidal and indeed have a mortality rate much greater than the general population (72,160,162). Below write several questions you might ask to determine a patient's suicidal feelings:

28. The characteristic motor presentation of depression is either _____ or _____. When decreased motor activity is severe, a _____ can develop.

29. The slowed speech, slowed responses to environmental stimuli and decreased motor behavior observed in many depressed patients is called psychomotor retardation. Although seemingly paradoxical, psychomotor retardation, hypoactivity, and agitation can be observed in the same patient.

20. affect, sad

21. agitation

22. hypoactivity

23. (Omega sign)   Singing   (Constricted affect)
   (Anxiety)   Hyperactivity   (Agitation)
   (Hypoactivity) (Veraguth's folds)   Flight-of-ideas

24. stupor

25. form, content

26. "How does the future look?"---"Do you think your difficulties will improve?"

    "Do you think your family needs you?" --- "Are you a worthwhile person?"

    "Do you think you can do anything about all this?"

    "Have you let people down?" --- "Are you a bad person?"

27. "Well, with all this going on, you must feel pretty badly. Do you ever get the feeling you'd like to go to sleep and not wake up?"

    "Do you ever get the feeling you'd be better off dead?"

    "Did you ever wish you could just end it all?"

    "Did you ever think of harming yourself?...Of killing yourself?... Have you tried?...Do you feel that way now?"

28. agitation, hypoactivity, stupor

29. No answer required

30.   The slowing down of speech, motor behavior, and general unresponsiveness of depressed patients, known as _____ _____, can become so severe that patients become mute, bedridden and immobile, unresponsive even to painful stimuli, but at times able to follow people with their eyes. This uncommon condition is called a depressive _____.

31.   Circle the words or phrases characteristic of depression:

Sad or anxious mood	Euphoria	Hyperactivity
Stupor	Omega sign	Grandiose delusional ideas
Constricted range of Affect	Feelings of hopelessness, worthlessness, guilt	
Suicide	Flight-of-ideas	

32.   The mood disturbance of some depressed patients can become so severe that feelings of hopelessness, worthlessness and guilt become the thought content of delusional ideas. Since these delusional ideas develop from a mood disorder, they are said to be _____. In contrast, autochthonous delusional ideas which do not develop from other psychopathology are said to be _____.

33.   Depressed patients not infrequently believe that they are terrible people, responsible for public tragedies or the deaths of others or that they have committed unpardonable sins, are doomed, are going to die or be killed or that they are already dead. Some believe they have a horrible disease such as a brain tumor or multiple cancers. Others think that some of their body parts are rotting away or that they have garbage in their intestines. These ideas develop from a profound mood disorder and are therefore called _____ _____ _____.

34.   Some depressed patients have perceptual disturbances. The content of the misinterpreted real stimuli, which is known as _____, reflects their depression. Noises and shadows become frightening figures or demons ready to punish them for their sins.

35.   Many depressed patients hallucinate. They hear "incomplete" voices calling them names or stating their sins. They smell their "evil" or taste their decay. Hallucinations and delusions are not uncommon among individuals with a major depression (8,9,88,177) and the presence of these signs should not discourage you from a diagnosis of depression in the presence of a sufficient number of other symptoms. As many of these delusions in depressive illness develop from the profound mood of sadness, they are said to be _____.

36.   Unlike the mental status examination, which only focuses upon _____ behavior, the diagnostic process must also consider historical information or _____ behavior.

37.   Patients with a major depression are most often seen within a few weeks to a few months of the onset of the episode. Because of the morbidity risks by sex in the general population, the majority of depressed patients will be _____.

30. psychomotor retardation, stupor

31. (Sad or anxious mood)   Euphoria   Hyperactivity
    (Stupor)   (Omega sign)   Grandiose delusional
                                                    ideas
    (Constricted range of affect)(Feelings of hope-
                                  lessness, worth-
                                  lessness, guilt)
    (Suicide)   Flight-of-ideas

32. secondary, primary

33. secondary delusional ideas

34. illusions

35. secondary

36. present, past

37. women

38.   Although all age groups, including children, can become depressed, it is rare for an individual to have a first depressive episode before age 15, or after age 60. Peak onset years are between 40 and 60
(141 pp. 72-74, p. 88, 177). The probabilities are strong that the
majority of depressed patients you will encounter will be middle-aged
and female. What is the likelihood of these depressions being associated with manic episodes? Explain your answer.

39.   Circle the items which increase the probability that your patient
is suffering from a major depression:

Omega sign	Psychomotor retardation
Euphoria	Age 48
Male	Female
Feelings of hopelessness	Recent suicide attempt
Hyperactivity	Flight-of-ideas

40.   Depressed patients will almost always have a sleep disturbance.
Early morning (2 or 3 a.m.) waking and inability to fall asleep again
is most typical, but any significant insomnia is consistent with the diagnosis of major depression.   Another characteristic feature of major
depression is a peak onset of between _____ years of age.

41.   Loss of sleep is typical of depression. Characteristically, patients
have _____ _____ insomia. Patients generally feel worse during
the early morning and somewhat better in the late afternoon or early
evening. This 24-hour mood cycle (worse in the morning; better in
the evening) is termed a "diurnal" mood swing.

42.   Loss of appetite, or anorexia, with weight loss (greater than
5 pounds) is also extremely common in major depression as is a
general loss of interest in daily activities. Although some characteristic
depressive behaviors are historical data and thus not part of the
mental status examination, their evaluation is essential for any
diagnostic determination.

43.   Place a D next to the items characteristic of depression:

Weepy and anxious	Teenager
Life is not worth living	Can't sleep
"I could conquer the world"	Doesn't feel like eating
50-year-old woman	Euphoric
Delusion of guilt	Suicide attempt

44.   Depressed patients often have multiple physical complaints: head--
aches, backaches, generalized weakness, heaviness in arms and legs,
constipation, and tiredness are commonly reported. These symptoms
are common in many systemic illnesses and in some coarse brain disorders. A psychiatric examination and evaluation are not complete without a complete physical examination and appropriate laboratory evaluation to insure the absence of other diseases with behavioral symptoms.

38. small - only 15% of affective disorders are bipolar

39. (Omega sign)   (Psychomotor retardation)
    Euphoria   (Age 48)
    Male   (Female)
    (Feelings of hopelessness)(Recent suicide attempt)
    Hyperactivity   Flight-of-ideas

40. 40 and 60

41. early morning

42. No answer required

43. Weepy and anxious D   Teenager
    Life is not worth living D   Can't sleep D
    "I could conquer the world"   Doesn't feel like eating D
    50-year-old woman D   Euphoric
    Delusion of guilt D   Suicide attempt   D

44. No answer required

45.   The key to clinical diagnosis is the process of changing probabilities. When all of the following clinical criteria are satisfied, the probability is enormous (26,74,85,126,132,136,137) that the patient is suffering from a major depression.

1. Sad or anxious mood

2. Three of the following (a through f)

   a. early a.m. waking (insomnia)
   b. diurnal mood swing (worse in the a.m.)
   c. anorexia with greater than 5 pound weight loss in 3 weeks
   d. psychomotor retardation or agitation
   e. suicidal thoughts or behavior
   f. feelings of guilt, self-reproach, hopelessness, worthlessness

3. No coarse brain disease or use of steroids or reserpine in the past month, no systemic illness known to cause depressive symptoms.

   The probabilities are also great that most individuals with the above condition will be _____ and _____ age. Approximately what percent of the general population is at risk for affective disorder? _____

46.   In the following case vignette, circle the words or phrases which relate to the diagnostic criteria for depression. Are sufficient criteria for depression satisfied? If not, which one(s) is/are missing?

   A 47-year-old woman is hospitalized because of increasing apprehension, fears of impending death, and thoughts that devils are bothering her. She sees no hope for her condition and feels she is a worthless person. For the 10 days prior to admission, she did not sleep and spent her days pacing. There was no weight loss, no change in her mood throughout the day, and no evidence of systemic illness.

47.   In the following case vignette, circle the words or phrases which relate to the diagnostic criteria for depression. Are sufficient criteria for depression satisfied? If not, which one(s) is/are missing?

   A 26-year-old woman was hospitalized because of sadness, trouble falling asleep, loss of appetite with a 7 pound weight loss and ideas that she "was a prostitute" and "sinful." She felt people had "bad thoughts" about her, that she was worthless, that there was no hope. Her sadness was worse during the early part of the day. On the day of admission, she attempted suicide.

48.   In the following case vignette, circle the words or phrases which relate to the diagnostic criteria for depression. Are sufficient criteria for depression satisfied? If not, which one(s) is/are missing?

   A 46-year-old woman is referred to you because she took an overdose of analgesics. She appears agitated, worried and anxious. An Omega sign is present. She is emaciated, and admits losing 60 pounds in the last 6 months. She expresses worry about a "lump" in her left axilla and says she has cancer. When you ask her about her suicide attempt, she says, "I didn't think there was any alternative." All physical examination findings and laboratory findings are within normal limits and her history is negative for drug abuse and for evidence of systemic illness, including cancer.

45. female, middle, 2%

46. A 47-year-old woman is hospitalized because of increasing (apprehension,) fears of impending death, and thoughts that devils are bothering her. She (sees no hope) for her condition and (feels she is a worthless person.) For the 10 days prior to admission, (she did not sleep) and spent her days (pacing.) There was (no weight loss,) (no change) in her mood throughout the day,) and (no evidence of suicidal thoughts.) Physical examination and laboratory findings are within normal limits and her history is negative for drug abuse and for evidence of systemic illness.

Yes, enough criteria are met to satisfy the diagnosis of depression.

47. A 26-year-old woman was hospitalized because of (sadness,) (trouble) (falling asleep,) loss of appetite with a 7 pound weight loss) and (ideas) (that she "was a prostitute" and "sinful.") She felt people had "bad thoughts" about her, that she was (worthless,) that there was (no) (hope.) Her (sadness was worse during the early part of the day.) On the day of admission, (she attempted suicide.)

No, there is no statement regarding physical examination, laboratory findings and medical or drug abuse history.

48. A 46-year-old woman is referred to you because she took an (overdose) (of analgesics.) She appears (agitated,) (worried and anxious.) An Omega sign is present. She is emaciated, and admits to (losing 60 pounds) (in the last 6 months.) She expresses worry about a "lump" in her left axilla and says she has cancer. When you ask her about her suicide attempt, she says, ("I didn't think there was any alternative.") All physical examination findings and laboratory findings are within normal limits and her history is negative for drug abuse and for evidence of systemic illness, including cancer.

Yes

49.   In the following case vignette, circle the words or phrases which relate to the diagnostic criteria for depression. Are sufficient criteria for depression satisfied? If not, which one(s) is/are missing?

A 33-year-old woman sought consultation because of insomnia (particularly in the early a.m.) which had persisted for two months. Her appetite had been poor, but no weight loss was evident. She described feeling "moody," particularly in the morning, feeling like crying, losing sexual desire, and feeling that the future "looks frightening." Physical examination and laboratory findings were within normal limits, and her history was negative for drug abuse and for evidence of systemic illness.

50.   Affective disorders can be separated into _____ and _____ groups. Individuals in both groups suffer from major depression, however, the _____ patients also experience episodes of mania.

51.   The depression of bipolar patients is clinically similar to that of unipolar patients (6,7). Only the presence or absence of past _____ episodes will determine the polarity of an individual patient's disorder. Of those individuals whose first episode is a depression, approximately 5 percent will become bipolar (44,98,176).

52.   As is true for depression, the hallmark of mania is an altered mood. In mania, euphoria and irritability are most commonly observed. Lability of affect is also frequently observed leading to rapid shifts from excessive jocularity to anger and occasionally to sudden bursts of tears and expressions of profound sadness. In depression, the common moods are _____ and _____ .

53.   When all the following clinical criteria are satisfied, the probability is enormous that the patient is experiencing a manic episode (8,9,24, 153,157,177,178) and thus has _____ affective disease.

1. Hyperactivity

2. Rapid/pressured speech

3. Euphoric or irritable mood

4. No emotional blunting

5. No coarse brain disease, no psychostimulant drug abuse in the prior month, no systemic illness known to cause manic symptoms

54.   In the following case vignette, circle the words or phrases which relate to the diagnostic criteria for mania. Are the criteria for mania satisfied? If not, which one(s) is/are missing?

A 22-year-old college student was found in his dormitory, mute and unresponsive. Later that night at the infirmary, he became agitated, hyperactive, assaultive and verbally overproductive. When hospitalized, he also exhibited a euphoric, as well as irritable, mood. His rate and pressure of speech was increased and he had flight-of-ideas. He had delusional ideas of grandiosity and admitted to hearing a whispered voice.

49. A 33-year-old woman sought consultation because of insomnia (particularly in the early a.m.) which had persisted for two months. Her appetite had been poor, but no weight loss was evident. She described feeling "moody," particularly in the morning, feeling like crying, losing sexual desire, and feeling that the future "looks frightening." Physical examination and laboratory findings were within normal limits, and her history was negative for drug abuse and for evidence of systemic illness.

Yes

50. bipolar, unipolar, bipolar

51. manic

52. sadness, anxiety

53. bipolar

54. A 22-year-old college student was found in his dormitory mute and unresponsive. Later that night at the infirmary, he became agitated, hyperactive, assaultive and verbally overproductive. When hospitalized, he also exhibited a euphoric, as well as irritable, mood. His rate and pressure of speech was increased and he had flight-of-ideas. He had delusional ideas of grandiosity and admitted to hearing a whispered voice.

No. There is no discussion of the presence or absence of coarse brain disease, psychostimulant drug abuse or possible systemic conditions. This patient does satisfy all the other criteria, but without a physical examination and careful history, even the best mental status examination is incomplete.

55. In the following case vignette, circle the words or phrases which relate to the diagnostic criteria for mania. Are the criteria for mania satisifed? If not, which one(s) is/are missing?

A 33-year-old woman is hospitalized because she has been hearing voices and believes she is "the center of the world." She is agitated, hyperactive and demonstrates several mannerisms, stereotypes and a moderate degree of posturing. Her mood is euphoric, her affect full, her speech rapid and pressured. She has a thought disorder. Physical examination and laboratory findings are within normal limits and her history is negative for drug abuse and for evidence of systemic illness.

56. In the following case vignette, circle the words or phrases which relate to the diagnostic criteria for mania. Are the criteria for mania satisfied? If not, which one(s) is/are missing?

A 48-year-old woman was transferred from another hospital because of depressed mood, an attempted suicide, early morning insomnia, crying spells and anorexia. She did not respond to electroconvulsive treatment. On admission, she was hyperactive and agitated. She became hostile, her speech was rapid and pressured. Her physical examination revealed hirsutism, masculinized body build, decreased muscle strength and tone and mild hypertension.

57. In the following case vignette, circle the words or phrases which relate to the diagnostic criteria for mania. Are the criteria for mania satisfied? If not, which one(s) is/are missing?

A 53-year-old woman was hospitalized because of agitation, constant "giddy laughter" and the thought that there was a plot to kill her family. She had put bandanas around the chairs at home and put objects in the windows as "symbols" to passers by. While she was being admitted, she sang, danced and joked. Her speech was rapid and pressured and she spent the first few days of hospitalization going from one activity to the next. Physical examination and laboratory findings were within normal limits and her history was negative for drug abuse and for evidence of systemic illness.

58. Draw lines to match the diagnostic criteria with the disorder:

	Hyperactivity
	Early morning waking
	Psychomotor retardation
Mania	Euphoria or irritable mood
	Sad or anxious mood
Depression	Feelings of guilt
	Suicidal thoughts

55. A 33-year-old woman is hospitalized because she has been hearing voices and believes she is "the center of the world." She is agitated, hyperactive and demonstrates several mannerisms, stereotypes and a moderate degree of posturing. Her mood is euphoric, her affect full, her speech rapid and pressured. She has a thought disorder. Physical examination and laboratory findings are within normal limits and her history is negative for drug abuse and for evidence of systemic illness.

Yes. The thought disorder was "flight-of-ideas." The rest is complete.

56. A 48-year-old woman was transferred from another hospital because of depressed mood, an attempted suicide, early morning insomnia, crying spells and anorexia. She did not respond to electroconvulsive treatment. On admission, she was hyperactive and agitated. She became hostile, her speech was rapid and pressured. Her physical examination revealed hirsutism, masculinized body build, decreased muscle strength and tone and mild hypertension.

No. Although all the inclusion criteria are met, the exclusion criteria are not complete. She has evidence of possible systemic illness and, upon further evaluation, adrenal hyperplasia was demonstrated.

57. A 53-year-old woman was hospitalized because of agitation, constant "giddy laughter" and the thought that there was a plot to kill her family. She had put bandanas around the chairs at home and put objects in the windows as "symbols" to passers by. While she was being admitted, she sang, danced and joked. Her speech was rapid and pressured and she spent the first few days of hospitalization going from one activity to the next. Physical examination and laboratory findings were within normal limits and her history was negative for drug abuse and for evidence of systemic illness.

Yes. Singing and dancing, decorating self and objects, delusions of persecution are all consistent with the diagnosis of mania.

58.

Mania — Hyperactivity
Early morning waking
Psychomotor retardation
Euphoria or irritable mood
Sad or anxious mood
Depression — Feelings of guilt
Suicidal thoughts

59. Place an M̲ next to the manic items and a D̲ next to the depressive items:

Rapid/pressured speech____   Psychomotor retardation____

Euphoria____   Sad mood____

Suicidal thoughts____   Hyperactivity____

Irritable mood____   Early a.m. waking____

Feelings of hopelessness____

60. A patient who talks to several people, one after the other, who goes from one place to another in quick succession, is said to be _____. This is a classical sign of _____.

61. In Part I, you learned that catatonia is a syndrome which, in 25 to 50 percent of cases, is a manifestation of major affective disease. In addition to specific motor behaviors we have considered, catatonia is characterized by periods of extreme hyperactivity and hypoactivity, also termed _____ and _____.

62. Mutism, stupor or excitement, although characteristic of _____, are not pathognomonic (diagnostic) signs. Other specific motor behaviors should be present before the diagnosis of _____ is made. List those motor behaviors.

63. Draw lines between matching items in the two columns:

Posturing   Severe hyperactivity

Excitement   Psychological pillow

Waxy flexibility   Slow resistance as patient allows examiner to place him in odd posture

Stupor   Increased motor frequency due to intense affect

Agitation   Severe hypoactivity often associated with generalized analgesia

64. Draw lines between matching items in the two columns:

Catalepsy   The furrowed brow of depression

Omega sign   The patient resists being moved with strength equal to that applied

Gegenhalten   Spending hours in one position

Veraguth folds   The sad eyes of depression

Grimacing   A facial posture

65. Draw a line between the matching items in the two columns:

Severe hypoactivity   Excitement

Tardive dyskinesia   Stupor

Severe hyperactivity   Drug induced brain damage

59. Rapid pressured speech M   Psychomotor retardation D
    Euphoria M   Sad mood D
    Suicidal thoughts D   Hyperactivity M
    Irritable mood M   Early a.m. waking D
    Feelings of hopelessness D

60. hyperactive, mania

61. excitement, stupor

62. catatonia, catatonia
    Catatonic motor behaviors: echopraxia, stereotype, automatic obed-
    ience (Mitgehen, Mitmachen), catalepsy,
    posturing, waxy flexibility

63. Posturing   Severe hyperactivity
    Excitement   Psychological pillow
    Waxy flexibility ———————— Slow resistance as patient allows examiner
                                    to place him in odd posture
    Stupor   Increased motor frequency due to intense
                                    affect
    Agitation   Severe hypoactivity often associated with
                                    generalized analgesia

64. Catalepsy   The furrowed brow of depression
    Omega sign   The patient resists being moved with
                                    strength equal to that applied
    Gegenhalten   Spending hours in one position
    Veraguth folds ———————— The sad eyes of depression
    Grimacing ———————————— A facial posture

65. Severe hypoactivity   Excitement
    Tardive dyskinesia   Stupor
    Severe hyperactivity   Drug induced brain damage

66. Draw lines between matching items in the two columns:

Stereotype	The patient repeats your movements
Echopraxia	Non-goal directed automatic, repetitive movement
Mitgehen	The patient repeats your words
Echolalia	Despite your verbal instructions to the contrary, the patient allows you to move his arm with light pressure

67. Draw lines between matching items in the two columns:

Mitmachen	Despite your verbal instruction to the contrary, the patient lets you posture his arm and when released, slowly moves it back to its original place
Stupor	Maintaining posture for long periods
Catalepsy	Severe hypoactivity

68. Draw lines between matching items in the two columns:

Veraguth's folds	Furrow between the eyebrows
Omega sign	Upward angle of inner canthus of eyes in depression
Waxy flexibility	Assuming odd body positions
Posturing	Slow resistance but allowing placement in odd body postures

69. Draw lines between matching items in the two columns:

Excitement	Increased non-goal directed motor activity---an expression of intense affect
Agitation	Extreme hyperactivity
Mitgehen	The patient repeats your words
Echolalia	Automatic obedience

70. In Part I, you learned that circumstantial speech, clang associations and flight-of-ideas are frequently observed in manic patients. Stereotype of speech, the automatic repetition of words or sounds at the end of a phrase termed _____, is observed in catatonia and thus also in mania.

71. Verbigeration is characterized by _____.
It is a form of verbal stereotypy and is often seen as part of the _____ syndrome. Circumstantial speech is often observed among patients with mania. Associations by the sound rather than the meaning of words, termed _____ associations are also observed in mania.

66.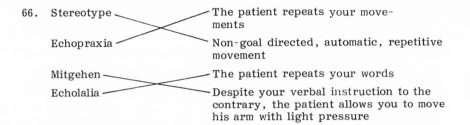

Stereotype — The patient repeats your movements

Echopraxia — Non-goal directed, automatic, repetitive movement

Mitgehen — The patient repeats your words

Echolalia — Despite your verbal instruction to the contrary, the patient allows you to move his arm with light pressure

67.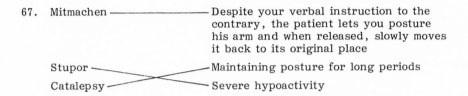

Mitmachen ——————— Despite your verbal instruction to the contrary, the patient lets you posture his arm and when released, slowly moves it back to its original place

Stupor — Maintaining posture for long periods

Catalepsy — Severe hypoactivity

68.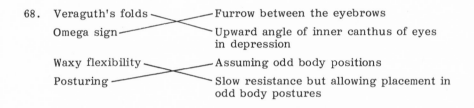

Veraguth's folds — Furrow between the eyebrows

Omega sign — Upward angle of inner canthus of eyes in depression

Waxy flexibility — Assuming odd body positions

Posturing — Slow resistance but allowing placement in odd body postures

69.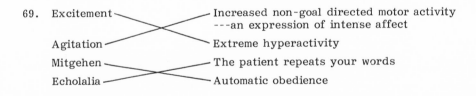

Excitement — Increased non-goal directed motor activity ---an expression of intense affect

Agitation — Extreme hyperactivity

Mitgehen — The patient repeats your words

Echolalia — Automatic obedience

70. verbigeration

71. stereotyped repetitions of phrases, words or sounds usually at the end of a sentence (neurological term is palilalia); catatonic, clang

295

72.   As many patients with mania exhibit signs and symptoms of catatonia, stereotypy of speech, termed_____, can also be observed among manic patients.

73.   Manics are often impulsive, intrusive and importunate. They have
boundless energy, need little sleep, but have little perseverance.
They will go on buying sprees or begin fanciful projects, but will fail
to complete the required work because they quickly lose interest and
begin a new task.   They continually interrupt interactions between
others, constantly making demands or repeating the same statements
which they insist you hear again. Their mood is often _____
or _____.

74.   Circle the behaviors typical of mania

Flight-of-ideas   Psychomotor retardation

Memory loss   Elation

Labile affect   Hypoactivity

Hyperactivity   Irritability

Impulsiveness   Shyness

Overtalkativeness

75.   Draw lines from the condition to the clinical items which reflect
diagnostic criteria. Not all clinical items need be used.

Feelings of guilt and self-reproach

Verbigeration

Rapid/pressured speech

Diurnal mood swing (worse in a.m.)

Emotional blunting

Mania   Psychomotor retardation

Euphoria

Sadness

Anorexia with more than 5 pound
weight loss

Depression   Early a.m. wakening

Irritability

Head decoration

Hyperactivity

Suicidal

Complete auditory hallucinations

72. verbigeration (or palilalia)

73. euphoric, irritable

74. (Flight-of-ideas)   Psychomotor retardation
     Memory loss   (Elation)
     (Labile affect)   Hypoactivity
     (Hyperactivity)   (Irritability)
     (Impulsiveness)   Shyness
     (Overtalkativeness)

75.

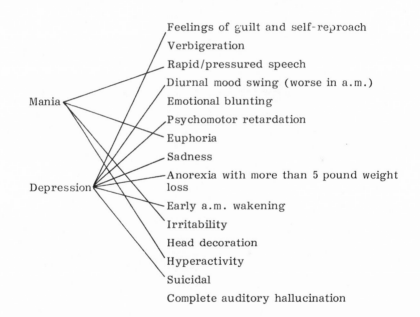

Mania

Depression

Feelings of guilt and self-reproach

Verbigeration

Rapid/pressured speech

Diurnal mood swing (worse in a.m.)

Emotional blunting

Psychomotor retardation

Euphoria

Sadness

Anorexia with more than 5 pound weight loss

Early a.m. wakening

Irritability

Head decoration

Hyperactivity

Suicidal

Complete auditory hallucination

76.   Read the following case vignette. Underline the words or phrases which relate to specific diagnostic criteria for mania and/or depression. Check those which are positive. Write your diagnosis below.

A 69-year-old woman was hospitalized stating "I am a bad woman ...the police are after me...they want to see me dead...I'm just rotten, that's all." She had a history of insomnia, crying episodes and complaining of feeling "terrible" in the morning but better as the day progressed. Her appetite had been good and her weight stable. At times, she felt she would be better off not awakening in the morning. Physical examination and laboratory findings were within normal limits and her history was negative for drug abuse and/or evidence of systemic illness.

77.   Read the following case vignette. Underline the words or phrases which relate to specific diagnostic cieteria for mania and/or depression and check those which are positive. Write your diagnosis below.

A 39-year-old man was hospitalized because of assaultiveness, irritability and severe agitation, and for saying: "I am a messenger of God...I have the secret for the cure of cancer because God told me." On admission, he was in a state of excitement. He was hyperactive and euphoric. His affective intensity was increased, his affect labile, shifting from irritability to euphoria to sadness with tears. His speech was rapid and pressured, he had flight-of-ideas. Physical examination and laboratory findings were within normal limits and his history was negative for drug abuse and for evidence of systemic illness.

78.   Read the following case vignette. Underline the words or phrases which relate to specific diagnostic criteria for mania and/or depression and check those which are positive. Write your diagnosis below.

A 49-year-old man was found by the police carrying a bow and arrow and pretending to be "Robin Hood." When seen in an emergency room, he was hyperactive and agitated, irritable and threatening. His speech was loud, rapid and pressured. He felt he was a "natural born leader," and for this reason law enforcement agencies were after him. Physical examination and laboratory findings were within normal limits and his history was negative for drug abuse and for evidence of systemic illness.

79.   Read the following case vignette. Underline the words or phrases which relate to specific diagnostic criteria for mania and/or depression and check those which are positive. Write your diagnosis below.

A 50-year-old woman sought consultation because she found herself unable to make herself "do things." She described recent "nervous and funny" feelings. She wanted to stay in bed all day, had trouble falling asleep and awakened early. She felt better in the morning and worse as the day progressed. During the past month she lost 20 pounds. She had suicidal thoughts. Physical examination and laboratory findings were within normal limits and her history was negative for drug abuse and for evidence of systemic illness.

76. A 69-year-old woman was hospitalized stating "I am a bad woman...
the police are after me...they want to see me dead...I'm just rotten
that's all." She had a history of insomnia, crying episodes and complaining of feeling "terrible" in the morning but better as the day
progressed. Her appetite had been good and her weight stable. At
times, she felt she would be better off not awakening in the morning.
Physical examination and laboratory findings were within normal limits and her history was negative for drug abuse and/or evidence of
systemic illness.

Depression
She demonstrates sadness (crying spells) plus insomnia, a diurnal
mood swing and suicidal tendencies (better off not awakening). She
satisfies the exclusion criterion.

77. A 39-year-old man was hospitalized because of assaultiveness and
irritability, severe agitation and for saying: "I am a messenger of
God...I have the secret for the cure of cancer because God told me."
On admission, he was in a state of excitement. He was hyperactive
and euphoric. His affective intensity was increased, his affect labile, shifting from irritability to euphoria to sadness with tears. His
speech was rapid and pressured, he had flight-of-ideas.
Physical examination and laboratory findings were within normal limits and his history was negative for drug abuse and for evidence of
systemic illness.

Mania

78. A 49-year-old man was found by the police carrying a bow and arrow
and pretending to be "Robin Hood." When seen in an emergency
room, he was hyperactive and agitated, irritable and threatening.
His speech was loud, rapid and pressured. He felt he was a "natural
born leader," and for this reason law enforcement agencies were after him. Physical examination and laboratory findings were within
normal limits and his history was negative for drug abuse and for
evidence of systemic illness.

Mania

79. A 50-year-old woman sought consultation because she found herself
unable to make herself "do things." She described recent "nervous
and funny" feelings. She wanted to stay in bed all day, had trouble
falling asleep and awakened early. She felt better in the morning
and worse as the day progressed. During the past month she lost
20 pounds. She had suicidal thoughts. Physical examination and
laboratory findings were within normal limits and her history was
negative for drug abuse and for evidence of systemic illness.

Depression
Her diurnal mood swing is the opposite of the classical description of
depression. Nevertheless, sufficient signs and symptoms are present
for the diagnosis. If you missed this one because of the reversed diurnal mood, remember: there are no pathognomonic signs.

299

80.   Patients with major affective disorder can be divided into those with only recurrent depressions, i.e., _____ disease and those with recurrent manias or with both manias and depressions, i.e., _____ disease.

81.   Which sex is at greater risk for affective disorder? (write your answer below)

82.   Which age group is at greatest risk for affective disorder? (write your answer below)

83.   The following behaviors have all been observed in patients with demonstrable affective disorder. Circle those which satisfy by definition or description diagnostic criteria for depression or mania and place a D next to each circled depressive criterion and an M next to each circled manic criterion:

Irritability	Feeling down in the dumps
Incomplete auditory hallucinations	Fecal smearing
Assaultive	Mutism, posturing, catalepsy
Thought broadcasting	Feels worse in morning; better in evening
Sits in a chair all day	Doing too many things at once in a rapid impulsive manner
When moves, does so slowly	Singing/dancing
Talking too much and too fast	Anxious mood
Repeats examiner's questions	Jumping from topic to topic
Would like to go to sleep and not wake up	Impulsive
Intrusive	Feelings of being dead

84.   It is not unusual for bipolar patients to exhibit depressive signs or symptoms during the course of a manic episode. Lability of affect is very common and a manic patient can quickly switch from a happy, singing, dancing, joking period to one of remorseful crying and hopelessness. Sometimes this shift is spontaneous, although a well-timed question from the examiner, "You know, you suddenly look sad...are you going to cry?" can bring on a flood of tears and statements about guilt, worthlessness and hopelessness on the heels of a string of loud coarse jokes, puns and laughs. List all the diagnostic criteria we have used for mania.

300

80. unipolar, bipolar

81. the female sex

82. middle age (40 to 60)

83. (Irritability) M   (Feeling down in the dumps) D
   Incomplete auditory hallucinations Fecal smearing
   Assaultive   Mutism, posturing, catalepsy
   Thought broadcasting   (Feels worse in morning; better)
                                        in evening / D
   (Sits in a chair all day) D   (Doing too many things at once in)
                                        a rapid impulsive manner / M
   (When moves, does so slowly) D   Singing/dancing
   (Talking too much and too fast) M   (Anxious mood) D
   Repeats examiner's questions   Jumping from topic to topic
   (Would like to go to sleep and)
    not wake up / D   Impulsive
   Intrusive   (Feelings of being dead) D

All the non-circled items are consistent with the diagnosis of affective disorder, particularly mania.

84. Criteria for Mania: (all of the following)

   1. Hyperactivity
   2. Rapid/pressured speech
   3. Irritable/euphoric mood
   4. No emotional blunting
   5. No coarse brain disease, no psychostimulant drug abuse in prior
      month, no systemic illness known to cause manic symptoms

301

85.   List all the diagnostic criteria we have used for depression. Although there is always room for improvement, and other sets of criteria (50,147) (similar but not identical) are in use, those you have
learned are reasonably reliable and have been partially validated by
clinical treatment response (1,5,8,9,154,157), laboratory data (2,4,
12,153,156), and family illness pattern (5,151,154).

Schizophrenia

86.   There are a number of differing points of view about the signs
and symptoms which define schizophrenia as a syndrome. Some psychiatrists (94) even say that schizophrenia cannot be defined according to criteria and is not a disease or a syndrome.
        However, many researchers have felt the need to develop sets of
criteria to differentiate the behaviors seen in affective diseases from
those produced by other conditions and from those observed in schizophrenics. The criteria which you will learn to use in this section
are reasonably reliable and have the advantage of having been, in
part, validated by laboratory data (2,3,153,156) clinical presentation
(5,152,154), treatment response (5,154) and family illness patterns
(5,152,154).
        The number of people called "schizophrenic" decreases dramatic-
ally when diagnostic criteria for schizophrenia are refined and subjected to tests for reliability and validity (159).
        Under the relatively old standard diagnostic criteria for schizo-
phrenia, nearly 40 percent of all psychiatric admissions were labeled
schizophrenic (166). (Some hospitals obviously using the grab-bag
approach achieved a 100 percent score!) With the more refined and
relatively new research diagnostic criteria, the diagnosis of schizophrenia is made in only 5 to 10 percent of all acute psychiatric admissions (159). This suggests a dramatic drop in the estimated morbidity
risk (EMR) for schizophrenia in the general population: from 1 percent to 0.3 percent (141 pp. 11-12,159). For affective disorders, the
EMR is about _____ percent. Compare this figure with those for schizophrenia. Which diagnosis are you most likely to make most frequently?

87.   In hospitals that use the diagnostic criteria I will be discussing
(or similar criteria), the diagnosis of affective disorder is made in
about 25 percent of acute admissions. Schizophrenia is diagnosed in 5
to 10 percent of the admissions (110,151,159). In England and Scot-
land where comparison studies have been made (38,89), affective disease is also the more frequent diagnosis. Many U.S. hospitals have
much looser criteria (or different concepts); in those hospitals, the
figures mentioned above are reversed. What is the estimated general
population morbidity risk for affective disorder and for schizophrenia
using modern research criteria?

85. Criteria for Depression (all of the following)
    1. Sad or anxious mood
    2. Three of the following:
       a. early a.m. waking
       b. diurnal mood swing (worse in a.m.)
       c. more than 5 pound weight loss in 3 weeks
       d. psychomotor retardation/agitation
       e. suicidal thoughts/behavior
       f. feelings of guilt, self-reproach/hopelessness/worthlessness.
    3. No coarse brain disease or use of steroids or reserpine in the past
       month, no systemic illness known to cause depressive symptoms

86. 2, affective disorders

87. 2 percent for affective disorder, 0.3 percent for schizophrenia

88. The criteria for schizophrenia are the following:

All four are required:

1. No diagnosable affective disorder

2. No coarse brain disease or hallucinogenic stimulant drug use or systemic illness known to cause psychiatric symptoms

3. Clear consciousness

4. One of the following is required
   a. Emotional blunting
   b. Formal thought disorder
   c. First rank symptom (any one)

Which of the above criteria is most similar to those used for depression and mania?

89. We have defined pathognomonic to mean a sign or symptom that occurs in only one condition. There are no pathognomonic signs in psychiatry. Thus, although the required presence of emotional _____, formal _____ _____ and _____ _____ symptoms (required as inclusion criteria) increase the probability of valid diagnosis for schizophrenia, you must also consider the criteria which preclude the diagnosis (exclusion criteria) because other disorders, such as temporal lobe epilepsy (42) also can present with schizophrenic symptoms.

90. The inclusion criteria for the diagnosis of schizophrenia are

_____ _____, _____ _____
_____, and _____ _____
symptoms.

91. In Part I, we discussed how the global impression of emotional blunting can be separated into component parts which are more easily evaluated during a mental status examination. Constricted range and decreased intensity are two component parts of emotional blunting. List as many others as you can recall:

92. The facial appearance in patients with emotional blunting is characterized by: _____.

93. Patients with emotional blunting speak in an unvarying _____ voice.

94. Patients with emotional blunting are often seclusive, avoiding social contact and are indifferent to their surroundings (hospital staff, visitors, relatives, physical environs).

"How do you like it here in the hospital?"

"Did you enjoy your visit with your family?"

These are questions which will often produce apathetic responses. Emotionally blunted individuals have a _____ range and a _____ intensity of affect. They have an _____ face, _____ eyes and they speak in a _____ voice.

304

88. 2. Coarse brain disease, drugs and systemic illness can each produce manic, depressive and schizophrenic syndromes.

89. blunting, thought disorder, first rank

90. emotional blunting, formal thought disorder, first rank

91. expressionless face, unblinking eyes, monotonous voice, no expressed concern for loved ones

92. an expressionless, unblinking look

93. monotonous

94. constricted, decreased, expressionless, unblinking, monotonous or unvarying

95.   Emotionally blunted individuals often are indifferent to, and express little affection for their family and friends. This emotional indifference leaves them unconcerned for their present situation and without plans or desires for the future. When asked how they feel about being in the hospital, or how they would feel if they had to remain hospitalized for many months, patients respond, "Well, I suppose I'll have to," "It's o.k. being here," "Well, I don't like it, but what can I do?". Once again, list as many characteristics of emotional blunting as you can.

96.   Circle the words or phrases associated with emotional blunting.

Apathetic mood   Profound sadness

Labile affect   Constricted affective range

Grandiose, euphoric mood   Expressionless face

Monotonous voice   Friendliness

97.   Check the words or phrases associated with emotional blunting.

Spending all day staring at the T.V., has little
to do with other patients   _____

Appears indifferent to being hospitalized and
has no future plans   _____

Stays by himself, but is not sad   _____

Greets all the visitors to the ward with a big
"Hello"   _____

Wants to help the hospital staff, is liked by
all   _____

Cries when a fellow patient suffers a heart
attack   _____

Laughs shallowly without humor   _____

95. constricted range, decreased intensity of affect, expressionless face, unblinking eyes, monotonous or unvarying voice, indifferent to and without affection for family and friends, unconcerned for their present situation, without plans or desires for the future.

96. (Apathetic mood)   Profound sadness
    Labile affect   (Constricted affective range)
    Grandiose, euphoric mood (Expressionless face)
    (Monotonous voice)   Friendliness

97. Spending all day staring at the T.V., has little
    to do with other patients   ___√___

    Appears indifferent to being hospitalized and has √
    no future plans   _____

    Stays by himself, but is not sad   ___√___

    Greets all the visitors to the ward with a big
    "Hello"   _____

    Wants to help the hospital staff, is liked by all _____

    Cries when a fellow patient suffers a heart
    attack   _____

    Laughs shallowly without humor   ___√___

307

98.   In Part I we discussed formal thought disorder and how the presence of these phenomena increases the probability of the diagnosis
of schizophrenia. Make a written list of the formal thought disorders
and when appropriate, draw the little "box-diagrams" to depict each.
Define the formal thought disorders that do not lend themselves to the
diagrammatic description.

98. A. Verbigeration (palilalia)

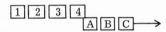

Stereotyped repetition of associations at end of phrase or sentence.

B. Talking past the point
(tangential speech)

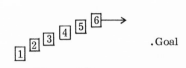

C. Neologisms

New words

D. Word approximations

Imprecise but closely related word,
e.g., "writer" for "pen"

E. Drivelling speech
(jargon agrammatism)

Double talk. Syntax is intact but
speech has no meaning.

F. Derailment

1 2 3 4
     A B C ⟶

(sudden switch from one associational line to a new parallel line)

G. Non-sequitur

Verbal response totally unrelated
to stimulus question or statement

H. Perseveration

Automatic usage of stock words or
phrases often without meaningful
connections to associational stream
of thought.

1 2 A 3 4 A 5 A ⟶ .Goal

If you had difficulty with 97 and 98, please go back to Part I and
review the section on Thought and Speech.

99.   In Part I, we discussed the first rank symptoms of Kurt Schneider. List these and briefly define each.

100.   Patients often have secondary delusional ideas involving telepathy, electronic surveillance, or power rays, to explain how their thoughts escape aloud from their heads so that others can hear them. This is the phenomenon of _____ _____.

101.   When a patient tells you something the content of which suggests apophany, you should ask the basic question "_____?"

102.   Once a patient has told you some of the details of his apophanous ideas, you can progress smoothly to the examination of first rank symptoms. If a patient responds positively to the question "You mean to say that you feel your thoughts leaking out of your head and they are as loud as my voice?", he is admitting to the first rank symptom of _____ _____.

103.   A 33-year-old man said his wall paper was filled with "radioactivity" which "took over" his body and made him do things against his will. He was experiencing the Schneiderian _____ symptom of _____ _____ _____.

104.   An irritable 35-year-old man complained that someone had bitten him in his leg and that the bite had injected "things" into his body which he could "feel" in his head and chest. These "things" were making noise and preventing him from concentrating. This man's complaint is an example of an _____ _____ _____. His belief that someone had placed these "things" in him by biting him on the leg is an example of a _____ delusional idea.

99. A. Phonemes (complete auditory hallucinations)
Clearly audible voices, sustained and perceived as coming from "outside" the self.

B. Thought broadcasting
The subjective, literal experience of feeling one's thoughts escaping aloud from one's head into the air for all to hear.

C. Experiences of influence
The subjective, literal experience of feeling oneself being controlled by some "outside" force or agency.

D. Experiences of alienation
The subjective, literal experience of feeling parts of one's body, or thoughts or feelings as being foreign bodies in no way connected to the self.

E. Delusional perceptions
The interpretation of a real perception into a personalized significant but arbitrary meaning. There is no meaningful connection between the real perception and the conclusion.

If you had any difficulty with this question, please return to Part I and review the section on First Rank Symptoms.

100. thought broadcasting

101. "How do you know?"

102. thought broadcasting

103. first rank, experience of influence

104. experience of alienation, secondary

105.   The 35-year-old man in the previous item also clearly heard voices coming from the "things" in his head and chest. These voices constantly commented upon his actions and often repeated his own thoughts. This is an example of a _____ _____

_____

106.   Draw lines between matching items in the two columns:

Thought broadcasting   "Someone is putting his thoughts in my head."

Phoneme   "My thoughts came out of my head like a radio."

Experience of alienation   Complete auditory hallucination

107.   As we discussed in Part I, schizophrenia and affective disorders have several symptoms in common. Hallucinations, delusions, catatonic motor features and first rank symptoms can occur in both groups of patients (5,24,88,109,143,147,152,154,157,158,177). To assure a more distinct separation of groups and thus a higher probability of diagnostic accuracy for each patient, the schizophrenic exclusion criterion of: "no diagnosable affective disorder" is used. If the patient has sufficient symptoms to satisfy the criteria for depression or mania, it is preferable to diagnose affective disorder even when there are some signs of schizophrenia present. It is always better to be a therapeutic optimist and first treat the condition with the better outcome (affective disease). Research data support the validity of the precedence of affective symptoms over schizophrenic symptoms (1,3,5-7,24,25,87,90, 96,110,150,154,155,157,158,176).

108.   Match the clinical item to the disorder in which it is most commonly observed by placing a check mark in the appropriate box (more than one checked category for any thought disorder is possible).

	Mania	Schizophrenia
Drivelling		
Flight-of-ideas		
Perseveration		
Non-sequiturs		
Derailment		
Clang associations		
Paraphasia		
Tangential speech		
Circumstantial speech		
Blocking		
Verbigeration		

105. complete auditory hallucination or phoneme

106.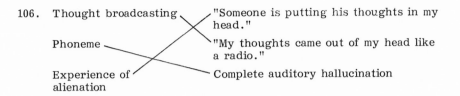

Thought broadcasting — "Someone is putting his thoughts in my head."

Phoneme — "My thoughts came out of my head like a radio."

Experience of alienation — Complete auditory hallucination

107. No answer required

108.

	Mania	Schizophrenia
Drivelling		√
Flight-of-ideas	√	
Perseveration		√
Non-sequiturs	√ with flight-of-ideas	√
Derailment		√
Clang associations	√	
Paraphasia		√
Tangential speech		√
Circumstantial speech	√	
Blocking		√
Verbigeration	√	√

313

109. Circle the words or phrases satisfying any of the diagnostic criteria for schizophrenia:

Hyperactivity	Emotional blunting
Flight-of-ideas	Psychomotor retardation
First rank symptoms	No coarse brain disease
Delusions and hallucinations	Euphoric
Talking past the point (tangential speech)	

110. Circle the words or phrases satisfying any of the diagnostic criteria for schizophrenia:

Irritability	Thought broadcasting
Perseveration	Feelings of hopelessness
Agitation	Lack of emotional warmth, drive or interest
Delusional perception	Seizures

111. Circle the words or phrases satisfying any of the diagnostic criteria for schizophrenia:

No affective disease	Comatose
Labile affect	Neologism
Experience of influence	Brain tumor
Head trauma	Memory deficit with adequate concentration

112. Circle the words or phrases that would <u>exclude</u> the diagnosis of schizophrenia:

Warm and friendly	Thought disorder
Catalepsy	Encephalitis
Paraphasia	Clouded consciousness
Phoneme	LSD use

113. Are sufficient criteria for the diagnosis of schizophrenia satisfied in the following case vignette? If not, which one(s) is/are not satisfied and why?

A 43-year-old man was hospitalized because of repeated calls to the police. During admissions, he insisted that his house was going to be bombed. When you examine him, he is alert and cooperative. He is mildly irritable, expresses no warm feelings concerning his family and does not relate to you. He has multiple delusional ideas. His speech includes talking past the point, several neologisms, paraphasia and several episodes of derailment. Pseudomemories are present, but no other memory disturbances can be observed. He exhibits no signs of affective disorder, physical examination and laboratory findings are within normal limits and he has no history of drug abuse or systemic illness.

109. Hyperactivity
Flight-of-ideas
(First rank symptoms)
Delusions and hallu-
cinations
(Talking past the point
(tangential speech))

(Emotional blunting)
Psychomotor retardation
(No coarse brain disease)
Euphoria

110. Irritability
(Perseveration)
Agitation
(Delusional perception)

(Thought broadcasting)
Feelings of hopelessness
(Lack of emotional warmth, drive or interest)
Seizures

111. (No affective disease)
Labile affect
(Experience of influence)
Head trauma

Comatose
(Neologism)
Brain tumor
Memory deficit with adequate concentration

112. (Warm and friendly)
Catalepsy
Paraphasia
Phoneme

Thought disorder
(Encephalitis)
(Clouded consciousness)
(LSD use)

113. Yes. Even though he has no first rank symptoms, his formal thought disorder and emotional blunting, in clear consciousness and in the absence of coarse brain, systemic disease or affective disorder satisfy sufficient criteria for the diagnosis of schizophrenia.

114.   Are sufficient criteria for the diagnosis of schizophrenia satisfied
in the following case vignette? If not, which one(s) is/are not satisfied and why?

A 44-year-old woman was hospitalized because she became belligerent. She is untidy but alert, paces, rocks and constantly moves
her fingers. Her affect is constricted and profoundly blunted.
She has a paucity of speech, rarely responding with more than
one or two words. There is no evidence of formal thought disorder
or first rank symptoms of Schneider. There are no signs of affective disease or memory dysfunction. Physical examination and
laboratory findings are within normal limits and there is no historical evidence of coarse brain disease, drug abuse or systemic illne
While hospitalized she remains, except for brief periods of irritability
aloof, placid and generally unresponsive to staff, other patients, or
ward activities.

115.   Are sufficient criteria for the diagnosis of schizophrenia satisfied
in the following case vignette? If not, which one(s) is/are not satisfied and why?

A 20-year-old man is hospitalized because of threatening behavior.
He is easily "upset." He often laughs for no obvious reason, also
snarls and makes gestures like those of a dog. He has attempted
to bite people.
On initial examination, he was mute, immobile and analgesic. Catalepsy was present. A second examination performed when he is
alert and no longer stuporous reveals him to have severe emotional blunting, paraphasic speech, and complete auditory hallucinations. Physical examination reveals evidence of an old craniotomy.
The patient had had a head injury as a child and suffered a sub-
dural hematoma which required evacuation.

116.   Are sufficient criteria satisfied for the diagnosis of schizophrenia
in the following case vignette? If not, which one(s) is/are not satisfied and why?

A 40-year-old woman is hospitalized because of her constant com-
plants to the police that she's been hearing voices in her attic.
When examined, she is alert and cooperative, though mildly irritable. She speaks in a monotone, has little emotional spontaneity
and relates poorly to the examiner. Affective range is restricted,
intensity decreased and little warmth can be elicited, even when
she talks about her children. She describes several clear voices
coming out of her attic which persist throughout the day. She
attributes this to some person sending a ray to her TV antenna.
Her speech is stilted (overly formal, somewhat dysrhythmic). Paraphasias are present.   There is no evidence of affective disorder or
memory dysfunctions. Physical examination and laboratory findings
are within normal limits and there is no evidence of drug abuse,
coarse brain disease or history of systemic disease.

316

114. Yes. In the absence of coarse brain disease, medical illness and affective disease, the presence of severe emotional blunting, even without formal thought disorder or first rank symptoms, shows a high
probability that this patient has schizophrenia.

115. No. He has emotional blunting and formal thought disorder, but the
exclusion criteria are not satisfied. This is an example of secondary
or symptomatic schizophrenia. That is, the patient has the syndrome
but with an obvious etiology (head injury).

The schizophrenia we have been discussing contrary to this case is
idiopathic. No one knows the etiology.

116. Yes. Sufficient criteria are satisfied for the diagnosis of schizophrenia.

317

117.   Match the diagnostic criteria with the diagnosis by writing the letter of the criterion in the space provided next to the appropriate disorder.

a. Formal thought disorder

b. Anxious/sad mood

Mania _____

c. Psychomotor retardation

d. No coarse brain disease

Depression _____

e. First rank symptoms

f. No systemic illness known to
produce similar picture

Schizophrenia _____

g. No drug abuse in month prior
to symptom onset

h. Euphoria

i. Hyperactivity

118.   Match the diagnostic criteria with the diagnosis by writing the letter of the criterion in the space provided next to the appropriate disorder.

a. Feels terrible in a.m., better
in afternoon

b. Cries all the time

Mania _____

c. No emotional rapport

d. Euphoric

Depression _____

e. Delusional idea of being evil

f. Tangential speech

Schiziphrenia _____

g. Jargon agrammatism

h. Hyperactivity

i. Slowed speech/motor behavior

j. Talks too much and too fast

318

117.

a. Formal thought disorder

b. Anxious/sad mood

Mania   d, f, g, h, i

c. Psychomotor retardation

d. No coarse brain disease

Depression b, c, d, f, g

e. first rank symptoms

f. No systemic illness known to produce similar picture

Schizophrenia a, d, e, f, g

g. No drug abuse in month prior to symptom onset

h. Euphoria

i. Hyperactivity

118.

a. Feels terrible in a.m., better in afternoon

b. Cries all the time

Mania   d, h, j

c. No emotional rapport

d. Euphoric

Depression   a, b, e, i

e. Delusional idea of being evil

f. Tangential speech

Schizophrenia   c, f, g

g. Jargon agrammatism

h. Hyperactivity

i. Slowed speech/motor behavior

j. Talks too much and too fast

119. Match the diagnosis criteria with the diagnosis by writing the letter of the criterion in the space provided next to the appropriate disorder.

a. Irritable, laughs and cries

b. Neologisms

c. Thought broadcasting

Mania _____

d. Anorexia with weight loss of 10 lbs. in 2 weeks

Depression _____

e. Early a.m. insomnia

f. Speech rapid and pressured

Schizophrenia _____

g. Not emotionally blunted

h. No coarse brain disease

i. Suicidal

j. Feels hopeless and worthless

k. Hyperactive

120. Over the years, schizophrenia has been classified into subgroups labeled: "paranoid," "catatonic," "hebephrenic," "simple," "chronic," "undifferentiated" and "schizo-affective" types (37). There is a growing body of evidence that the "schizo-affective" type should not be considered part of schizophrenia (3,30,36,106,119,146,154,155,161,163, 172,173). Some researchers consider it a separate condition (172,173) and others (30,36,106,119,146,161), including myself, consider most people with the diagnosis of "schizo-affective type" to have affective disorder. This theoretical problem will only be resolved by the clarification offered by further data. For our purposes, the definite diagnostic criteria we use and our therapeutic optimism suffice. A person who has signs and symptoms which satisfy the criteria for affective disorder does not, by definition, satisfy the criteria for schizophrenia and should be treated for affective disease. Individuals whose signs and symptoms approach but do not satisfy either set of criteria should first be treated for the condition with the best prognosis, i.e., affective disorder.

121. The variety of subgroups in the traditional view of schizophrenia reflects an attempt to identify the most characteristic feature of the subgroup. Thus, although observed to share many signs and symptoms with other schizophrenics, "catatonic schizophrenics" were unlike other schizophrenics in that they exhibited predominant catatonic features.

There is no evidence that patients satisfying the above criteria schizophrenia can be successfully separated into subgroups. They either have the condition or they don't! A patient who satisfies the criteria for schizophrenia is diagnosed as schizophrenic. Variations of other clinical phenomena are secondary and not pathognomonic (152,159). List the criteria for schizophrenia.

320

119.

Mania   a, f, g, h, k

Depression   d, e, g, h, i, j

Schizophrenia   b, c, h

a. Irritable, laughs and cries
b. Neologisms
c. Thought broadcasting
d. Anorexia with weight loss of 10 lbs. in 2 weeks
e. Early a.m. insomnia
f. Speech rapid and pressured
g. Not emotionally blunted
h. No coarse brain disease
i. Suicidal
j. Feels hopeless and worthless
k. Hyperactive

120. No answer required

121. All four required:
1. No diagnosable affective disorder
2. No coarse brain disease or hallucinogenic stimulant drug use or systemic illness known to cause psychiatric symptoms
3. Clear consciousness
4. One of the following is required
   a. Emotional blunting
   b. Formal thought disorder
   c. First rank symptom (any one)

122.   In the following case vignette, underline the words and/or phrases which satisfy any diagnostic criterion. Are there enough criteria satisfied to make a diagnosis? If so, what is your diagnosis?

A 39-year-old man was hospitalized because he had been banging on his neighbors' doors in the early morning hours. He complained to police that he couldn't sleep because the neighbors were "heckling" him and "dictating" his every movement and action by a "jolt in the skull." When you see him, the patient is cooperative and fully alert. After initial irritability, he does not exhibit any mood. His affect is restricted in range and he expresses little warmth. He is concerned about his neighbors and "some wise guys" who are "out to kill" him, and he feels it is unfair that he has been hospitalized. He has little interest in his wife (from whom he is separated) or his two children. "They made their beds," he says. The patient often responds to questions by talking about the same subject but not to the point. Occasionally his answers are unrelated to the questions. On those occasions, he uses the same words and phrases in his answer in an automatic fashion. He says that people are talking to him all the time. Their voices, sometimes whispered, sometimes very loud, are being "plugged" into his ear. There is no evidence of sadness, euphoria, motor disturbance or coarse brain disease. Physical examination and laboratory findings are within normal limits and his history is negative for drug abuse or systemic illness.

123.   In the following case vignette, underline the words and/or phrases which satisfy any diagnostic criterion. Are there enough criteria satisf to make a diagnosis? If so, what is your diagnosis?

A 49-year-old woman was hospitalized because she was repeatedly screaming "I don't know what I'll do..." and for staying in bed all day staring at the ceiling, crying, not eating and not sleeping at night. When you examine her, she is lying in bed, fully alert but dishevelled and dirty. She refuses to speak, turns away from you and hides her head. A little while later she is somewhat more cooperative. Her movements and speech are markedly slowed. There is no agitation. Her affect is restricted in range and intensity. Her mood is sad. She says "there is no use, I can't be helped...leave me alone, I want to die." She admits to hearing a muffled voice and occasionally seeing shadowy threatening figures. Physical examination and laboratory findings are within normal limits and she has no history of drug abuse or systemic illness.

122. A 39-year-old man was hospitalized because he had been banging on his neighbors' doors in the early morning hours. He complained to police that he couldn't sleep because the neighbors were "heckling" him and "dictating" his every movement and action by a "jolt in the skull." When you see him, the patient is cooperative and fully alert. After initial irritability, he does not exhibit any mood. His affect is restricted in range and he expresses little warmth. He is concerned about his neighbors and "some wise guys" who are "out to kill" him and he feels it is unfair that he has been hospitalized. He has little interest in his wife (from whom he is separated) or his two children. "They made their beds," he says. The patient often responds to questions by talking about the same subject but not to the point. Occasionally his answers are unrelated to the questions. On those occasions, he uses the same words and phrases in his answer in an automatic fashion. He says that people are talking to him all the time. Their voices, sometimes whispered, sometimes very loud, are being "plugged" into his ear. There is no evidence of sadness, euphoria, motor disturbance or coarse brain disease. Physical examination and laboratory findings are within normal limits and his history is negative for drug abuse or systemic illness.

Yes.
Schizophrenia
He satisfies all the exclusion criteria and exhibits emotional blunting (some irritability can be present), formal thought disorder (talking past the point, or tangentiality, non-sequiturs, perseveration), first rank symptoms (experience of control, phonemes).

123. A 49-year-old woman was hospitalized because she was repeatedly screaming "I don't know what I'll do..." and for staying in bed all day staring at the ceiling, crying, not eating and not sleeping at night. When you examine her, she is lying in bed, fully alert but dishevelled and dirty. She refuses to speak, turns away from you and hides her head. A little while later she is somewhat more cooperative. Her movements and speech are markedly slowed. There is no agitation. Her affect is restricted in range and intensity. Her mood is sad. She says "there is no use, I can't be helped...leave me alone, I want to die." She admits to hearing a muffled voice and occasionally seeing shadowy threatening figures. Physical examination and laboratory findings are within normal limits and she has no history of drug abuse or systemic illness.

Yes
Major Depression
The exclusion criteria are satisfied. She exhibits a sad mood, feelings of hopelessness, a desire to commit suicide and insomnia.

Although the classical sleep pattern of early a.m. wakening is most characteristic in a major depression, it is not uncommon for patients to have sleeping difficulties throughout the night.

124.   In the following case vignette, underline the words and/or phrases which satisfy any diagnostic criterion. Are there enough criteria satisfied to make a diagnosis? If so, what is your diagnosis?

A 43-year-old man was hospitalized because he was becoming progressively more seclusive and was putting metal screws into his legs. When you asked him about this he said "shorts....electronics" and then became unintelligible. His sleep was disturbed but there was no weight loss or appetite change. The patient was cooperative and fully alert. His motor behavior was normal except for some facial tics. He often closed his eyes. He scratched his body in a purposeless way. His affective range and intensity were decreased. He was mildly irritable and apathetic. He was unconcerned about being hospitalized or about the welfare of his family. He had no future plans. His speech was not pressured; it was mumbled and consisted mostly of nouns. When asked how he felt, he said "tipper, shorts....electronics...a blanket head is not yellow..." His memory was intact. Physical and laboratory findings were within normal limits and his history was negative for drug abuse and systemic illness.

125.   In the following case vignette, underline the words and/or phrases which satisfy any diagnostic criterion. Are there enough criteria satisfied to make a diagnosis? If so, what is your diagnosis?

A 50-year-old woman sought consultation because of "nervousness" and because she had thoughts about killing herself. During the preceding month she had lost interest in her work, spent progressively more time in bed, had difficulty sleeping throughout the night and had lost 20 pounds. There was no diurnal change in these behaviors. When examined, she was fully alert and cooperative. Her motor behavior was decreased in frequency and slow. Her affect was restricted, her mood sad. Physical examination and laboratory findings were within normal limits and her history was negative for drug abuse and systemic illness.

124. A 43-year-old man was hospitalized because he was becoming progressively more seclusive and was putting metal screws into his legs. When you asked him about this he said "shorts...electronics" and then became unintelligible. His sleep was disturbed but there was no weight loss or appetite change. The patient was cooperative and fully alert. His motor behavior was normal except for some facial tics. He often closed his eyes. He scratched his body in a purposeless way. His affective range and intensity were decreased. He was mildly irritable and apathetic. He was unconcerned about being hospitalized or about the welfare of his family. He had no future plans. His speech was not pressured; it was mumbled and consisted mostly of nouns. When asked how he felt, he said "tipper, shorts....electronics...a blanket head is not yellow..." His memory was intact. Physical and laboratory findings were within normal limits and his history was negative for drug abuse and systemic illness.

Yes
Schizophrenia
He satisfies the exclusion criteria and exhibits formal thought disorder (drivelling speech/jargon agrammatism) and emotional blunting.

125. A 50-year-old woman sought consultation because of "nervousness" and because she had thoughts about killing herself. During the preceding month she had lost interest in her work, spent progressively more time in bed, had difficulty sleeping throughout the night and had lost 20 pounds. There was no diurnal change in these behaviors. When examined, she was fully alert and cooperative. Her motor behavior was decreased in frequency and slow. Her affect was restricted, her mood sad. Physical examination and laboratory findings were within normal limits and her history was negative for drug abuse and systemic illness.

Yes
Major Depression
She satisfies the exclusion criteria and exhibits sadness and anxiety, psychomotor retardation, insomnia, weight loss and suicidal thoughts.

126.   In the following case vignette, underline the words and/or phrases
which satisfy any diagnostic criterion. Are there enough criteria
satisfied to make a diagnosis? If so, what is your diagnosis?

A 25-year-old man was hospitalized because he was extremely agitated, overtalkative and "incoherent." He was not sleeping and
had lost "a great deal of weight." He was dishevelled but fully
alert. He talked continuously and was unable to sit still. He
spoke rapidly in a dramatic matter, jumping from topic to topic.
His mood was euphoric. During his first few days in the hospital
he was constantly engaging staff members in conversation, asking
the same questions over and over again. He danced and sang in
the hallways. He decorated his head with bits of paper and cloth.
He ran from one ward activity to another, rarely completing a task
before starting a new one. He said people communicated with him
by their movements and the clothing they wore; that a nurse using
green ink was a sign that he was the "Son of God"; that God
spoke to him through the rays of the sun. The patient spoke on
several occasions for minutes on end using words that rhymed with
sun: "I am the son, see the sun, see a bun, hi hon', hi honey
bun..." Physical and laboratory findings were within normal limits and he had no history for drug abuse, coarse brain disease, or
systemic illness.

127.   In the following case vignette, underline the words and/or phrases
which satisfy any diagnostic criterion. Are there enough criteria
satisfied to make a diagnosis? If so, what is your diagnosis?

A 28-year-old woman was hospitalized because she kept saying
"God is punishing me. I am a bad girl." During the few weeks
before admission she became increasingly restless, did not sleep
well, ate excessively and smoked constantly (which was unusual
for her). She began to complain that people were talking about
her being a "bad mother." She said God spoke to her. The voice
was described as clear, coming from above and constant. At times
she seemed fearful and hid behind furniture; at other times she
giggled and laughed for no apparent reason and walked about with
cigarette ashes on her head. Just prior to hospitalization she was
observed hopping and jumping about, then holding her arms and
hands in a strange prolonged position and then kneeling down to
pray. When you first examined her, she became angry, agitated
and threw things about the room. Later, she walked up and down
the corridors, disrobing, masturbating, screaming, punching doors,
talking to the walls, going from one activity to the next, interrupting conversations, talking non-stop and rapidly. Physical examination and laboratory findings were within normal limits and she
had no history of coarse brain disease, drug abuse or systemic
illness.

126. A 25-year-old man was hospitalized because he was extremely agitated, overtalkative and "incoherent." He was not sleeping and had lost "a great deal of weight." He was dishevelled but fully alert. He talked continuously and was unable to sit still. He spoke rapidly in a dramatic manner, jumping from topic to topic. His mood was euphoric. During his first few days in the hospital, he was constantly engaging staff members in conversation, asking the same questions over and over again. He danced and sang in the hallways. He decorated his head with bits of paper and cloth. He ran from one ward activity to another, rarely completing a task before starting a new one. He said people communicated with him by their movements and the clothing they wore; that a nurse using green ink was a sign that he was the "Son of God"; that God spoke to him through the rays of the sun. The patient spoke on several occasions for minutes on end using words that rhymed with sun: "I am the son, see the sun, see a bun, hi hon', hi honey bun..." Physical and laboratory findings were within normal limits and he had no history for drug abuse, coarse brain disease or systemic illness.

Yes
Mania
He satisfies the exclusion criteria and exhibits rapid/pressured speech, euphoria and hyperactivity. He also has flight-of-ideas and clang associations.

His possible delusional perception, delusional ideas, auditory hallucinations, head decoration, singing, dancing, impulsive, intrusive, and importunate behaviors are all seen in manic episodes (24,88,96,157, 177).

127. A 28-year-old woman was hospitalized because she kept saying "God is punishing me. I am a bad girl." During the few weeks before admission she became increasingly restless, did not sleep well, ate excessively and smoked constantly (which was unusual for her). She began to complain that people were talking about her being a "bad mother." She said God spoke to her. The voice was described as clear, coming from above and constant. At times she seemed fearful and hid behind furniture; at other times she giggled and laughed for no apparent reason and walked about with cigarette ashes on her head. Just prior to hospitalization, she was observed hopping and jumping about, then holding her arms and hands in a strange prolonged position and then kneeling down to pray. When you first examined her, she became angry, agitated and threw things about the room. Later, she walked up and down the corridors, disrobing, masturbating, screaming, punching doors, talking to the walls, going from one activity to the next, interrupting conversations, talking non-stop and rapidly. Physical examination and laboratory findings were within normal limits and she has no history of coarse brain disease, drug abuse or systemic illness.

Yes
Mania
She satisfies exclusion criteria and exhibits rapid/pressured speech, hyperactivity (an excitement state) and an irritable mood. Her catatonic features, nudity, agitation, violence, public masturbation are all observed in severe mania (24,86,98,157,177).

327

DIAGNOSTIC CRITERIA - SUMMARY

128.   The following table was presented in Part I and summarizes the
observed relationships between the thought disorders we have examined and several major psychiatric conditions. These thought
disorders are not pathognomonic (the tabled relationships are not
absolute), but the presence of any one is suggestive of the condition in which it is most frequently observed.

	Mania	Catatonia	Schizophrenia	Chronic Mild-Moderate Coarse Brain Disease
Verbigeration		X	X	X
Clang assoc- iations	X			
Tangential speech			X	X
Fragmented speech	X	X	X	X
Word salad			X	X
Word approx- imations			X	X
Neologisms			X	X
Circumstantial speech	X			X

Circle the thought disorders which satisfy the diagnostic criteria
you have been studying for schizophrenia.

128.

	Mania	Catatonia	Schizophrenia	Chronic Mild-Moderate Coarse Brain Disease
Verbigeration		X	(X)	X
Clang assoc- iations	X			
Tangential speech			(X)	X
Fragmented speech	X	X	X	X
Word salad			(X)	X
Word approx- imations			(X)	X
Neologisms			(X)	X
Circumstantial speech	X			X

Phenomena in the Catatonic column are not circled because although they fit the diagnosis of "Catatonia," we have learned that catatonia is not a disease, but a syndrome associated with affective disorder, schizophrenia and coarse brain disease.

329

129.   Place a check mark in the appropriate box to indicate into which mental status section each behavior item best fits. Circle the checks which satisfy diagnostic criteria and put the first letter of the associated disorder next to the circled check (M - Mania, D - Depression, S - Schizophrenia).

	General Appearance	General Motor Behavior	Catatonia	Affect
Tardive dyskinesia				
Stupor				
Grimacing				
Manner				
Clear consciousness				
Blunting				
Posturing				
Body type				
Waxy flexibility				
Agitation				

130.   Place a check mark in the appropriate box to indicate into which mental status section each behavior item best fits. Circle the checks which satisfy diagnostic criteria and put the first letter of the associated disorder (M - Mania, D - Depression, S - Schizophrenia) next to the circled check.

	General Appearance	General Motor Behavior	Catatonia	Affect	Thought Disorder
Clang association					
Hyperactivity					
Posturing					
Flight-of-ideas					
Verbigeration					
Intense affect					
Lability of mood					
Euphoria					
Tangential speech					
Irritability					
Sadness					
Unkempt clothes					

129.

	General Appearance	General Motor Behavior	Catatonia	Affect
Tardive dyskinesia		√		
Stupor		(acceptable)	√	
Grimacing			√	
Manner	√			
Clear consciousness	(√)S			
Blunting				(√)S
Posturing			√	
Body type	√			
Waxy flexibility			√	
Agitation		(√)D		

130.

	General Appearance	General Motor Behavior	Catatonia	Affect	Thought Disorder
Clang association					√
Hyperactivity		(√)M			
Posturing			√		
Flight-of-ideas					√
Verbigeration			√		(√)S
Intense affect				√	
Lability of mood				√	
Euphoria				(√)M	
Tangential speech					(√)S
Irritability				(√)M	
Sadness				(√)D	
Unkempt clothes	√				

If you circled any of the others (except "unkempt clothes") and indicated an "M" or "D", you would have been correct in the sense
that these phenomena are often seen in affective disease. However,
they are not specific diagnostic criteria.

131.   Place a check mark in the appropriate box to indicate into which mental status section each behavior item best fits. Circle the checks which satisfy diagnostic criteria and put the first letter of the associated disorder (M - Mania, D - Depression, S - Schizophrenia) next to the circled check.

	General Appearance	General Motor Behavior	Catatonia	Affect	Thought Disorder
Thin					
Agitated					
Echolalia					
Grimacing					
Dishevelled					
Labile affect					
Anxiety					
Rambling speech					
Non-sequiturs					
Irritability					
Clouded consciousness					
Perseveration of associations					

131.

	General Appearance	General Motor Behavior	Catatonia	Affect	Thought Disorder
Thin	✓				
Agitated		⊘D			
Echolalia			✓		
Grimacing			✓		
Dishevelled	✓				
Labile affect				✓	
Anxiety				⊘D	
Rambling speech					✓
Non-sequiturs					⊘S
Irritability				⊘M	
Clouded consciousness	✓				
Perseveration of associations					⊘S

Clouded consciousness although not a criterion does exclude the diagnosis of the major psychoses: depression, mania and schizophrenia.

132.   Place a check mark in the appropriate box to indicate into which mental status section each behavior item best fits. Circle the checks which satisfy the diagnostic criteria and put the first letter of the associated disorder (M - Mania, D - Depression, S - Schizophrenia) next to the circled check.

	Appearance	Gen. Motor Behavior	Catatonia	Affect	Thought Disorder	Apophany
Euphoria						
Self-expo-sure						
Hyperactive						
Flight-of-ideas						
Posturing						
Delusional perception						
Heavy body build						
Singing and dancing						
Secondary delusional ideas						
40-year-old woman						
Clang assoc-iations						

334

132.	Appearance	Gen. Motor Behavior	Catatonia	Affect	Thought Disorder	Apophany
Euphoria				✓M		
Self-expo- sure	✓					
Hyperactive		✓M				
Flight-of- ideas					✓	
Posturing			✓			
Delusional perception						✓S
Heavy body build	✓					
Singing and dancing	✓	✓ acceptable				
Secondary delusional ideas						✓
40-year-old woman	✓					
Clang assoc- iations					✓	

Again, though the other phenomena are not diagnostic criteria, they can occur most frequently in affective disorder, particularly mania.

335

133.   Place a check mark in the appropriate box to indicate into which mental status section each behavior item best fits. Circle the checks which satisfy diagnostic criteria and put the first letter of the associated disorder (M - Mania, D - Depression, S - Schizophrenia) next to the circled check.

	General Appearance	Motor Behavior	Affect	Thought Process	Apophany	Perceptual Dysfunct.	First Rank Symptom
Delusional perception							
Delusional mood							
Delusional ideas							
Hyperactivity							
Incomplete auditory hallucination							
Flight-of-ideas							
Irritability							
Autochthonous delusional ideas							
Clang associations							
Euphoria							
Sadness							
Posturing							

133.	General Appearance	Motor Behavior	Affect	Thought Process	Apophany	Perceptual Dysfunct.	First Rank Symptom
Delusional perception					✓S		✓S
Delusional mood					✓		
Delusional ideas					✓		
Hyperactivity		✓M					
Incomplete auditory hallucination						✓	
Flight-of-ideas				✓			
Irritability			✓M				
Autochthonous delusional ideas					✓		
Clang associations				✓			
Euphoria			✓M				
Sadness			✓D				
Posturing		✓					

134. Place a check mark in the appropriate box to indicate into which mental status section each behavior item best fits. More than one check per symptom is possible.

	Mania	Catatonia	Schizophrenia	Coarse Brain Disease
Delusions				
Violence				
Inappropriate mood				
Thought disorder				
Poor personal hygiene				
Tardive dyskinesia				
Agitation				
Loose associations				
Illusions				
Hallucinations				
Persecutory delusions				
Bizarre behavior				

134.

	Mania	Catatonia	Schizophrenia	Coarse Brain Disease
Delusions	√	√	√	√
Violence	√	√	√	√
Inappropriate mood	√	√	√	√
Thought disorder	√	√	√	√
Poor personal hygiene	√	√	√	√
Tardive dyskinesia	√	√	√	√
Agitation	√	√	√	√
Loose associations	√	√	√	√
Illusions	√	√	√	√
Hallucinations	√	√	√	√
Persecutory delusions	√	√	√	√
Bizarre behavior	√	√	√	√

This item demonstrates the relative worthlessness of imprecise terms
and descriptions. Precise description of each of the phenomena
might have allowed you to assign them to particular columns. In
diagnosis, the same principle applies. The more precise your
descriptions, the more likely you are to make a correct diagnosis.

COARSE BRAIN DISEASE

135.   The DSM-III term "organic mental disorder" will not be used
in this text as it implies the existence of "inorganic" or metaphysical
brain syndromes, a notion which is contrary to basic biology and
the generally accepted idea that the brain is the organ of behavior
and that all behavior—pathological, deviant and normal—reflects
brain function. As a substitute for the DSM-III term, I will use
"coarse brain disease" to label clinical conditions which have
demonstrable etiology or pathophysiology. These brain disorders
are "coarse" in that their pathology is measurable with present
technology. They contrast with other mental disorders in which
the pathology is not yet measurable and in which the etiology or
pathophysiology is unknown.

About one out of five patients hospitalized on an acute psychiatric inpatient service has coarse brain disease (159,166,169). In
acute general medical surgical units approximately one out of nine
patients has coarse brain disease (111,169,170), usually a subacute
delirium. By convention, a delirium refers to a process which is
_____ in onset, and unlike the dementias, its response
to treatment is usually _____.

136.   The variety of acute and chronic coarse brain syndromes is too
great to be completely detailed in this text. I will discuss only a few
conditions, more as illustrations of the diagnostic process than as
comprehensive presentations of differing disorders. I will not discuss
the coarse brain disease affecting children. This important area is
beyond the scope of this book. It deserves a volume of its own.

137.   Pathological processes resulting in coarse brain disease can present as delirium, localized syndromes, or dementia. These conditions are not pathognomonic; single etiology can present as all three
during the course of the illness. Although a detailed mental status,
neurological and physical examination can narrow the possibilities,
a detailed history and laboratory investigation are essential for reasonable diagnostic accuracy (169).

340

135. rapid, good

136. No answer required

137. No answer required

138.   Many non-etiological factors influence the picture of a coarse brain disease process. Thus a single morbid process can produce a localized brain syndrome, an acute diffuse brain syndrome termed _____, and a chronic diffuse brain syndrome termed _____.

139.   Both the speed at which the morbid process involves the brain and the extent of the process can determine whether a neuro-virus, for example, will produce an acute diffuse process termed a _____, a chronic diffuse process termed _____, or a localized syndrome.

140.   Individual predisposition (vulnerability) can also determine the clinical presentation resulting from a morbid process. In a clinical presentation in which the brain vulnerability is great or the morbid process severe, an acute, diffuse process termed a _____ will often develop.

141.   During the daylight hours, many delirious patients appear to be without psychopathology. At night, however, what during the day was a mildly tired, somewhat restless patient becomes a confused, agitated nursing problem that brings house staff running from all corners of the building. A search for mild hints of delirium during the day can save you and the patient a sleepless night. Circle the words and phrases below indicating non-etiological factors which can influence the clinical picture of a coarse brain disease process:

Rapidly spreading morbid process   Middle class

Age and nutritional status of   Localizing morbid process
patient

Divorced with one child   Insidious onset

142.   The degree of cortical arousal will determine the clinical state or level of consciousness. List these different clinical levels:

143.   In all patients who are delirious, some degree of reduced cortical arousal (i.e., alteration in level of consciousness) is present (43,45,46,170). Check the descriptions below which are consistent with an altered state of cortical arousal (i.e., level of consciousness).

_____   Unresponsive even to painful stimulation

_____   Awake and appropriately answers all questions

_____   Keeps falling asleep, occasionally fails to respond to examiner's questions

_____   Unresponsive to questions unless examiner shakes patient and shouts

144.   Patients with a reduced level of consciousness often appear perplexed and their eyes wander and fail to focus. When the delirium is pronounced they may also be lethargic. Write a brief description of the behaviors of a lethargic patient.

145.   Delirious patients often appear confused and delayed in their responses. These behaviors reflect an underlying _____.

138. delirium, dementia

139. delirium, dementia

140. delirium

141. (Rapidly spreading morbid process*)   Middle class

    (Age and nutritional status of patient**)   (Localizing morbid process***)

    Divorced with one child   (Insidious onset*)

    *   speed of process
    ** individual's vulnerability
    *** localizing process

142. alertness, lethargy, semi-coma, coma

143.   √ Unresponsive even to painful stimulation

        Awake and appropriately answers all questions

      √ Keeps falling asleep, occasionally fails to respond to examiner's questions

      √ Unresponsive to questions unless examiner shakes patient and shouts

144. They have difficulty staying awake, keep on falling asleep and occasionally fail to respond to examiner's questions.

145. Alteration in cortical arousal or reduced level of consciousness.

146.   An alteration in the level of consciousness makes the processing of incoming stimuli difficult. Delirious patients commonly misinterpret the events about them, and are often suspicious and frightened. Because of their reduced level of consciousness, they often appear _____ and _____. Their responses are often _____, _____, or fail to occur at all.

147.   The following behaviors are observed in patients with an alteration in consciousness except (circle your answer):

    a. Perplexed

    b. Lethargic and sleepy

    c. Confused

    d. Rapid reaction time

    e. Delayed reaction time

148.   Any intense mood can lead to increased frequency of motor behavior termed _____. Delirious patients who are often anxious and occasionally terror-striken often demonstrate restlessness and an occasional severe increase in motor behavior, i.e., _____.

149.   Because of their reduced _____, delirious patients often have difficulty listening to, retaining and understanding data. A deficit in immediate recall, short-term, and recent memory is common. Mrs. Jones who "just can't seem to follow" your instructions regarding her medication schedule or dressing changes, etc., may not be a "bad patient." Evaluate her cognitive functioning! One out of nine Mrs. Joneses on an acute general medical surgical unit is suffering from some coarse brain morbid process.

150.   Circle the words or phrases characteristic of a delirious state.

Lethargic	Perplexed and suspicious
Restless	Talks too much
Omega sign	Confused
Delayed reaction time	Sleepy
Agitated	Fully awake
Emotional blunting	Recent memory deficit

151.   Three days after bowel surgery, over the course of a day, a patient becomes restless. She picks at her bed clothes and constantly tries to get out of bed. Most likely she has a _____.

152.   In conjunction with restlessness and agitation and a picture of "confusion," patients with acute diffuse cerebral dysfunction or a _____ often exhibit signs of sympathetic nervous system arousal. Their pulse is rapid; they are cold and clammy (peripheral vasoconstriction and increased sweating); they may hyperventilate; and they may have increases in blood pressure. Although cold - clamminess - rapid pulse - lethargy often signal "shock," they just as frequently imply _____.

344

146. perplexed, lethargic, confused, delayed

147. a. Perplexed
    b. Lethargic and sleepy
    c. Confused
    d. Rapid reaction time
    e. Delayed reaction time

148. agitation, agitation

149. level of consciousness

150. Lethargic   Perplexed and suspicious
     Restless   Talks too much
     Omega sign   Confused
     Delayed reaction time   Sleepy
     Agitated   Fully awake
     Emotional blunting   Recent memory deficit

151. delirium

152. delirium, delirium

153.   Delirious patients often misinterpret stimuli. A group of doctors and nurses discussing another patient become a conspiring group out to harm the delirious patient; shadows become menacing figures; changes in the daily routine become threats. Secondary delusional ideas can develop. Misinterpretation of actual real stimuli termed _____, and perceptions without real stimuli termed _____ are not uncommon. Delirious patients hallucinate in all sensory modalities. The most common sensory modality involved is visual.

154.   The perception of vague unformed sounds or lights without a real stimulus is an _____ _____. A hallucination that only occurs when a particular sensory modality is stimulated is a _____ _____. These phenomena are not infrequently observed in delirious patients.

155.   Circle the words or phrases characteristic of a delirious state.

Generally irreversible	Cannot focus well on incoming stimuli
Restless	Localized lesion
Diffuse	Deficit in short-term memory
Severe anxiety	Chronic
Acute	Sympathetic arousal
Elementary and functional hallucinations	Deficit in recent memory

156.   A 68-year-old man is brought to your clinic by his family because he has been shouting, not sleeping and saying "odd things that do not make sense." The patient enters the examining room furtively, looking about him in a perplexed manner. Although his eyes are widely open and his pupils somewhat dilated, he fails to focus on you as you speak. He is sweating and pale and unable to sit still. Despite a note by a physician that says the patient is "schizophrenic" you suspect a _____ _____.

157.   Delirious patients are often irritable, anxious, or suspicious. The moods often shift rapidly. This rapid shifting from one mood to another, or _____ _____ _____, is characteristic of many coarse brain disease processes.

158.   The patient in item #156 said odd things and did not make any sense when he spoke. The characteristic speech of delirium is unconnected associations which are non-goal directed. This is called _____ _____. Diagram this thought process disorder.

159.   Because of their reduced level of consciousness, delirious patients almost always exhibit some cognitive dysfunction associated with the frontal lobes. Concentration and global orientation are usually affected. Write a sentence on how you would test for concentration and global orientation.

153. illusions, hallucinations

154. elementary hallucination (pseudo hallucination acceptable, but not
     as accurate)
     functional hallucination

     If you had any difficulty with this question, please review the per-
     ceptual function section in Part I, starting with item 261.

155. Generally irreversible (Cannot focus well on incoming stimuli)
     (Restless)   Localized lesion
     (Diffuse)   (Deficit in short-term memory)
     (Severe anxiety)   Chronic
     (Acute)   (Sympathetic arousal)
     (Elementary and func-   (Deficit in recent memory)
      tional hallucinations)

156. Delirious state. (Upon examination, you discover the patient has
     had a myocardial infarction; he is hospitalized and treated; he
     should recover from both his infarction and his delirium.)

157. lability of affect

158. rambling speech

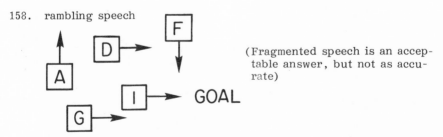

(Fragmented speech is an acceptable answer, but not as accurate)

159. Concentration is tested by asking the patient to do serial 7's, recall
     numbers forwards and backwards or spell simple 5-letter words back-
     wards; global orientation is tested by asking the patient to give the
     date, day of the week, year, locale.

347

160.   Write an M next to each item most characteristic of mania, an S
next to each item most characteristic of schizophrenia, a D next to
each item most characteristic of depression and a DL next to each
item most characteristic of delirium.

Early a.m. insomnia ____	Rambling speech ____
Neologisms ____	Flight-of-ideas ____
Hyperactivity ____	Delusions of guilt ____
Sympathetic arousal ____	First rank symptoms ____
Euphoria ____	Lethargy ____
Perplexity ____	Visual hallucinations ____

161.   Write an M next to each item most characteristic of mania, an S
next to each item most characteristic of schizophrenia, a D next to
each item most characteristic of depression and a DL next to each item
most characteristic of delirium.

Diurnal mood swing ____ (worse in a.m.)	Recent memory deficit ____
Clang associations ____	Paraphasias ____
Elementary hallucination ____	Psychomotor retardation ____
Thought broadcasting ____	Not alert ____
Hopelessness ____	Disorientation ____
Singing and dancing ____	

162.   Write an M next to each item most characteristic of mania, an S
next to each item most characteristic of schizophrenia, a D next to
each item most characteristic of depression and a DL next to each
item most characteristic of delirium.

Emotional blunting ___	Omega sign ____
Intrusive and importunate ____	Unfocused stare ____
Suicidal ____	Bright cheerful expression ____
Confused ____	Talks too much ____
Telling jokes and punning ____	Can't do serial 7's ____

163.   An acute, diffuse, usually reversible coarse cortical disease process
with some degree of reduced cortical arousal is termed a _____
A chronic, diffuse, usually irreversible coarse cortical disease process
is termed a _____.

164.   When a person insidiously develops a diffuse cortical brain dysfunction which is relatively unresponsive to treatment, he is said
to have a _____. This implies that pre-morbidly the person
was functioning reasonably well but that since the onset of the morbid process deterioration of function has occurred.

160. Early a.m. insomnia D
Neologisms S
Hyperactivity M
Sympathetic arousal DL
Euphoria M
Perplexity DL

Rambling speech DL
Flight-of-ideas M
Delusions of guilt D
First-rank symptoms S
Lethargy DL
Visual hallucinations DL

161. Diurnal mood swing D
(worse in a.m.)
Clang associations M
Elementary hallucinations DL
Thought broadcasting S
Hopelessness D
Singing and dancing M

Recent memory deficit DL

Paraphasias S
Psychomotor retardation D
Not alert DL
Disorientation DL

162. Emotional blunting S
Intrusive and importunate M
Suicidal D
Confused DL
Telling jokes and punning M

Omega sign D
Unfocused stare DL
Bright cheerful expression M
Talks too much M
Can't do serial 7's DL

163. delirium, dementia

164. dementia

165.   The following statements characterizing dementia are all true except (underline your answer):

    a. insidious onset with chronic course

    b. diffuse cortical dysfunction

    c. relatively unresponsive to treatment

    d. premorbid function is poor

    e. premorbid function is good

166.   A dementia can occur at any age. We are considering only some of the dementias which develop after puberty. Despite the etiology and age of onset, dementias have several common characteristics (139,169,171). List them.

167.   Circle the words or phrases most characteristic of dementia:

Acute	Insidious	Reversible
Chronic	Loss of previous function	Secondary to neoplasm
Localized	Widespread	

168.   Circle the words or phrases most characteristic of dementia:

Acute onset	Age-related
Multiple cortical areas involved	Involving only the frontal lobe
Usually irreversible	Poor functioning since birth
Insidious onset	

169.   Place a DE next to the items most characteristic of dementia and a DL next to the items most characteristics of delirium. You may have to indicate an item for both.

Insidious onset ____	Diffuse ____
Reversible ____	Loss of prior function____
Irreversible ____	Acute ____

170.   In major depression, slow speech and a paucity of thought are characteristic. In mania _____ speech and _____ _____ _____ are characteristic of the thought process. In delirium _____ _____ is characteristic of the thought process disorder. In dementia as in schizophrenia, _____ thought disorder is most often observed.

165. d

166. insidious onset, chronic course, widespread cognitive dysfunction,
relatively unresponsive to treatment, premorbid function is good

167. Acute   (Insidious)   Reversible

(Chronic)   (Loss of previous) Secondary to neoplasm
             function

Localized   (Widespread)

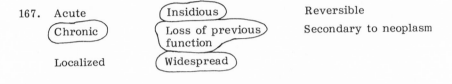

168. Acute onset   Age-related

(Multiple cortical areas involved)   Involving only the frontal lobe

(Usually irreversible)   Poor functioning since birth

(Insidious onset)

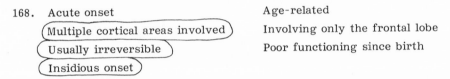

169. Insidious onset _DE_   Diffuse _DL,DE_
     Reversible _DL_   Loss of prior function _DL,DE_
     Irreversible _DE_   Acute _DL_

Again, keep in mind that the characterization of delirium as acute
and reversible and dementia as chronic and irreversible is _not_ without _many_ exceptions.

170. rapid, flight of ideas (too many thoughts), rambling speech, formal

171. In major depression, a restricted affect with a mood that is
_____ or _____ is characteristic. In mania, an expanded,
labile affect with moods of _____ or _____ is characteristic. In delirium, the mood most often seen is severe _____,
although irritability, suspiciousness and lability of affect are
not uncommon. In schizophrenia and often in dementia _____
_____ is the characteristic defect in affect. Demented
patients can also exhibit lability of affect.

172. The motor behavior seen in major depression is characteristically
_____. In mania, a major diagnostic motor sign is
_____. In delirium, often secondary to an intense mood, motor
_____ is seen. Although schizophrenics and people with
dementia tend to be awkward, and there are some characteristic gait
and other motor disturbances associated with individual dementing
processes, neither schizophrenia nor dementia has a characteristic
motor sign.

173. In major depression, mania and schizophrenia, orientation and
memory functions are usually intact. In delirium and dementia, orientation and memory function are _____ _____.

174. Part of the sad facial expressions of patients with major depression are the _____ sign and _____. Manics
often look bright-eyed, ecstatic; their skin is tight and flushed.
People in a delirium appear _____. The sign of emotional
blunting in schizophrenia is a face that is _____ and
_____. People who are demented may, like schizophre-
nics, have a _____ _____ face. People with
dementia may also have abnormal muscle tone (139,171) (which should
always be thoroughly tested). These patients can exhibit a sagging
facial expression when decreased tone is present.

175. The thought content associated with a major depression reflects
feelings of _____, _____, _____ and
_____. Manics often (but not always) have grandiose
ideas of great wealth, power, or stature. There is no characteristic
content in schizophrenia, delirium or dementia. "Bizarre" content
is not diagnostic.

352

171. sad, anxious, euphoria or irritability, anxiety, emotional blunting

172. hypoactive (slowed), hyperactivity, agitation

173. usually disturbed

174. Omega, Veraguth's folds, perplexed, expressionless, unblinking, expressionless

175. hopelessness, worthlessness, guilt, suicide

176. Complete the following chart by writing in each appropriate box the most characteristic clinical behaviors in each mental status area for each disorder.

	Depression	Mania	Schizophrenia	Delirium	Dementia
General Appearance					
Motor Behavior					
Affect					
Thought Processes					
Thought Content					
Memory and Orientation					

176.

Area	Depression	Mania	Schizophrenia	Delirium	Dementia
General Appearance	sad face Omega sign Veraguth's folds	bright-eyed flushed ecstatic	unblinking expression-less face	perplexed	unblinking expression-less face
Motor Behavior	slow hypoactive agitated	hyper-active	none	agitated	none sometimes gait or tonicity disturb-ance
Affect	sad or anxious restricted	euphoric irritable labile expansive	blunted	labile anxious	blunted or labile
Thought Processes	slow; paucity of thought	fast; flight-of-ideas	formal thought disorder	rambling	formal thought disorder
Thought Content	guilt hopeless-ness worthless-ness suicide	grandiosity	none	none	none
Memory and Concentration	mild or no deficit	mild or no deficit	mild or no deficit	deficit	deficit

FRONTAL LOBE SYNDROMES

Please review the sections on cognitive functions of the various lobes, Part I (items #335-397) before you proceed to this section.

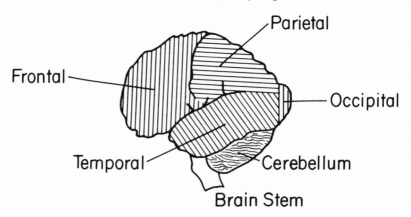

LATERAL (OUTSIDE) SURFACE OF BRAIN. LEFT HEMISPHERE

FOR REFERENCE TO ITEMS 177-281

177.   Coarse brain disease can present as an acute, diffuse, usually reversible process with some degree of reduced cortical arousal known as _____ , a chronic, diffuse, usually irreversible process or _____ , or a localized syndrome which can be either acute or chronic and which often results in significant behavioral changes and occasionally alteration of mood.

178.   In Part I you learned to evaluate cognitive function and relate specific dysfunctions to specific cortical regions. Localized brain disease will often result in syndromes composed of specific _____ dysfunction, specific _____ changes and some _____ alteration.

356

177. delirium, dementia

178. cognitive, behavioral, mood

179.   Unlike major depression, mania and schizophrenia, there are no
established, reliable and valid criteria for delirium and dementia.
DSM-III criteria (13) approach this standard, but further testing is
needed. List the criteria for the following:

Major Depression   Mania   Schizophrenia

180.   The frontal lobes rostral to (in front of) the motor areas have
executive function over other areas of the cerebral cortex (77 pp.
79-99, pp. 176-225). Unlike other cortical regions, the differentiation of the frontal lobes into dominant and non-dominant functions
is not clear-cut. Although language function is localized in the
_____ , usually the _____ frontal lobe, other frontal
lobe functions appear more diffuse.

179.

Major Depression	Mania	Schizophrenia
1. Sad or anxious mood	1. Hyperactivity	1. No diagnosable affective disorder
2. Three of the following (a through f)	2. Rapid/pressured speech	2. No coarse brain disease or hallucinogenic or stimulant drug use or systemic illness known to cause psychiatric symptoms
a. early a.m. waking	3. Irritable/euphoric mood	
b. diurnal mood swing (worse in a.m.)	4. No emotional blunting	
	5. No coarse brain disease, no psychostimulant drug abuse in prior month, no systemic illness known to cause manic symptoms.	3. Clear consciousness, memory and orientation intact (if one or both are impaired, this must be due solely to inattentiveness or poor concentration.
c. greater than 5 lb. weight loss in 3 weeks		
d. psychomotor retardation or agitation		4. One of the following:
e. suicidal thoughts or behavior		a. emotional blunting
f. feelings of guilt, self-reproach, hopelessness, worthlessness		b. formal thought disorder
		c. first rank symptoms (any one)
3. No coarse brain disease or use of steroids in the past month; no systemic illness known to cause depressive symptoms.		

180.   dominant, left

181.　　　In Part I, you learned to evaluate seven frontal lobe functions.
There were:

1. Global orientation
2. Concentration
3. Active perception
4. Motor regulation
5. Language
6. Judgment
7. Abstract thinking

What are the tasks you would ask of a patient to evaluate these
functions?

182.　　　List the frontal lobe functions which can be evaluated during the
mental status examination.

1. _____
2. _____
3. _____
4. _____
5. _____
6. _____
7. _____

In addition, the frontal lobes also regulate the functioning of other
cortical areas. They initiate, moderate and terminate complex higher
cortical functions.

183.　　　Circle the mental status tests of frontal lobe function:

Echophenomena	Calculations	Similarities
Copy simple shapes	"No ifs ands or buts"	Writing
Serial 7's	Recall words series	Repeat rhythms

184.　　　Draw lines between matching items in the two columns:

Identification of upside down objects	Motor regulation
Serial 7's	Language
"No ifs ands or buts"	Concentration
Similarities	Active perception
Draw circle	Abstract thinking

181. 1. Determine the date, place
      2. Do serial 7's
      3. Identify upside-down objects
      4. Perform motor tasks and observe the presence of perseveration, inertia
      5. Observe for the presence of Broca's aphasia (non-fluent, slow labored, dysarthric speech)
      6. Determine quality of patient's solution to real-life problems
      7. Test for ability to understand similarities or problem solve.

182. 1. Global orientation
      2. Concentration
      3. Motor regulation
      4. Judgment
      5. Language
      6. Active perception
      7. Abstract thinking

183.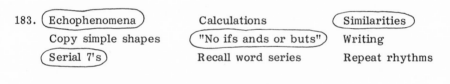

(Echophenomena)   Calculations   (Similarities)
Copy simple shapes   ("No ifs ands or buts") Writing
(Serial 7's)   Recall word series   Repeat rhythms

184.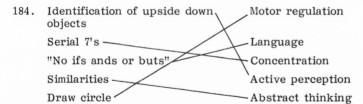

Identification of upside down objects   Motor regulation
Serial 7's   Language
"No ifs ands or buts"   Concentration
Similarities   Active perception
Draw circle   Abstract thinking

361

185.   Individuals with frontal lobe dysfunction often exhibit profound behavioral changes in addition to their inability to perform well on specific mental status tasks. Two major frontal lobe syndromes have been described: the convexity syndrome (affecting lateral or outside surfaces) and the orbito-frontal syndrome (affecting medial/orbital surfaces) (21,77,99 pp. 187-225, pp. 318-322, 115 pp. 131-134). The behaviors in these syndromes are often complex, but they reflect deficits in the basic functions of the frontal lobe and they can be elicited for diagnostic purposes. Once again, list the seven frontal lobe functions.

1. _____

2. _____

3. _____

4. _____

5. _____

6. _____

7. _____

186.   In Part I, I said that the frontal lobe acts like a futuristic computer which not only implements and monitors old programs but develops new programs as needed. This active planning requires drive, ambition, desire and the ability to follow through on these motivations. Although much of the energy and mood for this active planning originates in lower brain structures (limbic system and reticular activating system), it is expressed through the frontal lobes. Thus frontal lobe dysfunction can present as a loss of active planning, a loss of drive, ambition, desire and the ability to follow through on these motivations. Emotional blunting is an example of this loss and although it is a major diagnostic criterion for _____ it also reflects frontal lobe dysfunction and is the most obvious and frequent behavioral manifestation of the convexity (lateral surface) syndrome (21,77,115).

187.   The individual with lateral frontal lobe dysfunction termed the _____ appears apathetic and bland without initiative.

188.   Patients with the convexity syndrome often demonstrate a paucity of thought and a coarsening of personality characterized by an insensitivity to the feelings of others, being overly stubborn and set in one's ways and with a loss of concern for personal appearance, manners, present circumstances or future prospects. The convexity syndrome correlates with dysfunction in the _____ _____ _____.

189.   Lateral frontal lobe dysfunction producing the _____ _____ is characterized by a _____ of affect and a _____ of personality.

190.   In its typical form, the frontal lobe convexity syndrome is characterized by affective _____ and personality _____. In its less common form, the frontal lobe convexity syndrome is also characterized by catatonia and/or incontinence of urine and feces.

362

185. 1. Global orientation
     2. Concentration
     3. Motor regulation
     4. Judgment
     5. Language
     6. Active perception
     7. Abstract thinking

186. schizophrenia

187. convexity syndrome

188. lateral frontal lobe

189. convexity syndrome, blunting, coarsening

190. blunting, coarsening

191.   Circle the words or phrases consistent with a frontal lobe convexity syndrome:

Catalepsy   Euphoria   Unkempt and unclean

Paucity of thought   Construction apraxia Overly stubborn

"No ifs ands or buts" Emotional blunting

192.   The two major frontal lobe syndromes are the orbito-frontal syndrome (medial) and the _____ _____
        (_____).

193.   The cross-hatched area in the diagram would most likely result in which frontal lobe syndrome?

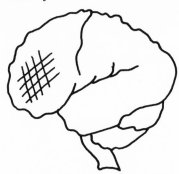

194.   The orbito-frontal syndrome usually reflects dysfunction in the medial and orbital surfaces of the frontal cortex (see the cutaway diagram A of the brain). In diagram B indicate where you might expect to find a lesion resulting in a frontal lobe convexity syndrome.

A   B

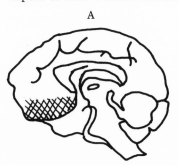   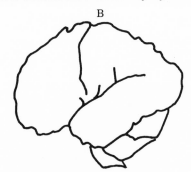

Medial Surface of   Lateral Surface of
Right Hemisphere   Left Hemisphere

195.   In the frontal lobe convexity syndrome the characteristic affective change is _____ _____. In the orbito-frontal syndrome, euphoria and irritability are most characteristic.

191.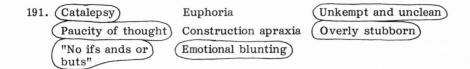
   Catalepsy   Euphoria   Unkempt and unclean
   Paucity of thought   Construction apraxia   Overly stubborn
   "No ifs ands or buts"   Emotional blunting

192. convexity syndrome (lateral)

193. convexity (lateral) frontal lobe syndrome

194.

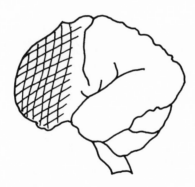

195. emotional blunting

196.   The euphoria seen in the orbito-frontal syndrome is often shallow, foolish and silly in quality. In Part I you learned a German
term for this mood: _____.

197.   Witzelsucht is the typical mood of the _____
_____ syndrome.

198.   Individuals with significant frontal lobe dysfunction often exhibit
a deficit in their ability to concentrate and attend to stimuli. They
become easily distracted by irrelevant stimuli. This inability to attend to stimuli or to persevere in a task can lead to uncontrolled associations. The patients will jump from topic to topic, commenting
upon everyone and everything in the immediate vicinity. This familiar thought disorder is _____. Although it is associated
with the disgnosis of _____ it can also be observed in individuals with disease of medial-orbital areas of the frontal lobe.

199.   Patients with dysfunction in the medial-orbital areas are often
unable to regulate their motor behavior. This can take the form of
intrusive and importunate behavior, hyperactivity, echophenomena
or rapid/pressured speech. (If you add this to flight-of-ideas, euphoria and irritability, you have a nice description of mania.) What
criterion for mania helps to distinguish a patient who is suffering
from manic-depressive illness from one with an orbito-frontal syndrome? (Hint: Think of the diagnostic criteria for mania.)

200.   The fact that patients with mania, depression, and
schizophrenia exhibit signs and symptoms similar in form to those
resulting from coarse brain disease, should not be surprising in light
of studies indicating that patients with those psychiatric conditions
have demonstrable brain dysfunction (2,4,51,76,84,115,136,153,156,
164,167). Although we have evidence for brain dysfunction in these
patients, no one knows the etiology of these conditions. What coarse
frontal lobe syndrome is likely to be confused with schizophrenia?
_____ and with mania? _____.

201.   Place a C next to the words or phrases characteristic of a frontal
lobe convexity syndrome and an O next to the words or phrases
characteristic of an orbito-frontal syndrome.

Apathy ____   Flight-of-ideas ____

Witzelsucht ____   Paucity of ideas ____

Unkempt/unclean ____   Distractible ____

Catalepsy ____   Intrusive and importunate ____

"No ifs ands or buts" ____   Overly stubborn ____

Hyperactive ____   Irritable ____

366

196. Witzelsucht

197. orbito-frontal

198. flight-of-ideas, mania

199. 1. No evidence of coarse brain disease. (Also, no evidence of stimulant drug use in the past month, or systemic illness known to cause similar abnormal changes).
2. The moods of mania are associated with a full affect, whereas the moods of the orbito-frontal syndrome are shallow and are associated with some emotional blunting.

200. convexity, orbito-frontal

201. Apathy C
Witzelsucht O
Unkempt/unclean C
Catalepsy C
"No ifs ands or buts" C
Hyperactive O

Flight-of-ideas O
Paucity of ideas C
Distractible O
Intrusive and importunate O
Overly stubborn C
Irritable O

202.   Identify the frontal lobe syndrome.

A 21-year-old man was brought to you by his parents for consultation because he sat in front of the television set throughout the day, had become progressively uncommunicative and was neglecting his personal hygiene. When examined, he sat in a stooped position, looking blankly at the floor. His face was without expression and he moved in a slow stiff manner. His hair was dishevelled, his clothes dirty and mucus stained. He picked his nose constantly during the examination. He was not embarrassed by his appearance, had no interests, did not seem to mind being examined and had no future plans. He spoke in short choppy sentences. When asked who else lived at home, he responded "mother, father, brother." He rarely used conjunctions or pronouns in his speech.

203.   Identify the frontal lobe syndrome.

A 54-year-old woman was hospitalized on a psychiatric ward because of assaultiveness. Following admission, she paced the halls engaging everyone she saw in conversation. When you tried to speak with her, she did not reply, but as soon as you moved on to another patient, she interrupted you with statements about her life, your appearance, the ward and other patients. Once she started to speak, you could interrupt her only with great difficulty. She then became angry, yelled and cursed at you. On one occasion, she tried to hit you but was restrained. On other occasions she laughed and joked but with little humor. She made silly comments about her hospitalization, although she thought her children had "railroaded" her. Despite your instructions to the contrary, she repeated your movements. She was disoriented. Her electroencephalogram and CT scan were both abnormal.

202. Convexity

203. Orbito-frontal

TEMPORAL LOBE SYNDROME

204.   You have learned about two frontal lobe syndromes, the
_____ _____ and the _____
_____ _____. Dysfunction in the temporal lobe also produces a distinct syndrome.

205.   Psychomotor epilepsy refers to a seizure process which manifests
itself in transient behavioral changes. Temporal lobe epilepsy is one
kind of psychomotor epilepsy specifically involving a seizure process
in one or both of the temporal lobes. Thus, whereas all temporal
lobe epilepsies are psychomotor, all psychomotor epilepsies are not
temporal lobe in origin (19,20,56,149). We will limit ourselves to the
temporal lobe syndromes (19,20,42,58,99 pp. 142-146, 115 pp. 29-45,
143,144).

206.   Temporal lobe seizures are of short duration (usually seconds,
occasionally minutes). Since they usually produce behavioral changes,
they are one form of _____ seizures.

207.   In addition to their _____ duration, temporal lobe seizures
produce an alteration in consciousness. This alteration is behav-
iorally manifested by a clouded or perplexed appearance.

208.   The characteristic duration of a temporal lobe seizure is
_____. Consciousness is _____ and usually manifested
by a _____ or _____ appearance.

209.   Patients with temporal lobe epilepsy typically have some memory
disturbance for the seizure and for events immediately preceding and
following the seizure. Although the memory deficit may span several
minutes or even hours, the usual seizure can be measured in
_____.

210.   When untreated, temporal lobe epilepsy tends to be recurrent.
These recurrent seizures have a characteristic duration, level of
consciousness and memory function. What are they?

370

204. convexity syndrome, orbito-frontal syndrome

205. No answer required

206. psychomotor

207. short

208. short, altered, clouded, perplexed

209. seconds

210. short duration, altered consciousness, memory deficit for the seizure and for events immediately preceding and following the seizure

211.   When a temporal lobe seizure is "typical" it presents little diagnostic difficulty. Some temporal lobe seizure disorders, however,
are preceded by prolonged behavioral changes, a prodromal period,
and/or followed by a postictal (post seizure) period, each of which
can last days or weeks. The total episode thus may easily last a
month and can be confused with schizophrenia, or less commonly
with mania. The typical seizure pattern, however, is characterized
by _____ .

212.   Temporal lobe seizures are of _____ duration, involve an
_____ in consciousness, result in some disturbance of
_____ and without treatment are _____ .
Which of these precludes the diagnosis of schizophrenia?

213.   During a temporal lobe fit patients often exhibit motor automatisms. Common motor automatisms are chewing and swallowing
movements or lip smacking. Patients may also suddenly get up
and walk around the room. Occasionally, more complicated
behaviors are observed. Patients may pour a glass of water,
write something, or put on an article of clothing. During this
period the patient is unresponsive and his speech is arrested
or stilted and stereotyped with stock words. Will the patient
recollect these behaviors?_____ Without adequate treatment,
will these behaviors most likely occur again?_____ What will
be the usual duration of the behaviors?_____

214.   The chewing and swallowing movements and lip smacking often
seen during temporal lobe fits are called _____ _____ .

215.   During a temporal lobe fit and while exhibiting motor automatisms,
the patient is _____ to your questions. When the fit is over he
has no _____ of the incident.

216.   Place an X over the brain area most likely involved in a patient
who exhibits motor automatisms, stock words and unresponsiveness
for several moments and then cannot remember these events.

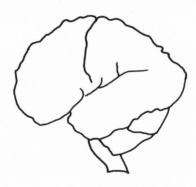

211. a short duration, alteration of consciousness, memory loss and recurrent episodes

212. short, alteration, memory, recurrent
alteration of consciousness, memory loss (acceptable as it "suggests"
coarse brain disease).

213. no, yes, short

214. motor automatisms

215. unresponsive, recollection

216.

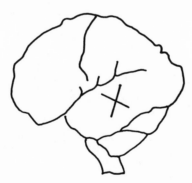

217.   Place an X over the brain area most likely involved in a patient who is apathetic, quiet, unkempt and who when asked to repeat "No ifs ands or buts" says: "No ifs buts."

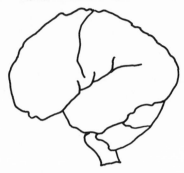

218.   The time period preceding the temporal lobe fit: the prodrome period, and the time following the fit: the postictal period, are usually much longer in duration than the actual seizure. Although patients often are unable to remember (are amnestic for) the fit, they can remember some of the events during the prodromal and postictal periods. Behaviors during these periods appear strange to the observer; they are often the cause of psychiatric hospitalization (143). Although transient, the behaviors observed during the psychomotor fit also can lead to psychiatric hospitalization. You have learned that stock words and motor _____ often occur and that during the fit the patient is _____ to external stimuli.

219.   Mood changes are associated with the temporal lobe syndrome. Sudden fear or violent angry outbursts can occur. These moods can develop during the period preceding the seizure; the _____, or during the period following the fit; the _____ period.

220.   Some evidence (16,51,52,62) suggests that psychomotor fits developing from seizures in the non-dominant temporal lobe are associated with depressive-like and manic-like episodes, whereas psychomotor fits developing from seizures in the dominant temporal lobe are associated with schizophrenic-like episodes. Usually the dominant temporal lobe is the _____.

221.   A patient with a depression secondary to seizure activity in the non-dominant temporal lobe most likely will have a lesion in the _____ hemisphere.

222.   A patient with a schizophrenic-like illness secondary to a seizure disorder most likely will have a lesion in the _____ hemisphere.

217.

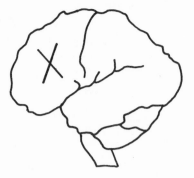

218. automatisms, unresponsive

219. prodrome, postictal

220. left

221. right

222. left (dominant)

223.   Perceptual disturbance and apophanous phenomena can also
occur in association with pre- and post-seizure periods. Olfactory,
tactile, visual and elementary auditory hallucinations are not uncommon. Patients also describe seeing whirling and moving lights and
changing colors; they may experience a darkening of vision and a
loss of three dimensional vision. Dysmegalopsia, when objects become larger, known as _____, or smaller, known as
_____, is also characteristic.

224.   Following a seizure, some epileptics suddenly leave their home
and drive or walk a significant distance, occasionally to another
town or city. This "automatic" travel occurs in an altered state of
consciousness and is called a fugue. As this fugue occurs after the
fit it is part of the _____ period. Not all fugue states,
however, reflect temporal lobe epilepsy.

225.   Memory disturbances are also commonly observed in temporal
lobe epileptics. False familiarity or _____, false unfamil-
iarity or _____, and anterograde amnesia are typical.

226.   Draw lines between matching items in the two columns. Items
on the left can be used more than once.

Convexity syndrome   Altered consciousness, memory
                          disturbance, motor automatisms

Temporal lobe epilepsy   Hyperactivity, over-talkativeness,
                          distractibility, irritable

Orbito-frontal syndrome   Rage reactions, stock words,
                          forced thinking, unresponsive,
                          recurrent

                          Apathetic, shallow moods, coars-
                          ening of personality

227.   Draw lines between matching items in the two columns. Items on
the left can be used more than once.

Orbito-frontal syndrome   Broca's aphasia, emotional blunting,
                          coarsening of personality

Convexity syndrome   Macropsia, jamais vu, amnesia,
                          transient episodes

Temporal lobe epilepsy   Lateral surface of frontal lobe,
                          paucity of ideas, overly stubborn

                          Importunate, intrusive, flight-of-
                          ideas

                          Perplexed, clouded, unresponsive,
                          fugue states

223. macropsia, micropsia

224. postictal

225. deja vu, jamais vu

226. Convexity syndrome   Altered consciousness, memory distur-
              bance, motor automatisms

   Temporal lobe epilepsy Hyperactivity, over-talkativeness,
              distractibility, irritable

   Orbito-frontal syndrome Rage reactions, stock words, forced
              thinking, unresponsive, recurrent

              Apathetic, shallow moods, coarsening
              of personality

227. Orbito-frontal syndrome Broca's aphasia, emotional blunting,
              coarsening of personality

   Convexity syndrome   Macropsia, jamais vu, amnesia, tran-
              sient episodes

   Temporal lobe epilepsy Lateral surface of frontal lobe, paucity
              of ideas, overly stubborn

              Importunate, intrusive, flight-of-ideas

              Perplexed, clouded, unresponsive,
              fugue states

377

228. Next to the appropriate word or phrase, place a T if it suggests a temporal lobe syndrome, a C if it suggests a frontal lobe convexity syndrome or an O if it suggests an orbito-frontal syndrome.

Anterograde amnesia ____   Dysmegalopsia ____

Apathy ____   Stock words or forced thinking ____

Deja vu ____   Broca's aphasia ____

Rage ____   Flight-of-ideas ____

Hyperactivity ____   Importunate, intrusive ____

Poor personal hygiene ____   Perplexed and clouded ____

229. In Part I you learned about a thought disorder in which associations are tightly linked, but take a circuitous route, filled with unnecessary associations, before reaching the goal. This disorder, termed _____, is often observed in chronic temporal lobe epileptics as part of their permanent, non-seizure behavior (16). This thought disorder is observable between, not during seizures.

230. Patients with chronic temporal lobe epilepsy develop other permanent behavioral changes in addition to circuitous speech, termed _____. One such behavior is a loss of sexual drive, as both frequency of sexual activity and interest in sex diminish. Decreased motor activity is termed hypoactivity, decreased sexual activity is termed _____ sexuality.

231. An individual with recurrent transient episodes of odd behaviors for which he has partial or complete memory deficit and who has lost interest in sex should be suspected of having _____ _____ _____.

232. Hypergraphia is a term to describe a voluminous increase in the amount one writes. Chronic temporal lobe epileptics can become hypergraphic. Frequently they maintain detailed notes or diaries of each day's experiences, their symptoms and thoughts about personal and world events. This writing is characterized by its perseverative, stilted style and by its endless use of unnecessary detail to make a point. This last characteristic is similar to the speech problem of these patients which is termed _____.

233. Patients with temporal lobe epilepsy without previous (premorbid) interest, can develop a perseverative fascination for vague philosophical and/or abstract religious topics. Over a period of a few years, interests can metamorphose from a few beers and a baseball game to the metaphysical universe and the nature of man. Ruminations on these subjects are typically without meaning. When these ruminations are recorded in an endless series of notebooks, the patient is said to also exhibit_____.

234. Permanent changes in one's pattern of speech, writing, thinking, and sexual activity can be observed in chronic temporal lobe epileptics. What are these changes? _____ _____, _____, _____ _____, _____.

228. Anterograde amnesia T   Dysmegalopsia T
      Apathy C   Stock words or forced thinking T
      Deja vu T   Broca's aphasia C
      Rage T   Flight-of-ideas O
      Hyperactivity O   Importunate, intrusive O
      Poor personal hygiene C   Perplexed and clouded T

229. circumstantial speech

230. circumstantial speech, hypo

231. temporal lobe epilepsy

232. circumstantial

233. hypergraphia

234. circumstantial speech, hypergraphia, over-abstract thinking, hyposexuality.

235.   Draw lines between matching items in the two columns. Items on the left can be used more than once.

Temporal lobe epilepsy	Stock words, forced speech, deja vu, dysmegalopsia, rage reaction
Convexity syndrome	Non-fluent aphasia, apathy, unkempt, urinary incontinence
Orbito-frontal syndrome	Circumstantiality, perceptual changes, transient odd behaviors
	Prodrome, depression with non-dominant dysfunction, episodes of unresponsiveness.
	Hypergraphia, religious conversion, hyposexuality
	Hyperactivity, flight-of-ideas, distractibility, poor concentration

236.   Next to the appropriate word or phrases, place a $\underline{T}$ if it suggests a temporal lobe syndrome, a $\underline{C}$ if it suggests a frontal lobe convexity syndrome, or an $\underline{O}$ if it suggests an orbito-frontal syndrome.

Lip-smacking ____   Witzelsucht ____

Transient ____   Overly stubborn ____

Fugue state ____   Stock words, forced speech ____

Urinary incontinence ____ Catalepsy ____

Paucity of ideas ____   Perplexed and clouded ____

Hyposexuality ____   Loss of drive and ambition ____

Dysmegalopsia ____   Deja vu, jamais vu ____

Unkempt, unclean ____   Amnesia for the event ____

Hyperactivity ____   Flight-of-ideas ____

Hypergraphia ____   Distractibility and poor concentration ____

237.   Identify the most likely area of cortical dysfunction.

A 28-year-old man was brought to the hospital by the police because he tried to break all the windows in a building across from his house. When the police found him, he was standing quietly and confused. Later that day, he had no recollection of the event but said this kind of experience had happened to him before.

235. Temporal lobe epilepsy ———— Stock words, forced speech, deja vu,
dysmegalopsia, rage reaction

Convexity syndrome ———— Non-fluent aphasia, apathy, unkempt,
urinary incontinence

Orbito-frontal syndrome ———— Circumstantiality, perceptual changes,
transient odd behaviors

Prodrome, depression with non-dominant
dysfunction, episodes of unresponsiveness

Hypergraphia, religious conversion,
hyposexuality

Hyperactivity, flight-of-ideas, distractibility, poor concentration

236. Lip smacking T
      Transient T
      Fugue state T
      Urinary incontinence C
      Paucity of ideas C
      Hyposexuality T
      Dysmegalopsia T
      Unkempt, unclean C
      Hyperactivity O
      Hypergraphia T

      Witzelsucht O
      Overly stubborn C
      Stock words, forced speech T
      Catalepsy C
      Perplexed and clouded T
      Loss of drive and ambition C
      Deja vu, jamais vu T
      Amnesia for the event T
      Flight-of-ideas O
      Distractibility and poor
      concentration O

237. temporal lobe - from the above information, it is impossible to de-
      termine right or left.

238.   Identify the most likely area of cortical dysfunction.

A 23-year-old man is referred to you because of episodic sadness, insomnia, anorexia with weight loss, and suicidal thoughts.
His fourth such episode occurred six months ago. Between
these episodes, he is generally in good health and feeling his
usual self except for transient periods of confusion during which
he nods his head in a rhythmic automatic fashion and smiles
in an odd way. His family says that during these episodes he
is unresponsive.

239.   Identify the most likely area of cortical dysfunction.

A 22-year-old man is brought to the clinic by his parents because
for the past year he has done nothing but sit in his room and
listen to records. He leaves his room only to eat and go to the
bathroom. He is slow moving, dirty, and dishevelled. He is
apathetic and denies any interest in anything other than listening to his records. His speech is slow, labored, and he has a
paucity of thoughts.

240.   Identify the most likely area of cortical dysfunction.

A 39-year-old man who sought hospitalization because he continually heard voices, coming from the ceiling, which discussed
his activities. These voices upset him and he contemplated suicide to "end their noise." Upon further questioning, he said
that he was also disturbed by sudden, brief periods when he
was unable to move his body but was forced (by some outside
"power") to speak and write things. His sister stated that she
had observed these episodes and that when one occurred, her
brother's speech was incomprehensible and he was unresponsive
to her efforts to communicate with him.

238. temporal lobe - probably non-dominant (because of associated depression)

239. convexity syndrome - lateral frontal lobe

240. temporal lobe epilepsy. Most likely in the dominant hemisphere because of associated speech disturbances and signs of a schizophrenic-like clinical picture.

PARIETAL LOBE SYNDROMES

241.   The parietal lobe is functionally organized to simultaneously synthesize symbolic, perceptual and motor processes. In general, the left or _____ parietal lobe controls verbal or symbolic abilities related to orientation and categorization whereas the right or _____ parietal lobe controls non-verbal motor perceptual abilities (40,99 pp. 147-186, 115 pp. 135-137).

242.   Dominant cerebral function generally refers to symbolic or _____ functions. Tests for specific dominant cerebral functions include:

Naming objects or testing for _____

Writing or testing for _____

Reading or testing for _____

Calculating or testing for _____

243.   Mental status cognitive function tasks to evaluate dominant parietal lobe function include _____ , _____ _____ , _____ , _____ , and _____ .

244.   In individuals with coarse brain disease, cortical dysfunction can range from a mild difficulty to the total absence of a particular function. The presence of acalculia, agraphia, finger agnosia and right-left disorientation point to a lesion in the _____ lobe. This condition is called Gerstmann's syndrome (40,57,112).

241. dominant, non-dominant

242. verbal
    anomia
    agraphia
    alexia
    acalculia

243. calculations, finger identification, right-left disorientation,
    reading, writing

244. dominant parietal

245.   Patients with dominant parietal lobe dysfunction often have difficulty grasping information as a whole or understanding difficult sentences (40,99 pp. 147-186). These patients lose the ability to organize and categorize. Sentences (thoughts) that require categorizing ("figuring out") are meaningless to patients suffering from this syndrome.

The following task tests the ability to organize and categorize:

Name these individuals: 1. "Your father's brother"

     2. "Your brother's father"

Testing for Gerstmann's syndrome also evaluates dominant parietal lobe function. If Gerstmann's syndrome is present, what dysfunctions would you expect to observe? (write them down)

246.   When told "Place your right hand on your left elbow," a patient hesitated, looked at both his hands, with great hesitation, he placed his left hand on his right ear. This response indicates the dysfunction of _____ and is suggestive of _____ _____ lobe dysfunction.

247.   An examiner pointed to a patient's fingers one at a time and asked: "What do you call this one?" Beginning with the right thumb, the patient responded: "Thumb...straight finger...second straight finger...index and outer or end finger." This is an example of _____ _____ and suggests dysfunction in the _____ _____ _____.

248.   Right/left disorientation and finger agnosia are two of four signs composing Gerstmann's syndrome. What are the other two?

249.   The lobe that simultaneously synthesizes non-verbal motor-perceptual abilities is the _____ _____ lobe.

250.   The inability to copy simple shapes is termed _____ and the inability to do simple tasks (such as dressing) is termed kinesthetic apraxia. These deficits are often observed in patients with non-dominant parietal lobe dysfunction (40,99 pp. 147-186).

251   Patients with non-dominant parietal lobe dysfunction may have difficulty in dressing themselves, making their beds, or feeding themselves. This inability to perform simple tasks is called a _____ _____.

252.   Patients with non-dominant parietal lobe dysfunction can have difficulty recognizing faces (17,107). What are some other difficulties due to non-dominant parietal lobe dysfunction?

253.   The non-recognition of faces is termed prosopagnosia. It reflects dysfunction in the _____ _____ _____.

245. acalculia, agraphia, finger agnosia, right-left disorientation

246. right-left disorientation, dominant parietal

247. finger agnosia, dominant parietal lobe.

248. dysgraphia, dyscalculia

249. non-dominant parietal

250. construction apraxia

251. kinesthetic (dressing) or motor apraxia

252. constructional apraxia, kinesthetic apraxia

253. non-dominant parietal lobe

254.   Finger agnosia is the non-recognition of one's fingers and is associated with dysfunction in the _____. The non-recognition of faces termed _____ is associated with dysfunction in the _____ _____ _____.

255.   Patients with prosopagnosia have difficulty recognizing _____. They may develop secondary delusional ideas concerning this "non-recognition" and may call family members and/or friends impostors or doubles and members of a "plot."

256.   A 27-year-old man said his mother was an impostor; that someone had "switched" her because her face was "different" from his "real" mother. This non-recognition, termed _____, has been given the psychiatric term Capgras' syndrome.

257.   The psychiatric term for the delusional idea that a familiar person is really an impostor is _____ syndrome.

258.   Many individuals with Capgras' syndrome actually have non-recognition of faces, termed _____, reflecting dysfunction in the _____ _____ _____ (11,17,75,107).

259.   Non-recognition of faces termed _____, is associated with dysfunction in the _____. The psychiatric term for this condition, when it is associated with secondary delusional ideas of familiar persons being "impostors" is _____.

260.   In addition to construction apraxia, dressing apraxia and prosopagnosia, patients with a dysfunction in the _____ lobe often guess in an uncontrollable manner when they are unable to recognize a correct perception. This replacement of direct correct perceptions by uncontrollable guesses is termed paragnosia (40).

261.   The following exchange took place between a patient and an examiner:

E: "Where are we now?"

P: (Looking about the emergency room) "I'm at McDonalds'."

E: "No, that's not right."

P: "A library?"

E: "No."

P: "A post office or a bus terminal?"

     This replacement of a direct perception by uncontrollable guesses is termed a _____.

254. dominant parietal lobe, prosopagnosia, non-dominant parietal lobe

255. faces

256. prosopagnosia

257. Capgras'

258. prosopagnosia, non-dominant parietal lobe

259. prosopagnosia, non-dominant parietal lobe, Capgras' syndrome

260. non-dominant parietal

261. paragnosia

262.   The following exchange took place between a patient and an examiner:

E: "You live with your parents?"

P: "My father, yes. I don't know who she is."

E: "What do you mean...Who she is? Isn't she your mother?"

P: "No way! Somebody else is inside of her. She's not the same. Her face is tilted or something."

This failure to recognize his mother's face is termed _____
The idea that someone else is inside her is the psychiatric syndrome termed _____ _____. The most likely area of cortical dysfunction is the _____ _____
_____.

263.   Another form of non-recognition associated with non-dominant parietal lobe dysfunction is the inability of an individual to recognize his own illness. This is termed anosognosia (168). Non-recognition of faces is termed _____ and non-recognition with wild guessing is termed _____.

264.   Denial, or non-recognition of illness, is termed anosognosia. It is associated with dysfunction in the _____
_____ _____.

265.   Check off tests of non-dominant parietal lobe function:

"Copy this object."   _____

"What finger is this?"   _____

"Put your shirt on."   _____

"Hold out your right hand...
Put your right hand on your
left ear."   _____

266.   Check off tests of dominant parietal lobe function:

"Copy the object."   _____

"Hold out your left hand...put
your left hand on your right
elbow."   _____

"Put your shoes on."   _____

"What finger is this?"   _____

262. prosopagnosia, Capgras' syndrome, non-dominant parietal lobe

263. prosopagnosia, paragnosia

264. non-dominant parietal lobe

265. "Copy this object."   ___√___
      "What finger is this?"   _____
      "Put your shirt on."   ___√___
      "Hold out your right hand...
      Put your right hand on your
      left ear."   _____

266. "Copy the object."   _____
      "Hold out your left hand...
      put your left hand on your
      right elbow."   ___√___
      "Put your shoes on."   _____
      "What finger is this?"   ___√___

267.　　The following exchange took place between a patient and an examiner:

E:　"How long has your left arm been paralyzed?"

P:　"It's not paralyzed! It's o.k."

E:　"I don't understand. You can't move it, can you?"

P:　"I pulled a muscle."

E:　"But you can't move it at all, not even your fingers!"

P:　"It's just temporary. I've not been sleeping."

E:　"You think you can't move it because you're tired?"

P:　"Yes."

E:　"There's nothing really wrong?"

P:　"Nothing."

　　　This patient's inability to recognize his paralyzed left arm is termed _____.

268.　　Patients with **parietal** lobe dysfunction may have trouble copying the examiner's movements. Ask the patient to do what you do.

1.　Extend left arm:

2.　Bend arm at elbow, hand open.

3.　Keep arm bent and make a fist.

4.　Repeat with right arm

　　　Inability to imitate these simple movements may indicate parietal lobe dysfunction opposite or contralateral to the arm/hand having difficulty (99 pp. 147-186). If a patient repeats your movements, despite instructions to the contrary, it is called _____ and indicates _____ lobe dysfunction.

269.　　Psychiatric patients often have difficulties copying simple figures even though they have no motor weakness. This is called _____ _____. When a patient cannot perform a simple motor task even though he has no motor weakness, he demonstrates a _____ _____.

270.　　Kinesthetic apraxia and construction apraxia are signs of dysfunction in the _____ _____ _____.

271.　　Capgras' syndrome is associated with the non-dominant parietal lobe dysfunction concerning non-recognition of faces or _____.

267. anosognosia

268. echopraxia, frontal

269. construction apraxia, kinesthetic (motor) apraxia

270. non-dominant parietal lobe

271. prosopagnosia

272.   Inability to recognize one's illness, termed _____,
is associated with non-dominant parietal lobe dysfunction.

273.   The substitution of a recognized perception by wild guesses
is termed _____.

274.   The presence of anosognosia, prosopagnosia, paragnosia,
construction apraxia, and kinesthetic apraxia strongly suggest
dysfunction in which cortical region? _____
_____ _____.

275.   Place a D-P for dominant parietal and N-P for non-dominant
parietal next to the appropriate items:

Construction apraxia _____   Kinesthetic apraxia _____

Right-left disorientation _____   Paragnosia _____

Finger agnosia _____   Acalculia _____

Capgras' syndrome_____   Dysgraphia _____

Anosognosia _____

276.   Identify the example of cortical dysfunction and give localization:

Unable to copy a cross   _____

Wild guesses replacing direct
perception   _____

Unable to recognize and name
fingers   _____

Unable to put left hand on
right ear   _____

Unable to imitate examiner's
hand and arm movements   _____

Unable to keep from imitating
examiner's arm movements   _____

Unable to dress oneself   _____

272. anosognosia

273. paragnosia

274. non-dominant parietal lobe

275. Construction apraxia N-P   Kinesthetic apraxia N-P
     Right-left disorientation D-P   Paragnosia N-P
     Finger agnosia D-P   Acalculia D-P
     Capgras' syndrome N-P   Dysgraphia D-P
     Anosognosia N-P

276. Unable to copy a cross   Construction apraxia, non-dominant
                                       parietal

     Wild guesses replacing
     direct perception   Paragnosia, non-dominant parietal

     Unable to recognize and
     name fingers   Finger agnosia, dominant parietal

     Unable to put left hand   Right/left disorientation,
     on right ear   dominant parietal

     Unable to imitate examiner's   Kinesthetic (motor) apraxia, contra-
     hand and arm movements   lateral parietal

     Unable to keep from imita-
     ting examiner's arm
     movement   Echopraxia, frontal

     Unable to dress oneself   Kinesthetic (motor) apraxia, non-
                                       dominant parietal

277.   Inability to do simple math (to calculate) is termed _____ and results from dysfunction in the _____ _____. It is one of our signs composing _____ syndrome. What are the other three?

278.   Check the appropriate box to indicate the brain region that relates best to each dysfunction.

Dysfunction	Frontal Lobe	Dominant Parietal	Non-Dominant Parietal
Acalculia			
Ideomotor apraxia			
Finger agnosia			
Echopraxia			
Poor concentration			
Construction apraxia			
Global disorientation			
Poor active perception			

277. acalculia, dominant parietal lobe, Gerstmann's, finger agnosia, right/left disorientation, dysgraphia

278.

Dysfunction	Frontal Lobe	Dominant Parietal	Non-Dominant Parietal
Acalculia		√	
Ideomotor apraxia	√ (if left hand only)	√	
Finger agnosia		√	
Echopraxia	√		
Poor concentration	√		
Construction apraxia			√
Global disorientation	√		
Poor active perception	√		

397

279.   Check the appropriate box to indicate the brain region that best relates to each dysfunction.

Dysfunction	Frontal Lobe	Dominant Parietal Lobe	Non-Dominant Parietal Lobe
Non-recognition of faces			
Acalculia			
Poor concentration			
Broca's aphasia			
Construction apraxia			
Agraphia			
Kinesthetic (dressing, motor) apraxia			
Echopraxia			
Can't do similarities			
Finger agnosia			
Can't define relationships			
Motor perseveration			
Dyslexia			
Can't identify upside-down objects			
Can't copy examiner's hand positions - both hands			
Can't do serial 7's			
Paragnosia			
Anosognosia			

279.

Dysfunction	Frontal Lobe	Dominant Parietal Lobe	Non-Dominant Parietal Lobe
Non-recognition of faces			√
Acalculia		√	
Poor concentration	√		
Broca's aphasia	√		
Construction apraxia			√
Agraphia		√	
Kinesthetic (dressing, motor) apraxia			√
Echopraxia	√		
Can't do similarities	√		
Finger agnosia		√	
Can't define relationships		√	
Motor perseveration	√		
Dyslexia		√	
Can't identify upside-down objects	√		
Can't copy examiner's hand positions - both hands		√	√
Can't do serial 7's	√		
Paragnosia			√
Anosognosia			√

280.   Identify the area of cortical dysfunction. List any cerebral dysfunctions you observe.

A 51-year-old woman was hospitalized because she called the police continuously complaining that strange people were "landing" on the beaches near her house in "an invasion". She also complained that there was someone masquerading as her son who came to her house and tried to convince her there was no invasion. Although she was standing in an active nursing station, her successive answers, when she was asked where she was, were: "post office...shopping center... library..." When she was told she was in a hospital, she laughed and said she was "never very good at geography and places".

281.   Identify the area of cortical dysfunction. List any cerebral dysfunctions you observe.

A 48-year-old man, college graduate, was hospitalized because of a false idea that he had murdered three people. When examined, he was unable to identify his fingers except for his thumbs. He could not do arithmetical problems involving carrying or borrowing steps; when asked to place his right hand on his left elbow, he placed his right hand on his right knee and repeated this error despite being told he was incorrect. He was able to print but he could no longer write in long hand.

400

280. non-dominant parietal lobe
Capgras' syndrome or prosopagnosia, paragnosia, anosognosia

281. Gerstmann's syndrome - dominant parietal lobe
finger agnosia, dyscalculia, right/left disorientation, dysgraphia

ANXIETY STATES (DSM-III TERM: ANXIETY DISORDERS)

282.   In a general medical practice nearly one-third of all patients seek help because of symptoms of anxiety (91 p. 31, 116). The morbidity risk for anxiety states in the general population has been estimated at 5% (35, 91 p. 31), making them one of the more common psychiatric conditions. The estimated general population morbidity risk for affective disorders is _____ and for schizophrenia is _____ .

283.   Anxiety is a fundamental mode of physiological response associated with emergency avoidance or attack (91, 143 pp. 85-103). Pathological anxiety, i.e., the anxiety states, is a group of disorders for which _____ of the general population is at risk.

284.   In man, at least, anxiety is both psychic, i.e., a subjective experience of a dysphoric mood, and somatic, i.e., with systemic signs and symptoms. The terms anxiety neurosis and anxiety states are synonymous. We will use the latter. What percent of the general population is at risk for these states? _____ . What percentage of patients coming to a general medical practitioner has complaints consistent with anxiety? _____ .

285.   In man, anxiety is both the subjective experience of a dysphoric mood, i.e., _____ anxiety, and the systemic signs and symptoms of anxiety, i.e., _____ anxiety.

286.   Acute anxiety is mediated by catecholamines, specifically adrenaline pathways. As yet, there is no known biochemical (physiological) understanding of chronic anxiety. An individual suffering from an acute anxiety attack experiences both the subjective experience of anxiety, _____ anxiety, and the physiological manifestation of a hyperadrenaline state known as _____ anxiety (91,116).

282. 2%, 0.3%

283. 4%

284. 5, 33

285. psychic, somatic

286. psychic, somatic

287.   Acute anxiety attacks can occur under stressful conditions in individuals without prior psychiatric history. When the stressful condition is resolved, the anxiety syndrome will also disappear and may never recur (35,91,116,175). The individual will remain symptom-free. This pattern of anxiety (or panic reaction) may not be an illness, but rather a response to stress inherent in all of us, with some individuals having greater liability, i.e., vulnerable to stress. As in all acute anxiety attacks, these stress reactions are biochemically mediated by _____ .

288.   Some acute anxiety attacks are merely exacerbations of chronic anxiety. Individuals with this pattern of symptoms will recover from the acute anxiety attacks but will remain ill with signs of chronic anxiety. The clinician cannot distinguish the isolated, stress-induced acute anxiety attack from the acute anxiety attack that is an exacerbation of a chronic condition (35,91,116, 117,143 pp. 85-103,175). Both types of acute attacks are clinically identical and both are biochemically mediated by _____(91,116).

289.   Some researchers (117) list 11 symptoms which are most frequently associated with acute anxiety. An <u>intense anxious mood</u> often associated with feeling of impending doom or death, a smothering or drowning feeling or <u>air hunger</u>, and a <u>discomfort</u>, tightness or pain in one's <u>chest</u> are three of the most common, and at least two of these three should be present to satisfy the diagnosis: acute anxiety attack. Can you clinically distinguish an acute anxiety attack which is an isolated stress response from one that is an exacerbation of a chronic condition?

290.   An intense anxious mood, air hunger and chest discomfort suggest the diagnosis of an _____ _____
_____ .

291.   To satisfy the diagnosis: acute anxiety attack, a patient should exhibit at least two of three major signs of anxiety. List these three signs:

   1.

   2.

   3.

287. adrenaline (catecholamine)

288. adrenaline (catecholamine)

289. No

290. acute anxiety attack

291. 1. Intense anxious mood
    2. Air hunger
    3. Chest discomfort

292.   Three major signs of acute anxiety are: _____
_____ _____, _____,
and _____. To satisfy the diagnosis: acute anxiety attack,
an additional three of the following eight signs should also be
present.

1. Lump in throat

2. Dizziness and/or faintness

3. Weakness and/or fatigue

4. Inward "shakiness"

5. Tremor

6. Paresthesias (pins and needles in fingers, toes and about
    the mouth)

7. Tachycardia (rapid heart beat) and/or palpitations

8. Vascular throbbing (usually with headaches)

293.   You are working at the emergency room and a 30-year-old man
is brought in on a stretcher. He is breathing rapidly, trembling,
holding his head and saying, "I'm going to die, I'm going to die."
He complains of chest tightness, air hunger, a tightness in his
throat and a coldness and numbness in his hands and feet. His
heart rate is 120 bpm, respirations 34 pm, blood pressure 140/85
mm Hg. His EKG, all laboratory tests and other physical findings
are all within normal limits. The most likely diagnosis is acute
anxiety attack. Circle the information which satisfies the criterion
"two out of three." Underline the information which satisfies the
criterion "three out of eight."

294.   Circle the words or phrases characteristic of acute anxiety.

Emotional blunting	Fear of impending doom	Paresthesias
Diurnal mood swing	Inward shakiness	Delusional mood
Dizziness	Vascular throbbing	Euphoria

295.   Circle the words or phrases characteristic of acute anxiety.

Smothering feeling	Verbigeration	Tremor
Fatigue	Air hunger	Flight-of-ideas
Lump in throat	Clang associations	Faintness
Tachycardia	Delusional perception	Chest pain

292. intense anxious mood, air hunger, chest discomfort

293. You are working at the emergency room and a 30-year-old man is brought in on a stretcher. He is breathing rapidly, trembling, holding his head and saying, "I'm going to die, I'm going to die." He complains of chest tightness, air hunger, a tightness in his throat and a coldness and numbness in his hands and feet. His heart rate is 120 bpm, respirations 34 pm, blood pressure 140/85 mm Hg. His EKG, all laboratory tests and other physical findings are all within normal limits.

294. Emotional blunting   Fear of impending doom   Paresthesias
     Diurnal mood swing   Inward shakiness   Delusional mood
     Dizziness   Vascular throbbing   Euphoria

295. Smothering feeling   Verbigeration   Tremor
     Fatigue   Air hunger   Flight-of-ideas
     Lump in throat   Clang associations   Faintness
     Tachycardia   Delusional perception   Chest pain

407

296.   Underline the three signs, two of which must be present to satisfy the first diagnostic criterion for acute anxiety attack. Then circle the eight signs, three of which must be present to satisfy the second diagnostic criterion for acute anxiety attack.

1. Dizziness

2. Tachycardia

3. Chest discomfort

4. Vascular throbbing

5. Air hunger

6. Tremor

7. Inward shakiness

8. Intense anxious mood

9. Lump in throat

10. Paresthesias

11. Weakness

297.   Intense anxious mood, air hunger, and chest discomfort are signs of acute anxiety. List the additional eight signs, three of which should also be present to satisfy the diagnosis of acute anxiety attack.

298.   List the 11 clinical signs associated with the diagnosis of acute anxiety attack. Circle those signs from which two of three are required and underline those signs from which three of eight are required.

299.   Because anxiety is a fundamental physiological response associated with "flight/fight" mechanisms, many of the physical signs and symptoms of anxiety in their milder form have adaptive value in stress situations. In its severe form, anxiety is experienced subjectively as a feeling of dysphoria, termed psychic anxiety and as physical symptoms termed _____ anxiety.

300.   Anxiety is a normal physiological response to stress and is associated with the _____ mechanism.

296. 1. (Dizziness)
     2. (Tachycardia)
     3. Chest discomfort
     4. (Vascular throbbing)
     5. Air hunger
     6. (Tremor)
     7. (Inward shakiness)
     8. Intense anxious mood
     9. (Lump in throat)
    10. (Paresthesias)
    11. (Weakness)

297. 1. Lump in throat
     2. Dizziness and/or faintness
     3. Weakness and/or fatigue
     4. Inward "shakiness"
     5. Tremor
     6. Paresthesias (pins and needles in fingers, toes and about the mouth)
     7. Tachycardia (rapid heart beat) and/or palpitations
     8. Vascular throbbing (usually with headaches).

298. 1. (Intense anxious mood)
     2. (Air hunger)
     3. (Chest discomfort)
     4. Lump in throat
     5. Dizziness and/or faintness
     6. Weakness and/or fatigue
     7. Inward "shakiness"
     8. Tremor
     9. Paresthesias (pins and needles in fingers, toes and about the mouth)
    10. Tachycardia (rapid heart beat) and/or palpitations
    11. Vascular throbbing (usually with headaches).

299. somatic

300. flight/fight

301.   Acute anxiety is biochemically mediated by _____.
This compound has specific effects on many body organs which
results in clinical signs we associated with somatic anxiety. However, the subjective feeling of dysphoria, termed _____
anxiety is not clearly related to any known biochemical substrate.

302.   In preparation for a flight/fight response, the organism requires optimal functioning:

   Bulging eyes (exophthalmos) and dilated pupils (mydriasis)
   insure optimal vision.

   As in most somatic signs of anxiety, exophthalmos and
mydriasis are responses to the compound_____.

303.   Peripheral vasoconstriction, resulting in pale and/or cold
skin, insures reduction of possible blood loss during an emergency,
flight/fight situation. Two other adrenaline responses insuring
optimal vision are:

304.   During flight/fight peripheral vasoconstriction insures _____
_____ _____. This may cause the skin to look
_____ and feel _____.

305.   In addition to insuring a reduction of blood loss via the
process of _____ _____, blood is also shunted
to the larger muscles preparing them for emergency action.

306.   During a flight/fight situation, what happens to the body's
blood?

307.   During a flight/fight situation, what happens to the eyes?

308.   In hopes of bluffing the enemy, mammals try to increase their
apparent size by standing their hair "on end" (pilerection). Humans, with the same number of hair follicles as apes, but with fine
hair, also pilerect their hair when stressed. We term this "goose
bumps" or "goose flesh" and it is another sign of the body's
preparation for _____.

309.   Increased adrenaline, released under stress, also results in
increased cardiac rate and output and increased respiratory rate.
Thus, more blood can be pumped to the working muscles and more
oxygen provided for fuel. What other changes occur in the
vascular system?

310.   In preparation for flight or fight the organism needs to be fully
alert. Muscle tone increases (sometimes causing tremors) to pre-
pare for action. What else happens to the muscles?

301. adrenaline, psychic

302. adrenaline

303. exophthalmos (bulging eyes), mydriasis (dilated pupils)

304. reduced blood loss, pale, cold

305. peripheral vasoconstriction

306. It is shunted to large muscles and peripheral vasoconstriction occurs.

307. They bulge and the pupils are dilated.

308. flight/fight

309. Blood is shunted to the larger muscles and away from the periphery
via peripheral vasoconstriction.

310. Blood is shunted to the larger ones.

311.   Circle those words or phrases consistent with a state of preparedness for flight/fight.

Tachycardia   Flushed

Sleepiness   Pallor

Goose flesh   Muscle tremors

Rapid breathing   Pin-point pupils

Dilated pupils   Wide-eyed

312.   Draw lines to match the items in the two columns.

Peripheral vasoconstriction   Goose bumps

Increased muscle tone   Pale and cold

Mammalian bluff   Tremors

More fuel to work   Increased rate of breathing
                                     and increased heart rate

313.   Now you will no longer be surprised to see a pale anxious patient who is rapidly and continuously looking about the room in a wide-eyed, alert manner; you will recognize the trembling and "goose flesh" in a _____ situation.

314.   There are several other clinical signs which can occur in acutely anxious patients. Adrenaline increases cardiac_____ and _____. This can lead to transient hypertension (systolic), irregular heart beat (cardiac arrhythmias), palpitations (feeling one's heart beat) and vascular throbbing often with head-aches.

315.   Circle the signs and symptoms which result from the cardio-vascular changes associated with a flight/fight situation.

Tachycardia   Palpitations

Lethargy   Irregular heart beat

Flushed skin   Diarrhea

Pale skin   Cold skin

Exophthalmos   Transient systolic hypertension

Pilerection   Mydriasis

Muscular tremors   Vascular throbbing

316.   Additional adrenaline responses include sweating, dry mouth, urgency and/or urinary incontinence, increased intestinal motility, and diarrhea. They are obviously not all adaptively advantageous and occur in the extreme when an effective _____ preparation and reaction cannot take place. In humans, this in-effective response is associated with the mood of anxiety.

317.   Sweating and a dry mouth are often experienced when anxiety is great. Because of the other adrenaline responses you have learned about, will the skin feel hot and moist or cold and moist?

412

311. 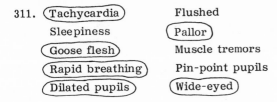 Flushed
     Sleepiness   (Pallor)
     (Goose flesh)   Muscle tremors
     (Rapid breathing)   Pin-point pupils
     (Dilated pupils)   (Wide-eyed)

312.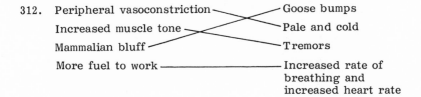

Peripheral vasoconstriction —— Goose bumps
Increased muscle tone —— Pale and cold
Mammalian bluff —— Tremors
More fuel to work —————— Increased rate of breathing and increased heart rate

313. flight/fight

314. rate, output

315. (Tachycardia)   (Palpitations)
     Lethargy   (Irregular heart beat)
     Flushed skin   Diarrhea
     (Pale skin)   (Cold skin)
     Exophthalmos   (Transient systolic hypertension)
     Pilerection   Mydriasis
     Muscular tremors   (Vascular throbbing)

316. flight/fight

317. cold and moist

318.   Increased intestinal motility with cramping and diarrhea and
increased urinary output (because of increased cardiac output)
with urgency and urinary incontinence can occur when anxiety
levels are extremely high. Thus, although the flight/fight mechanism has great adaptive value, it can in some individuals be subverted
into acute anxiety attacks which can become recurrent. What percent of the general population is at risk for such a disorder? _____
What percent of general medical practice patients seek help for
symptoms consistent with this disorder? _____ Can you
clinically distinguish the spontaneous isolated acute anxiety attack
from the acute anxiety attack which is an exacerbation of a chronic
anxiety state? _____

319.   List the diagnostic criteria for acute anxiety.

Two of the following three: _____

                                 _____

                                 _____

Three of the following eight: _____

                                 _____

                                 _____

                                 _____

                                 _____

                                 _____

                                 _____

                                 _____

320.   Circle all the signs associated with acute anxiety.

Abdominal cramps   "Runny nose"

Lethargy   Dilated pupils

Goose flesh   Hypertension

Bed wetting   Rapid breathing

Dry mouth   Muscle tremors

Clouded consciousness   Dizziness

Air hunger   Paucity of thought

Chest discomfort   Cold, moist skin

Dysmegalopsia   Palpitations

Vascular throbbing   Wide-eyed

Diarrhea   Witzelsucht

Sleepiness

318. 5%, 33%, No

319. Two of the following three:

Intense anxious mood
Air hunger
Chest discomfort

Three of the following eight:

Dizziness
Tachycardia
Vascular throbbing
Tremor
Inward shakiness
Lump in throat
Paresthesias
Weakness

320. (Abdominal cramps)
Lethargy
(Goose flesh)
(Bed wetting)
(Dry mouth)
Clouded consciousness
(Air hunger)
(Chest discomfort)
Dysmegalopsia
(Vascular throbbing)
(Diarrhea)
Sleepiness

"Runny nose"
(Dilated pupils)
(Hypertension)
(Rapid breathing)
(Muscle tremors)
(Dizziness)
Paucity of thought
(Cold, moist skin)
(Palpitations)
(Wide-eyed)
Witzelsucht

321.　　For convenience's sake (rather than on the basis of data) we can divide chronic anxiety states into two groups: 1) the phobic anxiety states and 2) the simple anxiety states. Phobic anxiety states are associated with an exaggerated fear usually of a non-dangerous object or situation. Simple anxiety states are termed as such because they are present without phobias. The pathological mechanisms underlying chronic anxiety are not known. Acute anxiety is mediated by the _____ pathways.

322.　　Chronic anxiety states can be divided into conditions with or without an associated exaggerated fear (usually of a non-dangerous object or situations). Such an "exaggerated fear" is termed a

_____.

323.　　Chronic anxiety states can be divided into _____

_____ states and _____ _____
states.

324.　　Chronic anxiety states associated with exaggerated fears (usually of a non-dangerous object or situation) are termed

_____ _____ _____.

325.　　Phobic anxiety states can be separated into:

1. Specific animal phobias

2. Specific situational phobias

3. Phobic-anxiety-depersonalization syndrome (PAD).

4. Agoraphobia

　　Specific animal and situational phobias differ only in content not in form and will be considered together. Both conditions can present as acute anxiety attacks but only when the affected individual is in proximity to the phobic object or situation. They are chronic only in the sense that even after many years the affected individual will always develop severe anxiety when in the phobic setting. Describe the signs you might find in a phobic person in proximity to the phobic object or situation.

326.　　Acute animal and acute situational phobias differ from each other only in _____. Write the definition of a phobia.

327.　　Acute animal phobias are exaggerated fears of such animals as: dogs, cats, horses, rabbits, mice, snakes, flies, and spiders. In a room where the phobia-producing animal is caged and totally harmless, the phobic patient nevertheless responds with acute anxiety. The patient is aware of the exaggeration of his response, knows it is unwarranted, perceives it as a symptom but cannot do anything about it other than avoid the object or situation. Acute situational phobias are exaggerated fears of situations such as public speaking or riding a train, car, plane, or boat or being in a high place or a small space. Here also, the patient is aware of the unwarranted exaggeration of his response, perceives it as a symptom but cannot stop the anxiety response when placed in the phobic situation or when the phobic situation is anticipated (47, 91,103,104,122,175).

416

321.	catecholamine (adrenaline)

322.	phobia

323.	phobic anxiety, simple anxiety

324.	phobic anxiety states

325.	1.	Intense anxious mood often associated with the feeling of impending death or doom
	2.	Smothering or drowning feeling, or air hunger
	3.	Chest discomfort, tightness or pain
	4.	Lump in throat
	5.	Dizziness and/or faintness
	6.	Weakness and/or fatigue
	7.	Inward "shakiness"
	8.	Tremor
	9.	Paresthesias
	10.	Tachycardia and/or palpitations
	11.	Vascular throbbing

326.	content. A phobia is an exaggerated fear, usually of a non-dangerous object or situation.

327.	no answer required

328.   Acute animal and situational phobias often begin in childhood
between the ages of 5 and 7 (47,103-105,122,175). Usually they
resolve spontaneously; occasionally they persist into adult life
(47,104,122,175). What is the phobic patient's attitude about his
phobia?

329.   Specific animal and situational phobias are most often circumscribed, i.e., there is little exaggerated anxiety outside the phobic
situation (104,122). At what age is the onset of these conditions
most likely to occur?

330.   An individual with a specific animal or situational phobia is
most frequently free from unusual anxiety when away from the
phobia inducing object or situation. Only in proximity to the phobic
object or situation does the individual develop exaggerated anxiety.
Because of their restricted nature which are object or situation-
specific, these phobias are said to be _____.

331.   Individuals with specific animal or situational phobias rarely
are fearful of more than one object or situation. They rarely have
more than one phobia, they are monophobic (104,122). Because
they have little unusual anxiety, except in the phobic situation,
their phobias are said to be _____.

332.   Individuals with a single isolated exaggerated fear are said to
be _____. If their anxiety is limited to the phobic
object or situation, it is said to be _____. In tests of
physiological response to stress, anxiety levels at rest and psychological profiles, individuals with specific animal or situational
phobias cannot be differentiated from normal controls (47,91,103,
104,122). These phobias have an excellent response to treatment
(47,91,103-105,122).

333.   Each of the following statements about individuals with specific
animal and situational phobias is true except (underline your
answer):

a)   They exhibit little excessive anxiety away from the
     phobic object or situation

b)   Physiologically and psychologically they cannot be
     differentiated from normal controls

c)   Their phobias are treatment responsive

d)   Their phobias usually developed around ages 5 to 7

e)   They usually have several phobias

334.   Circle the words or phrases most characteristic of specific
animal and situational phobias:

Good response to treatment   Circumscribed

Abnormal psychological profile   Often begins in later life

Often monophobic   Anxiety symptoms different
                                    from normal anxiety

418

328. He realizes it is an exaggerated or unwarranted fear but he cannot stop the anxiety response except by avoiding the phobic object or situation.

329. childhood, ages 5 to 7

330. circumscribed

331. circumscribed

332. monophobic, circumscribed

333. a) They exhibit little excessive anxiety away from the phobic object or situation
     b) Physiologically and psychologically they cannot be differentiated from normal controls
     c) Their phobias are treatment responsive
     d) Their phobias usually developed around ages 5 to 7
     e) They usually have several phobias

334. (Good response to treatment)   (Circumscribed)
     Abnormal psychological profile   Often begins in later life
     (Often monophobic)   Anxiety symptoms different
                                            from normal anxiety

419

335.   Agoraphobia is a phobic anxiety state which appears to be qualitatively different from the circumscribed monophobic and easily treatable _____ _____ and _____ phobias (35,47,91,122,143 pp. 85-103, 145, 175).

336.   Agoraphobia literally means "fear of the marketplace" (47,102-105,122,145). It has come to mean an exaggerated fear of any open (out-of-doors) space. Specific animal and situational phobias typically develop around ages _____ to _____. In contrast, agoraphobia usually develops between the ages of 15 and 35. The peak decade is 20 to 30 (47,102-105,122,143 pp. 85-103,145).

337.   Specific animal/situational phobias characteristically develop in childhood. Agoraphobia characteristically develops between ages _____ to _____ with a peak between ages 20 and 30.

338.   An individual who becomes phobic around age 25 is more likely to have which condition (circle one)?

          Specific animal phobia

          Specific situational phobia

          Agoraphobia

339.   The typical agoraphobic can often describe the exact moment of onset of the condition: "I was going shopping, and I suddenly felt weak...I thought I was going to fall or faint and had to go home." Several further trips out-of-doors with similar reactions and growing anxiety usually follow this rather benign onset. Within a year, most such individuals are house-bound, fearful of leaving for any reason, and panic-stricken if forced by circumstances to travel even one or two blocks. Unlike individuals with specific animal and situational phobias, agoraphobics continue to have high levels of anxiety (generalized anxiety) even when home, away from the phobic situation. Thus their anxiety is not limited and their phobia cannot be said to be _____.

340.   The sex distribution is not strikingly skewed in individuals with specific animal and situational phobias. However, more than two-thirds of agoraphobics are women (128). What is the phobic situation for agoraphobics?

341.   Individuals with the specific animal and situational phobias can/cannot (circle one) be differentiated from the normal controls on physiological tests of resting anxiety levels, nor in their response to stress and psychological profile, whereas agoraphobics are markedly different from the norm, significantly more anxious at rest, less adaptable to repeated stress and more "neurotic" and "introverted" on psychological testing (47,102-105,122,143 pp. 85-103,145). To top off a bad picture, their response to treatment is poor (47,102,105,122,143 pp. 85-103,145,165).

420

335. specific animal, situational

336. 5, 7

337. 15 to 35

338. specific animal phobia
     specific situational phobia
     (agoraphobia)

339. circumscribed

340. fear of any open, out-of-door space

341. cannot

342.   Circle those words or phrases most consistent with agoraphobia:

Female   Circumscribed anxiety   Onset 15 to 35

Onset 5 to 7   Peak onset 20 to 30   Male

Generalized anxiety   Good response to   Poor response to
                      treatment   treatment

Psychologically and
physiologically
abnormal

343.   Although the content varies from individual to individual, people
with specific animal/situational phobias characteristically have only
one phobia. They are _____. Although agoraphobics are
also monophobic their phobic content is always _____
and their anxiety is not _____.

344.   Place an A next to the words or phrases characteristic of
agoraphobia and an S next to the words or phrases characteristic
of specific animal (or situational) phobia:

Onset in childhood_____   Circumscribed _____

Fear of spiders_____   Fear of public speaking_____

Poor treatment response _____   Good treatment response_____

                                     Fear of open spaces _____

2/3 are women_____   Differs physiologically
                                     from norm_____

Much generalized anxiety _____

345.   Both agoraphobics and individuals with specific animal or
situational phobias can develop acute anxiety attacks. These acute
attacks are indistinguishable in these two patient groups and only
a careful history will determine the diagnosis. What are the characteristics of specific animal/situational phobias that differentiate
them from agoraphobics? Write down the distinguishing features
for each condition in the following categories: (1) sex ratio,
(2) age of onset, (3) generalization of anxiety, (4) content of
phobias, (5) physiological and psychological profile, and (6) response to treatment.

346.   The last phobic state we will consider is called phobic-anxiety-
depersonalization (PAD) syndrome. The sex-ratio is similar to
agoraphobia, 75 percent of the people suffering from PAD are

_____.

347.   Like individuals with agoraphobia, people with PAD syndrome
can be differentiated from the normal control on physiological
measures of resting anxiety, response to repeated stress, and psychological profile (102,129,143 pp. 85-103,145). These differences
from the norm are in contrast to _____ phobics who cannot be
distinguished from controls.

422

342. (Female)   Circumscribed anxiety   (Onset 15 to 35)

   Onset 5 to 7   (Peak onset 20 to 30)   Male

   (Generalized anxiety)   Good response to treatment   (Poor response
   (Psychologically and   to treatment)
   physiologically
   abnormal)

343. monophobic, fear of open space, circumscribed

344. Onset in childhood S   Circumscribed S
      Fear of spiders S   Fear of public speaking S
      Poor treatment response A   Good treatment response S
      2/3 are women A   Fear of open spaces A
      Much generalized anxiety A   Differs physiologically from
                                       norm A

345.
      1. Sex ratio almost equal   1. 2/3 women
      2. Onset in childhood (5 to 7   2. Onset in young adulthood
          years)   (15 to 35, peak 20 to 30)
      3. Circumscribed anxiety   3. Generalized anxiety
      4. Content varies yet   4. Content always fear of open
          monophobic   spaces
      5. Physiologically and   5. Physiologically and psycho-
          psychologically same as   logically different from nor-
          normal controls   mal controls
      6. Responsive to treatment   6. Unresponsive to treatment

346. female

347. specific animal/situation

423

348.   Unlike specific animal and situational phobias, agoraphobia and PAD syndromes most frequently begin between the ages of _____ and _____ (102,129,143 pp. 85-103, 145).

349.   Onset of agoraphobia and PAD syndrome before puberty or after age _____ is extremely rare, and when it occurs you should always first consider other neuropsychiatric and systemic conditions.

350.   In the PAD syndrome, the P stands for _____, the A stands for _____ and the D for _____.

351.   The typical PAD syndrome begins with a stress event, resulting in sudden intense anxiety or "emotional shock" (fainting is common). This is followed by a period of depersonalization of varying duration, sometimes hours or days, sometimes weeks or months during which the patient feels "detached," "as if in a dream," "foggy around the edges," "as if in slow motion," "above in the air watching myself." Exacerbations of depersonalization will then occur periodically through-out the course of the illness. From its name, you could also ex-pect two other chronic or exacerbating behaviors. They are _____ and _____.

352.   Sometime after the initial "shock" and depersonalization episode, the person with PAD syndrome develops increasing daily tension. This anxiety is generalized and pervasive. Periodic, acute anxiety attacks is not an uncommon course. As this anxiety is generalized, PAD syndrome, as well as agoraphobia, differs markedly from simple animal/situational phobias where the anxiety is _____.

353.   In the PAD syndrome phobias usually develop. Multiple phobias (situational or animal) are common, are often transient, and are never the core complaint. Since patients with PAD syndrome have multiple phobias they differ markedly from simple animal/situational phobics who have a disorder termed _____.

354.   The PAD syndrome course can be diagrammed as follows:

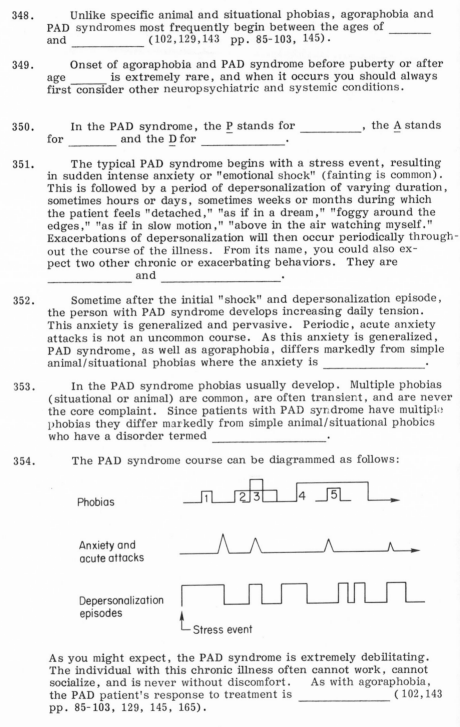

Phobias

Anxiety and acute attacks

Depersonalization episodes

Stress event

As you might expect, the PAD syndrome is extremely debilitating. The individual with this chronic illness often cannot work, cannot socialize, and is never without discomfort. As with agoraphobia, the PAD patient's response to treatment is _____ (102,143 pp. 85-103, 129, 145, 165).

424

348. 15, 35

349. 35

350. phobic, anxiety, depersonalization

351. phobias, anxiety

352. circumscribed

353. monophobic

354. poor

425

355.   PAD syndrome is familial (it runs in families) with 20 percent of patients having a positive family history (47,102,129,141 pp. 103-106, 143 pp. 85-103, 145). As in agoraphobia, the usual age of onset range is _____ to _____ with the peak decade being _____ to _____.

356.   Complete the following table by checking the appropriate box to match the clinical statement to the syndrome with which it is most likely associated. Some clinical statements can be checked more than once.

	Specific Animal/ Situational Phobia	PAD Syndrome	Agoraphobia
Onset in childhood			
Physiologically abnormal			
Good treatment response			
Little generalized anxiety			
Monophobic			
Episodes of depersonal- ization			
Episodes of acute anxiety			
Poor treatment response			
Circumscribed anxiety			
Approximately 70-80% are women			
Onset in early adulthood			
Psychic and somatic anxiety			
Much generalized anxiety			

357.   The anxiety state called neurasthenia has many synonyms. Some of these are "neurocirculatory asthenia," "cardiac neurosis," "effort syndrome," "anxiety neurosis," "Da Costa's syndrome," "vasoregulatory asthenia," "nervous tachycardia," "vasomotor neurosis," "nervous exhaustion," "irritable heart," and "soldier's heart." This multitude of names describes a single syndrome which I will arbitrarily call neurasthenia. As neurasthenia is usually not associated with phobias, it is called a "simple" anxiety state (27,35,117,143 pp. 85-103, 175). The three phobic anxiety states you have learned are:

358.   Neurasthenia is characterized by almost daily anxiety (psychic and somatic), fatigue or easy fatigability and occasional acute anxiety attacks. Why is neurasthenia called a "simple" anxiety state?

426

355. 15,35; 20,30

356.

	Specific Animal/ Situational Phobia	PAD Syndrome	Agoraphobia
Onset in childhood	√		
Physiologically abnormal		√	√
Good treatment response	√		
Little generalized anxiety	√		
Monophobic	√		√
Episodes of depersonalization		√	
Episodes of acute anxiety	√	√	√
Poor treatment response		√	√
Circumscribed anxiety	√		
Approximately 70-80% are women		√	√
Onset in early adulthood		√	√
Psychic and somatic anxiety	√	√	√
Much generalized anxiety		√	√

357. simple animal/situational, agoraphobia, PAD syndrome

358. Because it is usually not associated with phobias

359.   Neurasthenia usually develops after puberty (15 to 35 years most commonly) (35,117,143 pp. 85-103,165,175) it is familial (34,140,141 pp. 103-106,174) and is more common in women (female:male ratio is 2:1) (93). This age of onset range, family history pattern and sex ratio is similar to _____ and _____.

360.   Individuals with neurasthenia can be differentiated from normal controls on physiological tests of resting anxiety levels, response to stress and psychological profile (27,47,91,116,117,143 pp. 85-103, 122). This differentiation from the normal population is similar to that of agoraphobics and patients with PAD syndrome. In what other ways are neurasthenics similar to these other patient groups? Be specific.

361.   Individuals with neurasthenia respond poorly to treatment (47, 104,105,122,143 pp. 85-103). Although without phobias, neurasthenia is more like the PAD syndrome and agoraphobia than specific _____/_____ phobias.

362.   Patients with daily anxiety and fatigue termed _____ often perform poorly under stress or exercise and have a reduced physical work capacity (91,116,117).

363.   The response to treatment of specific animal and situational phobias is _____; agoraphobia, PAD syndrome and neurasthenia have a _____ response to treatment.

364.   90 percent of patients with simple animal/situational phobias respond well to treatment (47,103-105,122,145); whereas only 25 to 40 percent of patients with agoraphobia, PAD syndrome and neurasthenia respond well to treatment (27,47,102-105,122,129,143 pp. 85-103, 145,165). This separation of responsivity is not surprising as the animal/situational phobics are physiologically and psychologically _____ whereas the latter group of disorders are physiologically and psychologically _____.

365.   What is the most likely diagnosis for this patient?

A 27-year-old woman was shopping on a crowded street when she suddenly felt "light-headed" and had to lean on the wall of a building. She suddenly became fearful that if she started walking again, she would again become "light-headed," stumble and be "pushed to the ground by the crowd." Although she returned home without further incident, over a period of time, she became increasingly fearful of stepping out of doors and after a few months was limited to walking a few blocks to the local grocery store, or to travelling by car if someone else drove. At home she described being tense and restless with frequent headaches and palpitations. She had two "attacks" of hyperventilation associated with extreme fear and "air hunger." Physical examination and laboratory data were within normal limits except for slight rapidity of speech and a tremor in the upper lip. The mental status examination was within normal limits.

359. agoraphobia, PAD syndrome

360. Same age of onset range: 15-35
Same sex ratio: mostly female 70-80%
Familial
Generalized anxiety
Associated with acute anxiety attacks

361. animal/situational

362. neurasthenia

363. good, poor

364. normal, abnormal

365. agoraphobia

366.   What is the most likely diagnosis for this patient?

A 24-year-old man, without previous psychiatric history or significant medical history was brought to an emergency room because,
while reading at home he suddenly developed a pounding in his
chest, a tightness or lump in his throat, trouble breathing, a shaky
feeling, blurred vision, dizziness, headache, "nervousness" and a
feeling that he was going to die. On examination he was tremulous,
sweating, had dilated pupils (reactive), cold extremities, tachycardia
and systolic hypertension. The remainder of the physical and laboratory results were within normal limits.

367.   What is the most likely diagnosis for this patient?

A 42-year-old woman was seen in consultation because of her intense
fear when in the presence of any small furry animal (a rat, mouse,
hamster). When she was not in proximity to such animals, she was
without unusual anxiety and functioned well. She denied any other
complaints.

368.   What is the most likely diagnosis for this patient?

A 54-year-old woman was seen in the emergency room because she
complained of "uncomfortable breathing," chest tightness, blurred
vision, tachycardia and "nervousness" of 2 hours' duration. Physical examination and laboratory findings were all within normal limits except for a sinus tachycardia of 108. She admitted to several
of these "attacks" per year for the past 30 years. She also gave a
history of being tired most of the time and of having a "nervous
heart."

369.   What is the most likely diagnosis for this patient?

A 24-year-old woman received word that her husband was injured in
an automobile accident. Upon hearing the news she felt faint and
fell to the floor without losing consciousness. Although her husband's
injuries were minor, she experienced a dizzy felling "almost dream-
like" for several days. One week later, she was found at home lying
on the floor for no apparent reason. She said she was frightened.
During the next six months she became progressively less able to
perform her housework. She was tense and restless, cried easily,
and on occasion woke up during the night extremely frightened, complaining of difficulty in breathing. She became fearful of her children's pet canary saying "it will poke me in the eye"; she also was
fearful of riding in a car or of taking a bus. She experienced additional "dream-like...unreal" episodes. Physical examination and laboratory findings were within normal limits.

370.   What is the most likely diagnosis for this patient?

A 7-year-old boy was walking down the street when a sudden crash
severely startled him. As he turned towards the sound, he saw
that an automobile had struck a policeman's horse and knocked it to
the ground. The boy cried and said he was "frightened" and was
taken home where he soon felt better. Despite no unusual behavior
at home, at school or at play, he continued to complain of fearfulness
whenever he saw a horse on television, in a book or in the street.

366. acute anxiety attack

367. specific animal phobia

368. acute anxiety attack and neurasthenia

369. phobic-anxiety-depersonalization syndrome

370. specific animal phobia

371.   Many patients with signs and symptoms of anxiety are not suffering from an anxiety state but from a systemic illness or another
psychiatric condition. Below is a list of some of the conditions associated with the presence of anxiety. A description of each is beyond the scope of this book, but before you diagnose anxiety state,
keep these other possibilities in mind, and remember that a psychiatric examination includes a physical examination and a complete history of systems.

Depression	Thyroid disease
Pheochromocytoma	Early essential hypertension
Cerebral arteriosclerosis	Parkinson's disease
Temporal lobe epilepsy	Post-concussion syndrome
Angina	Cardiac arrhythmias
Presenile dementias	Influenza
Caffeine sensitivity	Hepatitis
Mononucleosis	

371. no answer required

MINOR DEPRESSION (DSM-III TERM: DYSTHYMIC DISORDER)

372.   Earlier in Part II you learned the criteria for major depression. What are they?

373.   Major depression when associated with mania is termed _____ affective disorder. Major depression without any history of mania is termed _____ affective disorder.

374.   Major depression refers to the condition also called endogenous depression. In contrast to major depression, _____ depression refers to the conditions also called neurotic or reactive depression. These terms should be considered only as clinical labels and not as indicators of etiology.

375.   Psychiatrists who use the term neurotic/reactive depression, i.e.,_____ depression, usually mean an abnormal psychological response in a vulnerable individual (143 pp. 77-81). What this vulnerability is, whether it exists, what stimuli are required for the response and what the mechanism is of this response are all unknown factors. I will consider only the clinical presentation of the condition (48,74,85,126,128).

376.   Endogenous or _____ depression and neurotic/reactive or _____ depression cannot be separated by the presence or absence of a precipitating event (53). However, the symptom content of neurotic/reactive depressions often reflects the present life situations of the patient.

434

372. (All required)
  1. Sad or anxious mood
  2. Three of the following:
     A. early a.m. waking
     B. dirunal mood swing (worse in the a.m.)
     C. more than a 5 lb. weight loss in 3 weeks
     D. retardation/agitation
     E. suicidal thoughts/behavior
     F. feelings of guilt/self-reproach/hopelessness/worthlessness
  3. No coarse brain disease or use of steroids or reserpine in past month, no systemic illness known to cause depressive symptoms.

373. bipolar, unipolar

374. minor

375. minor

376. major, minor

377.   Without treatment, the average duration of an endogenous or
_____ depression is 9 months. Without treatment, the average
duration of a neurotic/reactive or _____ depression is 4 to 6
weeks.

378.   The sleep pattern in major depression is classically _____
_____ awakening. In contrast, the sleep pattern in minor depression is difficulty in falling asleep.

379.   The eating pattern in major depression is clinically _____
_____ with associated weight _____. In contrast, the
eating pattern in minor depression is classically a normal or increased appetite with weight gain.

380.   Anorexia with more than a 5 lb. weight loss and early a.m. wakening are characteristic of _____ depression. Normal or increased appetite and inability to fall asleep (initial insomnia) are characteristic of _____ depression.

381.   One characteristic of a major depression is: feeling worse in the
_____ and better in the _____. Minor depressions do
not have this diurnal mood swing.

382.   Patients with major depression rarely exhibit mood changes in
response to environmental stimuli. They remain sad. Patients with
minor depression will often have a lifting of their mood in response
to the environment, i.e., their mood reacts to changes in the
environment. They _____ _____ have a diurnal mood
swing.

383.   Patients with minor depression rarely exhibit the profound psychomotor retardation or severe agitation often seen in patients with
_____ depression.

384.   Draw lines to the phrases in column B with the condition in column A.

                    A   B

                                           Early a.m. wakening
        Minor depression   Weight gain
                                           Initial insomnia
        Major depression   Anorexia and weight loss
                                           Diurnal mood swing
                                           Psychomotor retardation

377. major, minor

378. early a.m.

379. anorexia, loss

380. major, minor

381. a.m., evening

382. do not

383. major

384.

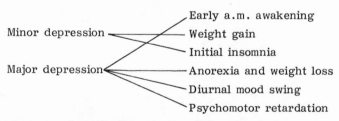

Please keep in mind that "classical" or "characteristic" pattern does not mean always and is not pathognomonic.

385.   Major or minor depression?

A 28-year-old woman was hospitalized because she ingested an overdose of aspirin in a suicide attempt. She described a long-standing
dissatisfaction with her work and a three-week-old feeling of pes-
simism and helplessness. She was anxious and was unable to fall
asleep at night. Although she said she was not hungry, she had
gained 7 lbs. during the past month. Her anxiety was associated with
angry spells which occurred throughout the day. In the hospital
she was demanding, manipulative, and often angry with the staff for
not meeting her demands.

386.   Major or minor depression?

A 34-year-old man came to an emergency room complaining that he
was fearful of killing himself because his wife wanted a divorce. His
wife told him this three weeks ago and since then he had been unable
to fall asleep, go to work or think about anything else. He gained
several pounds during this period.

387.   Major or minor depression?

A 44-year-old woman was seen in consultation because of inability
to work. She expressed a feeling of sadness, she had no energy
or interest and she felt that her life was over. She could not eat,
lost 10 lbs. during the past month and was unable to sleep. She described feeling somewhat better in the late afternoon or evening.

385. minor

386. minor

387. major - However, systemic illness, coarse brain disease and drug
      usage must be evaluated before a definitive diagnosis can be made.

OBSESSIONAL CONDITIONS

388.   Obsessions are persistent, distressing and unwanted thoughts or impulses which the sufferer knows are foolish, but which cannot be resisted. Compulsions are acts resulting from obsessions. An individual with an obsessional condition may repeat the same act over and over again. When asked about it, he will invariably say he is troubled by "having" to do it, but if he tries not to act upon his obsessive thought, his anxiety becomes too great and he succumbs. In contrast, some patients who have repetitive behavior do so in an automatic fashion. They do not find these behaviors distressing and unwanted and do not think of them as foolish. Such a behavior is termed _____ and is a feature of the syndrome termed
_____.

389.   Unwanted, persistent and distressing thoughts, i.e.,
_____, are signs of a rare condition occurring in less than 5 percent of all psychiatric patients (61). It occurs about equally in both sexes (79,86,118).

390.   When an individual acts upon his obsessional thoughts and impulses, he is said to have a _____.

391.   Most obsessional conditions begin before age 25 (79,86). Just as in the anxiety states, it is rare to see an individual whose obsessional condition (or any "neurotic" condition for that matter) began after age _____.

392.   Obsessional conditions have an early onset and are chronic (79, 86,118). As they occur in less than 5 percent of all psychiatric patients, they are fortunately also _____.

393.   Obsessional conditions have an _____ onset of illness, are chronic and rare. They seem to be familial but the data are unclear (22,80,127).

440

388. stereotype, catatonia (If you had difficulty with this question, please review the section on catatonia in Part I, items 61 through 94)

389. obsessions

390. compulsion

391. 35

392. rare

393. early

394.   The fact that a person has an obsessive thought is more significant than what his thought is about. The content of the obsession
or compulsion is not nearly as important as the _____
of the psychopathology.

395.   Obsessive thoughts often involve a fear of hurting oneself or
another person; a fear of being hurt in a particular manner; a fear
of contamination or disease; a fear of saying distressing, obscene,
blasphemous or nonsensical words or phrases. Ruminations (obsessive thoughts) about common daily activities such as dressing or house
maintenance are also characteristic of the condition. The more the
person tries to resist these thoughts the more anxious he becomes
until finally he must act (93). Such acts are called _____.

396.   Most normal children and many healthy adults have some obsessional behaviors: following a set routine for "good luck," avoiding
sidewalk cracks, rechecking things already well checked. There is
no standard demarcation line between the range of normality of these
behaviors and the abnormal. But individuals with obsessional conditions will invariably have significant levels of anxiety, occasionally
phobias, and, not infrequently, major or minor depressions (59,86,
118,148). Write the definition of an obsession:

Write the definition of a compulsion:

397.   Circle the obsessions:

"I keep thinking I'm going to put   "I can't get that tune out of my
a pencil in my eye."   head."

"I checked the lock three times   "I'm afraid that if I don't pick
to be sure."   up my clothes, something ter-
                                       rible will happen."

"I touch my nose, then my elbow,
and swallow. Then I feel better."

398.   Circle the compulsions:

"Every time I see a string, I   "I check the door 5 times, the
pick it up and put it in my   windows 5 times, under my bed
pocket, for fear that if I don't   5 times and in the closet 5 times.
I will die."   If I lose count I must do it over
                                       again."

"I keep thinking I'm going to   "If I don't call for the weather
harm someone. It's frightening   report every day I get frightened
but also silly."

"I know its foolish, but I keep
thinking something is going to
fall on my head and hurt me."

442

394. form

395. compulsions

396. An <u>obsession</u> is a persistent, distressing and unwanted thought or impulse.
A <u>compulsion</u> is an act resulting from an obsession.

397. "I keep thinking I'm going to put a pencil in my eye."

"I checked the lock three times to be sure."

"I touch my nose, then my elbow, and swallow. Then I feel better."

"I can't get that tune out of my head."

"I'm afraid that if I don't pick up my clothes, something terrible will happen."

398. "Every time I see a string, I pick it up and put it in my pocket, for fear that if I don't I will die."

"I keep thinking I'm going to harm someone. It's frightening but also silly."

"I know its foolish, but I keep thinking something is going to fall on my head and hurt me."

"I check the door 5 times, the windows 5 times, under my bed 5 times and in the closet 5 times. If I lose count I must do it all over again."

"If I don't call for the weather report every day I get frightened."

HYSTERIA (DSM-III TERM: SOMATOFORM DISORDERS)

399.   Hysteria is a term dating back several hundreds of years. It refers to the concept of "wandering uterus." (Today, it is often used by male physicians and psychologists to describe a female patient who annoys them.) In addition to being sexist, the term and concept are controversial because they often indiscriminately refer to the following conditions (66,143 pp. 103-119):

1. Hysterical reaction (similar if not indistinguishable from an acute anxiety attack)

2. Conversion hysteria (conversion reaction)

3. Hysterical personality

4. Briquet's syndrome

400.   A hysterical reaction usually refers to a condition characterized by severe agitation, severe anxiety, and a lot of screaming (68,121). In all other clinical manifestations, the condition appears identical to a severe acute anxiety attack. What are the signs of an acute anxiety attack? (List them)

401.   Conversion hysteria, also known as conversion reaction, or conversion symptom, are medically unexplained symptoms affecting the voluntary musculature or the organs of a special sense (e.g., eyes, ears). They often suggest neurological disease but no tissue pathology can be demonstrated. Examples include: paralysis, blindness, deafness, aphonia (inability to speak), difficulty in breathing, "fits," "spells," anesthesia, amnesia, and unconsciousness (68,121). Conversion hysteria should not be confused with the term "hysterical reaction" which is characterized by severe _____ and severe _____ and a lot of screaming.

444

399. no answer required

400. 1. Intense anxious mood often associated with the feeling of impending doom or death
2. Smothering or drowning feeling or air hunger
3. Chest discomfort, tightness or pain
4. Lump in throat
5. Dizziness and/or faintness
6. Weakness and/or fatigue
7. Inward "shakiness"
8. Tremor
9. Paresthesias
10. Tachycardia and/or palpitations
11. Vascular throbbing

401. agitation, anxiety, screaming

402.   Unexplained systemic symptoms such as headaches, backaches and other pains should not be included under the heading: conversion symptoms. "Conversion" phenomena are characterized by symptoms affecting the _____ musculature and organs of

_____ _____.

403.   Conversion symptoms suggest neurological disease. Can tissue pathology be demonstrated?

404.   As in most of the so-called "neurotic" disorders, more women than men are affected with conversion symptoms (71). The usual body parts (organs) affected are _____.

405.   There are a group of systemic medical conditions (e.g., ulcerative colitis, asthma, peptic ulcers, eczema) termed psychophysiological disorders (83) (the old term is psychosomatic, the new term is: "psychological factors affecting physical illness") which are dysfunctions with demonstrable tissue pathology. How does this contrast with conversion symptoms? Write your answer.

406.   Organ symptoms most often associated with psychophysiological disorders are those innervated by the autonomic nervous system (e.g., smooth involuntary muscles of bowels, blood vessels, skin) (123). How does this contrast with the organs most often associated with conversion symptoms? Write your answer.

407.   A "psychological/emotional" or physiological vulnerability to chronic stress has been hypothesized as a major causative factor in the development of psychophysiological disorders, hence the prefix "psycho." These systemic illnesses are often associated with high daily (generalized) levels of psychic and somatic anxiety and patients with these conditions can present with acute anxiety attacks (83,123, 130,135). What are the diagnostic criteria for such attacks?

408.   Psychophysiological disorders can be distinguished from conversion symptoms by the organs affected and the tissue pathology observed. What specifically are these differences between the two conditions?

409.   Most individuals receiving the diagnosis of "hysterical personality" are women (28,180). Onset for these behaviors usually occurs before age 15 (28,66,68,121,180). "Hysterical personality" is not "hysterical reaction" which is characterized by severe _____, severe _____, and a lot of _____ and which appears identical to acute anxiety.

402. voluntary, special sense

403. no

404. voluntary musculature, organs of special sense

405. Conversion symptoms have no demonstrable tissue pathology.

406. In conversion symptoms the organs of special sense and the voluntary musculature are most often involved.

407. Two of the following three: 1. Intense anxious mood
                                       2. Air hunger
                                       3. Chest discomfort

Three of the following eight: 1. Tachycardia
                                       2. Tremor
                                       3. Vascular throbbing
                                     4. Inward "shakiness"
                                     5. Lump in throat
                                   6. Paresthesias
                                   7. Dizziness
                                   8. Weakness

408. (1) Psychophysiological disorders affect organs innervated by the
autonomous nervous system whereas conversion symptoms involve
organs of special sense and the voluntary musculature; and
(2) Tissue pathology has been demonstrated only for psychophysiological disorders.

409. anxiety, agitation, screaming

410.   Individuals with hysterical personalities are said (28) to be:

1. Dramatic and histrionic
2. Egocentric and vain
3. Passive and manipulative
4. Sexually provocative
5. Dependent and demanding
6. Emotionally labile and excitable but shallow
7. Obsessive-compulsive

These behaviors are constant and usually begin before the age of

_____.

411.   The term hysterical personality does not imply either a hysterical reaction or a conversion symptom, although many psychiatrists
believe these conditions occur more frequently in individuals with a
hysterical personality than among the general population (2b, 71, 180).
A hysterical reaction is similar to an _____ _____
_____. A conversion symptom suggests a _____
disease for which no pathology can be demonstrated.

412.   A 22-year-old woman comes to see you because she is having
difficulties at work and with her fiancee. She relates her life events
in a dramatic and histrionic manner. When you suggest an alternative to her handling of a situation she becomes angry and then
bursts into tears. This behavior quickly abates as she becomes aware
that you are unresponsive to her outburst. She then proceeds to
cross her legs in a seductive manner. Circle the most likely diagnosis:

a) Hysterical reaction

b) Conversion reaction

c) Psychophysiological disorder

d) Hysterical personality

413.   Although often described as "dramatic," "histrionic" and "excitable" individuals with hysterical personalities also are described
as emotionally shallow with fleeting moods. What is the characteristic
age of onset of these behaviors and which sex is affected most frequently?

414.   Obsessive-compulsive behaviors have been described as part of
the hysterical personality. What is the difference between an obsession and a compulsion?

415.   Individuals with hysterical personalities are described as sexually
provocative. They are also described as emotionally _____
with _____ moods.

416.   Individuals with hysterical personalities are said to be passive,
but also manipulative. They are also sexually _____.

410. 15

411. acute anxiety attack, neurological

412. d

413. before age 15, women

414. An obsession is a persistent, distressing and unwanted thought or
impulse.
A compulsion is an act resulting from an obsession.

415. shallow, fleeting

416. provocative

417.   Circle the words and/or phrases characteristic of a hysterical personality.

Blind without pathology	Egocentric and vain
Stubborn	Sexually provocative
Dramatic and histrionic	Passive and manipulative
Intellectual	Shy

418.   Circle the words and/or phrases characteristic of a hysterical personality.

Altruistic	Dependent and demanding
Obsessive-compulsive	Mature
Emotionally labile	Dramatic
Asexual	Independent
Moods fleeting and shallow	Excitable

419.   Individuals with a hysterical personality tend to exhibit more frequently than others, behaviors which look like neurological disease of the voluntary musculature or organs of special sense but for which no pathology can be demonstrated. These behaviors are called _____.

420.   Draw lines to match the phrases in column B with the condition in column A. Conditions in column A can be used more than once.

A

Conversion hysteria

Hysterical reaction

Psychophysiological disorder

Hysterical personality

B

Voluntary muscles and organs of special sense involved but no pathology demonstrated

Agitation, screaming and anxiety

Egocentric, dramatic and excitable behaviors

Involuntary muscles involved

Ulcerative colitis, asthma, peptic ulcer

Mimics neurological symptoms but no medical explanation for symptoms

Dysphoria, air hunger, paresthesias, tremor, tachycardia and inward shakiness

Manipulative, sexually provocative, dependent and demanding

450

417. Blind without pathology   (Egocentric and vain)

       Stubborn   (Sexually provocative)

       (Dramatic and histrionic)   (Passive and manipulative)

       Intellectual   Shy

418. Altruistic   (Dependent and demanding)

       (Obsessive-compulsive)   Mature

       (Emotionally labile)   (Dramatic)

       Asexual   Independent

       (Moods fleeting or shallow)   (Excitable)

419. conversion symptoms (or conversion reaction or conversion hysteria)

420.

A	B
Conversion hysteria	Voluntary muscles and organs of special sense involved but no pathology demonstrated
Hysterical reaction	Agitation, screaming and anxiety
	Egocentric, dramatic and excitable behaviors
Psychophysiological disorder	Involuntary muscles involved
	Ulcerative colitis, asthma, peptic ulcer
Hysterical personality	Mimics neurological symptoms but no medical explanation for symptoms
	Dysphoria, air hunger, paresthesias, tremor, tachycardia and inward shakiness
	Manipulative, sexually provocative, dependent and demanding

421.   Although the reliability and validity of the concept of "hysterical personality" is unclear, Briquet's syndrome (DSM-III term:
"Somatization Disorder") has been shown to be a specific condition
(66,68,70,73,95,114). Many individuals with the label "hysterical
personality" satisfy diagnostic criteria for Briquet's syndrome (73).
For the research diagnosis of Briquet's syndrome, the patient must
have 25 medically unexplained chronic symptoms, for a "definite"
diagnosis, or 20 to 24 symptoms for a "probable" diagnosis in at
least 9 of the 10 following groups (114,121).

Group 1

Headaches
Sickly most of life

Group 2

Blindness
Paralysis
Anesthesia
Aphonia
Fits or convulsions
Unconsciousness
Amnesia
Deafness
Hallucinations
Urinary retention
Ataxia
Other conversion
  symptoms

Group 3

Fatigue
Lump in throat
Fainting spells
Visual blurring
Weakness
Dysuria

Group 4

Breathing difficulty
Palpitation
Anxiety attacks
Chest pain
Dizziness

Group 5

Anorexia
Weight loss
Marked fluctu-
  ations in weight
Nausea
Abdominal bloating
Food intolerances
Diarrhea
Constipation

Group 6

Abdominal pain
Vomiting

Group 7

Dysmenorrhea
Menstrual
  irregularity
Amenorrhea
Excessive bleeding

Group 8

Sexual indifference
Frigidity
Dyspareunia
Other sexual difficulties
Vomiting nine months
  of pregnancy, or hos-
  pitalized for hyperem-
  esis gravidarum

Group 9

Back pain
Joint pain
Extremity pain
Burning pains of the sexual
  organs, mouth, or rectum
Other bodily pains

Group 10

Nervousness
Fears
Depressed feelings
Need to quit working or
  inability to carry on
  regular duties because
  of feeling sick
Crying easily
Feeling life was hopeless
Thinking a good deal
  about dying
Wanting to die
Thinking of suicide
Suicide attempts

Briquet's syndrome is thus characterized by multiple symptoms in
multiple organ systems for which there are no "medical" explanations.
What other condition have you studied in which organ symptoms occur
without medical explanation?

421. Conversion reactions

422.   List the behavior associated with the label "hysterical personality."

1.
2.
3.
4.
5.
6.
7.

423.   The "definite" diagnosis of Briquet's syndrome requires the presence of _____ medically unexplained symptoms in at least
_____ of 10 organ systems groups.

424.   The diagnosis of hysterical personality and Briquet's syndrome
is much more commonly made in which sex? _____ Both conditions have an early onset with most behaviors present before age 15.

454

422. 1. dramatic and histrionic
      2. egocentric and vain
      3. passive and manipulative
      4. sexually provocative
      5. dependent and demanding
      6. emotionally labile, excitable but shallow
      7. obsessive-compulsive

423. multiple (25), 9

424. women

425.   Briquet's syndrome is a disorder resulting in _____
        symptoms in multiple _____. Below are the 10 categories in which
        _____ symptoms in _____ categories must occur for a defin-
        itive research diagnosis.

Group 1

Headaches
Sickly most of life

Group 2

Blindness
Paralysis
Anesthesia
Aphonia
Fits or convulsions
Unconsciousness
Amnesia
Deafness
Hallucinations
Urinary retention
Ataxia
Other conversion
    symptoms

Group 3

Fatigue
Lump in throat
Fainting spells
Visual blurring
Weakness
Dysuria

Group 4

Breathing difficulty
Palpitation
Anxiety attacks
Chest pain
Dizziness

Group 5

Anorexia
Weight loss
Marked fluctuations
    in weight
Nausea
Abdominal bloating
Food intolerances
Diarrhea
Constipation

Group 6

Abdominal pain
Vomiting

Group 7

Dysmenorrhea
Menstrual irreg-
    ularity
Amenorrhea
Excessive
    bleeding

Group 8

Sexual indifference
Frigidity
Dyspareunia
Other sexual difficulties
Vomiting nine months of
    pregnancy, or hospital-
    ized for hyperemesis
    gravidarum

Group 9

Back pain
Joint pain
Extremity pain
Burning pains of the sexual
    organs, mouth, or rectum
Other bodily pains

Group 10

Nervousness
Fears
Depressed feelings
Need to quit working
    or inability to carry
    on regular duties be-
    cause of feeling sick
Crying easily
Feeling life was hopeless
Thinking a good deal
    about dying
Wanting to die
Thinking of suicide
Suicide attempts

426.   Studies suggest that about 2 percent of the female population
        has diagnosable Briquet's syndrome (180). Associated conversion
        symptoms are common (71), but conversion symptoms are also seen
        in many other psychiatric and systemic conditions (49). Moreover,
        in any large series of cases of conversion symptoms, only a minority
        have Briquet's syndrome. Althought multiple hospitalizations, sur-
        gical procedures, and dramatic symptoms are common among women
        with Briquet's syndrome, a medical explanation for these symptoms
        _____ be demonstrated.

425. multiple, organ systems, 25, 9

426. cannot

427.   Briquet's syndrome runs in families (14,179). About 20 percent of first-degree female relatives of patients also have the condition. This risk is many times greater than the ____ percent seen in the general female population.

428.   Draw lines to match the phrase in column B with the condition in column A.

A	B
Briquet's syndrome	Unexplained loss of function in organs of special sense
Hysterical reaction	Multiple symptoms in multiple systems
Hysterical personality	Acute anxiety attack
Conversion symptom	Egocentric, dramatic, manipulative, demanding and excitable

429.   Draw lines to match the phrase in column B with the condition in column A.

A	B
Briquet's syndrome	Paralysis without medical cause
Hysterical personality	25 symptoms in 9 system groups
Hysterical reaction	Tachycardia, "air hunger", fear of impending doom, agitation
Conversion symptom	Sexually provocative, obsessive-compulsive, passive and manipulative

430.   Draw lines to match the phrase in column B with the condition in column A.

A	B
Briquet's syndrome	"Fits and spells" without medical cause
Hysterical personality	Multiple hospitalizations, multiple surgery, familial
Hysterical reaction	Difficulty breathing, dizziness, vascular throbbing, fear, tremors, systolic hypertensions
Conversion syndrome	Histrionic, vain, dependent, emotionally labile

427. 2%

428. Briquet's syndrome — Unexplained loss of function in organs of special sense

Hysterical reaction — Multiple symptoms in multiple systems

Hysterical personality — Acute anxiety attack

Conversion symptom — Egocentric, dramatic, manipulative, demanding and excitable

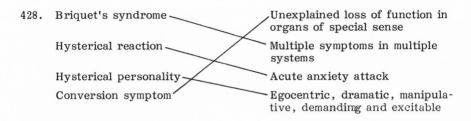

429.   A   B

Briquet's syndrome — Paralysis without medical cause

Hysterical personality — 25 symptoms in 9 system groups

Hysterial reaction — Tachycardia, "air hunger", fear of impending doom, agitation

Conversion symptom — Sexually provocative, obsessive-compulsive, passive and manipulative

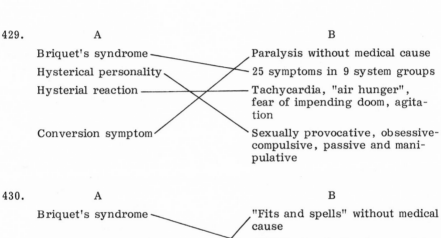

430.   A   B

Briquet's syndrome — "Fits and spells" without medical cause

Hysterical personality — Multiple hospitalizations, multiple surgery, familial

Hysterical reaction — Difficulty breathing, dizziness, vascular throbbing, fear, tremors, systolic hypertensions

Conversion syndrome — Histrionic, vain, dependent, emotionally labile

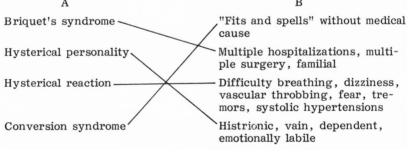

SOCIOPATHY (DSM-III TERM: ANTISOCIAL PERSONALITY DISORDER)

431.　　　　The adult personality can be defined as the affective and cognitive behaviors of the physiologically mature individual. An abnormal personality (i.e., personality disorder) implies (1) a deviation from the average personality (a mathematical, not a biological reality) or (2) a morbid process (a disease) resulting in a particular affective and cognitive pattern of behavior which alters the usual personality. In other words, some personalities are on the fringes of normal personality patterns, just as some people without illness are on the fringe of normal height (very tall or very short). When these fringe personality patterns result in discomfort to the individual or society, the individual is labeled abnormal, deviant or disordered, although no illness is present. Other personality patterns may be the result of disease (just as some people are on the fringe of normal height because of pituitary or other lesions).

　　　　Using the above model of affective and cognitive behavior patterns (personality) we would conclude that an individual with a very forceful assertive, outgoing personality although differing from the norm (and therefore statistically abnormal) most likely, is or is not (circle one) suffering from an illness.

432.　　　　Personality refers to _____ and _____ behavior patterns in the physiologically mature individual.

433.　　　　Personality patterns can be on the fringes of the normal range of behaviors. By definition, these patterns are statistically _____ but not necessarily due to illness.

434.　　　　Psychiatry has not yet been successful in identifying personality deviations with or without true illness and has not yet determined a scientifically reliable and valid category of personality deviation. One exception is Briquet's syndrome, another is sociopathy. Sociopathy (also known as psychopathic personality, sociopathic personality, antisocial personality) is a pattern of affective and cognitive behaviors characterized by: recurrent antisocial, delinquent and criminal behavior beginning before age 20 (often before puberty) (31,124).

460

431. is not

432. affective, cognitive

433. deviant (abnormal)

434. no answer required

435. The adult personality is the pattern of _____ and _____ behaviors in the physiologically _____ individual.

436. Sociopathy is a pattern of affective and cognitive behaviors, beginning before age 20 which is characterized by recurrent antisocial, delinquent and _____ behavior (31,124).

437. In one series of studies, nearly 80 percent of male felons exhibited recurrent antisocial and delinquent behavior before age 20. These were diagnosable _____ individuals (63-65).

438. Sociopathy is characterized by recurrent _____, _____, and _____ behavior beginning before age _____.

439. Sociopathy, or early onset recurrent _____, _____ and _____ behavior has been reported in 15 percent of male and 3 percent of female psychiatric patients (181) and may have a range of from 2 to 9 percent in the general population (64,97).

440. Sociopathy begins in childhood or early adolescence. It is extremely rare for sociopathic behavior patterns to develop after age _____.

441. Briquet's syndrome is most commonly seen in women. In contrast, sociopathy is most commonly seen in _____.

442. Sociopathic behaviors include recurrent childhood difficulties such as fighting, running away from home, failure in school, and truancy (31,124). In which sex would you expect to most frequently observe these behaviors?

443. Sociopaths often have a history of childhood hyperactivity (108, 124). However, keep in mind that not all adult sociopaths were hyperactive children and that most hyperactive children do not become sociopaths. In addition to hyperactivity, sociopaths usually have difficulties in the home and at school. What are these difficulties?

444. Sociopaths have stormy interpersonal histories. This includes poor job history, early heterosexual experiences with early marriage but a high divorce rate, adult promiscuity and a high prevalence of prostitution and homosexuality (31,33,124). These behaviors are usually present before the age of _____.

445. Sociopaths have an increased prevalence of conversion symptoms (71), Briquet's syndrome (33,101,124) and alcoholism (31,33,101,124). Their I.Q.'s have been reported to be low-normal or borderline (33, 39, 97) and they are described as cold and callous (31, 120, 133). From the list of their behaviors, what would you predict to be their relationships with legal authority?

462

435. affective, cognitive, mature

436. criminal

437. sociopathic

438. antisocial, delinquent, criminal, 20

439. antisocial, delinquent, criminal

440. 20

441. men

442. males

443. running away, school failure, and truancy

444. 20

445. Poor - with a history of trouble with the police; criminality

446. Circle the behaviors below which are associated with sociopathy:

Increased risk for alcoholism   Obsessive-compulsive behaviors

Egocentric   Increased risk for conversion symptoms

Briquet's syndrome   Cold and callous

Phobias   Psychophysiological disorder

447. A 50-year-old woman developed for the first time recurrent anti-social behavior, lost her job, and left her family. Is she likely to have sociopathy? _____ Explain your answer:

448. Sociopathic behaviors include (31,33,39,63-65,97,108,120,124, 133,181):

1. Childhood hyperactivity (Keep in mind that not all adult socio-paths were hyperactive children, and that not all hyperactive children become sociopaths).

2. Early fighting ·

3. Poor school adjustment (failure, truancy)

4. Running away from home in childhood and adolescence

5. Early heterosexual experiences, early marriage

6. Adult promiscuity, high divorce rate, high prevalence of pros-titution and homosexuality

7. Poor job history

8. Increased prevalence of conversion symptoms, Briquet's syn-drome and alcoholism

9. Low-normal or borderline I.Q.

10. Trouble with the police

11. Cold and callous affect

To sum up: Sociopaths exhibit recurrent _____,
_____ and _____ behavior.

449. There appears to be a strong relationship between sociopathy and Briquet's syndrome (33,101,124). The family illness patterns of the two conditions are similar and in a group of individuals selec-ted for one of these disorders you will find a greater than expected number who also demonstrate the other condition (33,63-65,67,101). Sociopathy and Briquet's syndrome may be the same disorder expres-sed differently in the two sexes; sociopathy being more common in _____ and Briquet's syndrome more common in _____.

450. Sociopathy is familial (i.e., more family members of sociopaths have sociopathy than you would expect from general population fig-ures). The families of sociopaths also have more than expected ill members with Briquet's syndrome. When ill, the male family members usually have _____, and the female family members usu-ally have _____ (29,32,41,63,64,67,69,124,134).

446. (Increased risk for alcoholism)   Obsessive-compulsive behaviors

Egocentric   (Increased risk for conversion)
                                          symptoms

(Briquet's syndrome)   (Cold and callous)

Phobias   Psychophysiological disorder

447. No. More common in men and almost always begins before age 20.

448. antisocial, delinquent, criminal

449. males, females

450. sociopathy, Briquet's syndrome

451.   Circle the words or phrases characteristic of sociopathy.

Early fighting   High I.Q.

Warm and friendly   Truancy

Poor job history   Alcoholism

Criminality   Hallucinations and delusions

452.   Circle the words or phrases characteristic of sociopathy.

Catatonic motor features   Running away from home

Shy and introverted   Delinquency

High divorce rate   Conversion symptoms

Thought disorder   Cold and callous

453.   Circle the words or phrases characteristic of sociopathy.

School failure   Childhood hyperactivity

Onset at age 30   Prostitution

Verbigeration   Early marriage

Criminality   More common in females

Familial

451. (Early fighting)   High I.Q.
        Warm and friendly   (Truancy)
     (Poor job history)   (Alcoholism)
     (Criminality)   Hallucinations and delusions

452. Catatonic motor features   (Running away from home)
     Shy and introverted   (Delinquency)
     (High divorce rate)   (Conversion symptoms)
     Thought disorder   (Cold and callous)

453. (School failure)   (Childhood hyperactivity)
     Onset at age 30   (Prostitution)
     Verbigeration   (Early marriage)
     (Criminality)   More common in females
     (Familial)

467

ALCOHOLISM

454.   Alcoholism refers to excessive use of alcohol resulting in medical,
social, interpersonal, vocational or legal problems. We have discussed
psychiatric conditions where the risk for alcoholism is increased.
These are _____ _____
and _____.

455.   Alcoholism is usually progressive and chronic, occasionally with
exacerbation and remissions. However, not all heavy drinkers are
alcoholics because by definition: alcoholism is excessive drinking
which results in physical, social and/or industrial dysfunction. Circle the descriptions which fit the above definition of alcoholism:

Lost job because of drinking	Two martinis before lunch and dinner and a brandy at night	Arrested for public intoxication
Consuming a six-pack of beer a day	Cirrhosis of the liver in a heavy drinker	Loss of driver's license because of driving while intoxicated
Three highballs after work, several mixed drinks on weekends	Constant family arguing over husband's drinking	

456.   The risk for alcoholism in the general male population is 3 to 5
percent and in the general female population is 1 percent (18,55,100,
138,142). The risk is highest among the young, urban dwellers, low
socioeconomic groups, Black Americans and non-Baptists (23,125).
France and the Soviet Union are countries with particularly high
alcoholism rates (131). Write the definition of alcoholism.

457.   Sociopathy and alcoholism are associated with the _____
sex. Affective disorder is associated with the _____ sex.

454. affective disorder, sociopathy

455. Lost job because of drinking | Two martinis before lunch and dinner and a brandy at night | Arrested for public intoxication

Consuming a six-pack of beer a day | Cirrhosis of the liver in a heavy drinker | Loss of driver's license because of driving while intoxicated

Three highballs after work, several mixed drinks on weekends | Constant family arguing over husband's drinking

456. Excessive drinking resulting in physical, social and/or industrial dysfunction.

457. male, female

458.   The usual onset of alcoholism in males is in the teens or early 20's. For females, it is somewhat later. An onset after age 45 is unusual (113). You should consider the presence of other conditions, particularly affective disorders in individuals with _____ onset of alcoholism.

459.   There appear to be clinical stages of alcoholism (15,81,82). These stages do not imply causation, nor does the individual patient pass through all stages in sequence (60). Staging is merely a method of clinical shorthand. A Stage I alcoholic will respond positively to most of the following questions:

1. Has your family ever objected to your drinking?

2. Have you ever thought you drank too much in general?

3. Have others ever said you drank too much for your own good?

4. Have you ever felt guilty about drinking?

5. Do you have a drink almost every day?

6. Have you ever lost friends because of drinking?

Behaviors consistent with a positive response to most of the above questions usually begin in the teens or early _____ and are most often seen in the _____ sex.

460.   Family objection, self-concern, statements of concern from others, guilt feelings about drinking, daily drinking and loss of friends due to drinking are all the positive responses of a stage ____ alcoholic.

461.   Circle the words or phrases associated with Stage I alcoholism.

Loss of friends due to drinking   DT's

Daily drinking   Guilt about drinking

Liver disease   Drinking before breakfast

Family objections to drinking   Drinking hair tonic

462.   Circle the words or phrases associated with Stage I alcoholism.

Self-concern about drinking too much   Benders

Drunk driving   Statements of concern from others

Family objections   Memory loss

458. late

459. 20's, male

460. I

461. (Loss of friends due to drinking)   DT's
     (Daily drinking)   (Guilt about drinking)
     Liver disease   Drinking before breakfast
     (Family objections to drinking)   Drinking hair tonic

462. (Self-concern about drinking   Benders
     too much)
     Drunk driving   (Statements of concern from
                                           others)
     (Family objections)   Memory loss

471

463.   A Stage II alcoholic will respond positively to most of the following questions:

1. Did you every get into trouble at work because of drinking?

2. Did you ever lose your job on account of drinking?

3. Did you ever have trouble with driving a car because of drinking? (accident, speeding, suspended or lost license)

4. Have you ever been arrested, even for a few hours, because of drinking and/or disturbing the peace?

5. Have you ever gone on benders? (48 hours of drinking associated with default of usual obligations. This must have occurred more than once).

Behaviors consistent with a positive response to most of these questions are associated with the _____ sex, onset in _____ or early _____, medical, social and interpersonal problems which are usually chronic.

464.   Circle the words or phrases characteristic of alcoholics or high risk for alcoholism.

Male	Elderly	Urban dweller
Farmer	Non-Baptist	Affective disorder
Schizophrenia	Sociopathy	Black American
Young	French	

465.   Trouble at work, loss of job, trouble with driving, arrest due to drinking and benders are all positive responses to questions of a stage _____ alcoholic.

466.   Circle the word or phrase associated with stage II alcoholism:

Trouble at work	DT's
Liver disease	Arrested because of drinking
Benders	Car accident after drinking

467.   Place an I next to the words or phrases characteristic of stage I alcoholism and a II next to the words or phrases characteristic of stage II alcoholism.

Benders ___	Feels guilty about drinking ___
Family objections to drinking ___	Loss of friends due to drinking ___
Arrested for drinking ___	Drunk driving ___
Loss of job due to drinking ___	Others complain of drinking ___

463. male, teens, 20's

464. (Male)   Elderly   (Urban dweller)
     Farmer   (Non-Baptist)   (Affective disorder)
     Schizophrenia (Sociopathy)   (Black American)
     (Young)   (French)

465. II

466. (Trouble at work)   DT's
     Liver disease   (Arrested because of drinking)
     (Benders)   (Car accident after drinking)

467. Benders II_   Feels guilty about drinking I_
     Family objections to drinking _I_   Loss of friends due to drink-
                                          ing I_
     Arrested for drinking II_   Drunk driving II_
     Loss of job due to drinking _II_ Others complain of drinking I_

473

468.   A stage III alcoholic, in addition to responding positively to stage I and II questions, will also respond positively to the following:

1. Have you ever wanted to stop drinking and couldn't?

2. Have you ever tried to control your drinking, by trying to drink only under certain circumstances?

3. Did you ever drink before breakfast?

4. Did you ever drink unusual things such as hair tonic, paint solvent and rubbing alcohol?

Behaviors consistent with a positive response to most of these questions are associated with (circle the appropriate words or phrases):

Male	Female	Teenager
Middle aged	20's	Urban dweller
Rural	Upper socioeconomic class	Affective disorder
Black American	Farmer	Non-Baptist
Baptist	Schizophrenia	Russian/French
Medical problems	Legal problems	Socioeconomic problems
Sociopathy		

469.   Inability to stop drinking, trying to control drinking by only drinking at certain times, drinking before breakfast and drinking unusual things such as hair tonic are all positive responses of a stage _____ alcoholic.

470.   Circle the words or phrases associated with stage III alcoholism.

Drinking before breakfast	Family objections to drinking
Loss of friends because of drinking	Drinking unusual things
Wanting to stop drinking but unable	Drunk driving
Benders	

471.   Place a I next to the words or phrases characteristic of stage I alcoholism, a II next to the words or phrases characteristic of stage II alcoholism and a III next to the words or phrases characteristic of stage III alcoholism.

Benders ___	Drinking before breakfast ___
Family objection to drinking ___	Drinking paint solvent ___
Wants to stop drinking but can't ___	Loss of job because of drinking ___
Loss of driver's license because of drinking ___	Guilt feelings about drinking ___

468. (Male)   Female   (Teenager)
      Middle aged   (20's)   (Urban dweller)
      Rural   Upper socioecono-   (Affective disorder)
                      mic class
      (Black American) Farmer   (Non-Baptist)
      Baptist   Schizophrenia   (Russian/French)
      (Medical problems) (Legal problems) (Socioeconomic problems)
      (Sociopathy)

469. III

470. (Drinking before breakfast)   Family objections to drinking
      Loss of friends because of   (Drinking unusual things)
      drinking
      (Wanting to stop drinking)   Drunk driving
      but unable
      Benders

471. Benders II   Drinking before breakfast III
      Family objections to   Drinking paint solvent III
        drinking I   Loss of job because of drinking II
      Wants to stop drinking   Loss of friends over drinking I
        but can't III   Guilt feelings about drinking I
      Loss of driver's license   Trying to limit drinking to certain cir-
        because of drinking II   cumstances III

475

472.   A stage IV alcoholic, in addition to responding positively to questions about stage I through III, will also respond positively to the following questions:

1. Have you ever gotten into fights when drinking?

2. Have you ever had memory losses when drinking (blackouts)?

3. To men only: Have you ever experienced impotence associated with drinking?

4. Have you ever had DT's, shakes, liver disease or other medical complications of drinking?

Behaviors consistent with a positive response to most of the questions are associated with (circle the appropriate words or phrases):

Female	Male	Sociopathy	Age 70
Teenager	Early 20's	French	City dweller
Farmer	Baptist	Non-Baptist	Affective disorder
Black American	Legal problems		

473.   Fighting when drinking, DT's, liver disease, memory loss when drinking and impotence when drinking are all associated with stage _____ alcoholism.

474.   Place the proper stage number (I, II, III, IV) next to the characteristic behavior of that stage:

Fighting when drinking ___   Benders ___

Drunk driving ___   Unable to stop drinking ___

Loss of friends because   Liver disease due to drinking ___
of drinking ___

Loss of job because of   Blackouts when drinking ___
drinking ___

DT's ___   Impotence when drinking ___

Family objections to   Drinking before breakfast ___
drinking ___

Guilt feelings about   Arrested because of drinking ___
drinking ___

Drinking hair tonic ___   Trouble at work because of
                                     drinking _____

Trying to control circum-   Others object to drinking ___
stances of drinking ___

472. Female   (Male)   (Sociopathy)   Age 70
     (Teenager)   (Early 20's)   (French)   (City dweller)
     Farmer   Baptist   (Non-Baptist)   (Affective disorder)
     (Black American)   (Legal problems)

473. IV

474. Fighting when drinking IV
Drunk driving II
Loss of friends because of
   drinking I
Loss of job because of
   drinking II
DT's IV
Family objections to
   drinking I
Guilt feelings about
   drinking I
Drinking hair tonic III
Trying to control circum-
   stances of drinking III

Benders II
Unable to stop drinking III
Liver disease due to drinking
   IV
Blackouts when drinking IV
Impotence when drinking IV
Drinking before breakfast II
Arrested because of drinking
   III
Trouble at work because of
   drinking II

Others object to drinking I

CLINICAL EVALUATIONS

You can now put your accumulated knowledge to practical use: You have just been asked to examine the following nine patients. They were referred to you because everyone is amazed by your diagnostic skills. Proceed with the patients the way you did in the last section of Part I.

CASE I

A 39-year-old white man is brought to the emergency room by the police because he became assaultive and agitated, and when confronted, he said: "I am a messenger of God...I have a secret for the cure of cancer because God told me."

His last statement is a _____ idea. Because it develops from an auditory hallucination it is _____.

The patient appears in good physical health, has good personal hygiene and is alert. His gait is normal, but he demonstrates increased frequency of motor behavior, termed _____, and during your examination he becomes involved in several surrounding events in the emergency room.

This behavior is termed _____.

The patient's eyes are open wide and are bright. His facial skin is taut, flushed and he has a perpetual smile upon his face, altered only by an angry expression when you appear not to understand him.

His affect is expanded in _____, increased in _____, and his mood, reflected in his facial expression, is _____.

CASE I

A 39-year-old white man is brought to the emergency room by the police because he became assaultive and agitated, and when confronted, he said "I am a messenger of God...I have a secret for the cure of cancer because God told me."

His last statement is a delusional idea. Because it develops from an auditory hallucination it is secondary.

The patient appears in good physical health, has good personal hygiene and is alert. His gait is normal, but he demonstrates increased frequency of motor behavior, termed agitation, and during your examination he becomes involved in several surrounding events in the emergency room.

This behavior is termed hyperactivity.

The patient's eyes are open wide and are bright. His facial skin is taut, flushed and he has a perpetual smile upon his face, altered only by an angry expression when you appear not to understand him.

His affect is expanded in range, increased in intensity, and his mood, reflected in his facial expression, is euphoric (and angry).

479

He is very concerned about his present situation, expresses warm feelings for his family, and elaborates plans for the future.

These suggest that he does not have _____ _____

His speech is rapid and he is difficult to interrupt. Occasionally he intrudes into the conversations of other staff members in the emergency room.

An example of _____/ _____ _____.

His thoughts jump from topic to topic and at times he appears to be carrying on two trains of thought simultaneously.

An example of _____- _____-_____.

He expresses his idea that he is God's messenger and admits to hearing God's voice which comes to him frequently during the day, from above, and is clear and often continuous.

An example of _____ _____ _____ which is one of the _____ _____ _____ _____ _____.

The patient is unable to do serial 7's or spell the word "world" backwards.

An example of difficulty in _____ which is also a measure of _____ _____ dysfunction.

All other cognitive functions appear within normal limits.

Physical examination and laboratory findings are within normal limits and there is no history of coarse brain disease, systemic illness or drug abuse.

This man satisfies the diagnostic criteria for _____ _____.

List these criteria:

He is very concerned about his present situation, expresses warm feelings for his family, and elaborates plans for the future.

These suggest that he does not have emotional blunting

His speech is rapid and he is difficult to interrupt. Occasionally he intrudes into the conversations of other staff members in the emergency room.

An example of rapid/pressured speech .

His thoughts jump from topic to topic and at times he appears to be carrying on two trains of thought simultaneously.

An example of flight-of-ideas.

He expresses his idea that he is God's messenger and admits to hearing God' voice which comes to him frequently during the day, from above, and is clear and often continuous.

An example of complete auditory hallucination or phoneme which is one of the first-rank symptoms of Schneider.

The patient is unable to do serial 7's or spell the word "world" backwards.

An example of difficulty in concentration which is also a measure of frontal lobe dysfunction.

All other cognitive functions appear within normal limits.

Physical examination and laboratory findings are within normal limits and there is no history of coarse brain disease, systemic illness or drug abuse.

This man satisfied the diagnostic criteria for mania.

List these criteria:

1. Hyperactivity
2. Rapid/pressured speech
3. Irritable/euphoric mood
4. No emotional blunting
5. No coarse brain disease, no psychostimulant drug abuse in prior month, no systemic illness know to cause manic symptoms.

CASE II

A 27-year-old white man is brought
to see you because after a family argu-
ment, he broke a mirror and a window.

The man is somewhat uncooperative and
belligerent. He is thin, wears braces
on his teeth, is unshaven and is untidy.
He is alert. He exhibits a fixed, unblinking expression (he has not received
neuroleptics). His gait is normal and he
is not agitated or hyperactive, nor does
he exhibit catatonic motor behaviors.

Except for irritability, he expresses no
mood or variability in his affect. He
does not express any feelings for his   These suggest _____
parents or his only sibling, denies any   _____.
interests and expresses no future plans.

Although his speech is stilted, he is difficult
to interrupt; but his speech is not rapid.   An example of _____
On occasion he responds to your questions   _____.
with unrelated statements.

He uses the word "drotter" in a   An example of _____.
private way.

The patient describes seeing "imaginary"   This non-vivid perceptual
girl friends in his mind's eye. He des-   symptom is termed a visual
cribes them as wearing maroon dresses   _____.
and glasses.

He says that on occasion they speak
to him and "control" his thoughts.

Their speech is whispered and comes   An example of _____
from inside his head.   _____ _____.

And they control his thoughts by some   An example of _____
"mechanism" which produces a "tingling"   _____, one of the
sensation in his brain forcing him to   _____ _____
think certain thoughts.   _____ _____
                                               _____.

Physical and laboratory findings are   Your diagnosis is
within normal limits. There is no   _____
history or evidence of coarse brain
disease, drug abuse or systemic illness.

482

A 27-year-old white man is brought
to see you because after a family argu-
ment, he broke a mirror and a window.

The man is somewhat uncooperative and
belligerent. He is thin, wears braces
on his teeth, is unshaven and is untidy.
He is alert. He exhibits a fixed, unblinking expression (he has not received
neuroleptics). His gait is normal and he
is not agitated or hyperactive, nor does
he exhibit catatonic motor behaviors.

Except for irritability, he expresses no
mood or variability in his affect. He
does not express any feeling for his   These suggest emotional
parents or his only sibling, denies any   blunting.
interests and expresses no future plans.

Although his speech is stilted, he is difficult
to interrupt; but his speech is not rapid.   An example of non-sequiturs.
On occasion he responds to your questions
with unrelated statements.

He uses the word "drotter" in a   An example of neologism
private way.

The patient describes seeing "imaginary"   This non-vivid perceptual
girl friends in his mind's eye. He des-   symptom is termed a visual
cribes them as wearing maroon dresses   pseudo-hallucination
and glasses.

He says that on occasion they speak
to him and "control" his thoughts.

Their speech is whispered and comes   An example of incomplete
from inside his head.   auditory hallucination.

And they control his thoughts by some
"mechanism" which produces a "tingling"   An example of experience of
sensation in his brain forcing him to think   influence, one of the first-
certain thoughts.   rank symptoms of Schneider.

Physical and laboratory findings are   Your diagnosis is schizo-
within normal limits. There is no history   phrenia
or evidence of coarse brain disease,
drug abuse or systemic illness.

List the criteria:

CASE III

A 46-year-old white woman, a former nurse, is hospitalized saying "I can't evacuate my bowels." She claims to have been well until about a year prior to admission. At that time she began experiencing constipation, poor appetite, weight loss of 20 pounds, initial and middle insomnia and feeling "down in the dumps." She denies any crying, diurnal mood variation or suicidal ideation.

These symptoms suggest _____.
Are they sufficient for the diagnosis? _____

When you ask her what she thinks the problem is, she points to her abdomen and says "it's blocked up." She states that she has not moved her bowels at all for six months.

You examine her. She is undernourished, yet alert. Her face is masklike and she persistently nods her head in a rhythmical fashion, unrelated to your questioning. Her mouth periodically grimaces. She repeatedly puts her hand up to her neck or smooths down her hair. When you ask about this behavior she replies "it's a habit."

Repetitive automatic behaviors are termed _____.

Her motor movements are slow (motor retardation).

Are enough symptoms now present for a diagnosis?

_____

484

List the criteria:

1. No diagnosable affective disorder
2. No coarse brain disease or hallucinogenic stimulant drug use or systemic illness known to cause psychiatric symptoms.
3. Clear consciousness, memory and orientation intact. (If one or both are impaired, this must be due solely to inattentiveness or poor concentration).
4. One of the following:
   a. emotional blunting
   b. formal thought disorder
   c. first rank symptoms (any one).

CASE III

A 46-year-old white woman, a former nurse, is hospitalized saying "I can't evacuate my bowels." She claims to have been well until about a year prior to admission. At that time she began experiencing constipation, poor appetite, weight loss of 20 pounds, initial and middle insomnia and feeling "down in the dumps." She denies any crying, diurnal mood variation or suicidal ideation.

These symptoms suggest major depression.
Are they sufficient for the diagnosis? No

When you ask her what she thinks the problem is, she points to her abdomen and says "it's blocked up." She states that she has not moved her bowels at all for six months.

You examine her. She is undernourished, yet alert. Her face is mask-like and she persistently nods her head in a rhythmical fashion, unrelated to your questioning. Her mouth periodically grimaces. She repeatedly puts her hand up to her neck or smooths down her hair. When you ask about this behavior she replies "it's a habit."

Repetitive automatic behaviors are termed stereotypes.

Her motor movements are slow (motor retardation).

Are enough symptoms now present for a diagnosis? No

(We still have not observed her mood or determined the presence or absence of coarse brain disease, drug abuse or systemic illness).

The patient's affect is restricted in
_____ , low in _____ and is
stable. She shows mild concern about
her bowel problems but is otherwise
apathetic. She is not concerned about
being hospitalized and says she would
be willing to stay six months to "find
out" about her "bowels" but she has
no future plans. She expresses no
warm feelings for anyone and relates
poorly to you.

She is _____
_____ .

Her speech is slow in rate, with long,
almost blank, pauses between question and answer.

Combined with her motor retardation, she exhibits
_____ -_____
retardation.
Can you now make the diagnosis Major Depression?___

Despite your efforts to change the
subject she continually returns to
statements concerning her bowels.
She does not have thought disorder.
She denies any perceptual disturbances or first rank symptoms of
_____ .

This is _____
_____ .

She is aware that she is in a hospital, knows its name, but can only
tell you it is the early part of the
month. She knows the year.

This is mild
_____ .

When asked to draw a circle with
each hand, she responds:

These responses are examples
of _____
_____ .

right hand   left hand

When asked to identify the following object, she does so but
only after turning her head to
the side.

This is a test for _____
_____ . Is her
response normal? _____

She cannot do serial 7's or serial
3's and cannot spell the word
"world" backwards.

This is an example of ____
_____ .

The patient's affect is restricted in range, low in intensity and is stable. She shows mild concern about her bowel problems but is otherwise apathetic. She is not concerned about being hospitalized and says she would be willing to stay six months to "find out" about her "bowels" but she has no future plans. She expresses no warm feelings for anyone and relates poorly to you.

She is emotionally blunted.

Her speech is slow in rate, with long, almost blank, pauses between question and answer.

Combined with her motor retardation, she exhibits psychomotor-retardation.

Can you now make the diagnosis Major Depression? No

(She does not have a sad or anxious mood)

Despite your efforts to change the subject, she continually returns to statements concerning her bowels. She does not have thought disorder. She denies any perceptual disturbances or first rank symptoms of Schneider.

This is perseveration of theme.

She is aware that she is in a hospital, knows its name, but can only tell you it is the early part of the month. She knows the year.

This is mild disorientation.

When asked to draw a circle with each hand, she responds:

These responses are examples of motor perseveration.

right hand  left hand

When asked to identify the following object, she does so but only after turning her head to the side.

This is a test for active perception. Is her response normal? No

and cannot spell the word "world" backwards.

This is an example of poor concentration.

When you ask her to place her
hand on her nose when you place
your hand on your chest, she
repeatedly, despite instructions
to the contrary, places her hand
on her chest.

This is an example of
_____.

The last four tasks suggest
she has _____
_____ _____.

She cannot identify her fingers and
has right-left disorientation. Although she is a registered nurse,
she says she cannot write script,
and is only able to print with
difficulty.

These behaviors are consistent with dysfunction in the
_____ _____.
Along with _____
they make up the condition
known as _____
syndrome.

Her efforts to copy simple figures
result in the following:

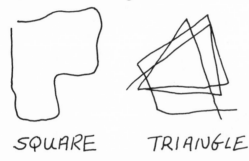

SQUARE   TRIANGLE

These are examples of
_____
and reflect dysfunction in
the _____ _____
_____.

She can name them and spell the names.
She is able to repeat a four word series.
She can recall two words after 5 minutes.

A test of _____ _____.
A test of _____ -
_____.

She is unable to remember dates and
sequences of important events prior
to six months ago.

An example of poor _____ -
_____ _____.

Her physical examination and laboratory
data are within normal limits. There is
no history of drug abuse, but other informants describe her illness as dating
back several years.

Your diagnosis is?
_____

When you ask her to place her hand on her nose when you place your hand on your chest, she repeatedly, despite instructions to the contrary, places her hand on her chest.

This is an example of echopraxia.

The last four tasks suggest she has frontal lobe dysfunction.

She cannot identify her fingers and has right-left disorientation. Although she is a registered nurse, she says she cannot write script, and is only able to print with difficulty.

These behaviors are consistent with dysfunction in the dominant parietal lobe. Along with acalculia they make up the condition known as Gerstmann's syndrome.

Her efforts to copy simple figures result in the following:

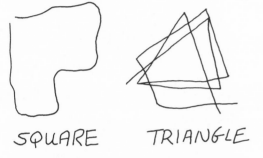

SQUARE   TRIANGLE

These are examples of construction apraxia and reflect dysfunction in the non-dominant parietal lobe.

She can name them and spell the names. She is able to repeat a four word series. She can recall two words after 5 minutes.

A test of immediate recall. A test of short-term memory.

She is unable to remember dates and sequences of important events prior to six months ago.

An example of poor long-term memory.

Her physical examination and laboratory data are within normal limits. There is no history of drug abuse, but other informants describe her illness as dating back several years.

Your diagnosis is? Dementia

CASE IV

A 33-year-old white woman comes to see you because "I haven't been sleeping."

For the past two months she has had difficulty falling asleep and staying asleep. Her appetite has been poor for the past two days but she denies any weight loss.

She describes feeling especially "moody" in the morning, that she has lost her sexual drive and that she always feels like crying but cannot do so. She states the future "looks frightening" and "bleak."

Her husband states that she has also been saying that she was afraid their son was "going blind" although there was no reason for this fear, and that during the past week she was telling him "I'm a whore...I'm no good...You're doing things to me."

You observe her to be neat and alert, but unfriendly, at times uncooperative, and somewhat suspicious. She moves slowly, is unsmiling, looks sad and has creases between her eyebrows which you recognize as an _____ _____. At times she puts her head down on her arms and says "it's useless."

Her affect is restricted in _____ , mood is sad, dejected, suspicious and slightly hostile.

She speaks slowly in a soft voice, frequently failing to complete her sentences.

This behavior combined with her motor behavior is recognizable _____ _____.

She suddenly states that the man living with her is "fatter" than her real husband and is "someone else."

This you know to be _____ syndrome, also called _____, or non-recognition of faces and associated with dysfunction in the area of the brain known as the

_____ _____ _____ _____.

490

CASE IV

A 33-year-old white woman comes to see you because "I haven't been sleeping."

For the past two months she has had difficulty falling asleep and staying asleep. Her appetite has been poor for the past two days but she denies any weight loss.

She describes feeling especially "moody" in the morning, that she has lost her sexual drive and that she always feels like crying but cannot do so. She states the future "looks frightening" and "bleak."

Her husband states that she has also been saying that she was afraid their son was "going blind" although there was no reason for this fear, and that during the past week she was telling him "I'm a whore...I'm no good...You're doing things to me."

You observe her to be neat and alert, but unfriendly, at times uncooperative, and somewhat suspicious. She moves slowly, is unsmiling, looks sad and has creases between her eyebrows which you recognize as Omega sign. At times she puts her head down on her arms and says "it's useless."

Her affect is restricted in range, mood is sad, dejected, suspicious and slightly hostile.

She speaks slowly in a soft voice, frequently failing to complete her sentences.

This behavior combined with her motor behavior is recognizable as psychomotor retardation.

She suddenly states that the man living with her is "fatter" than her real husband and is "someone else."

This you know to be Capgras' syndrome, also called prosopagnosia, or non-recognition of faces and associated with dysfunction in the area of the brain known as the non-dominant parietal lobe.

491

She has no thought disorder and
denies perceptual disturbances and
Schneiderian _____

_____ _____.

She cannot concentrate and cannot
properly copy a cross or a key but the
remainder of her cognitive testing   An example of _____
is within normal limits.   _____.

Physical examination and laboratory
data are within normal limits. There is
no evidence of coarse brain disease
although she does have some cognitive
dysfunction as you have already observed.

There is no history or evidence of
drug abuse.

Your diagnosis is _____ _____.

List the criteria:

CASE V

A 27-year-old white woman called the
police and said "I want to kill myself."
The police responded and brought her
to see you.

She says she has wanted to kill herself
for a long time. She finds life to be
empty, but has never had "sufficient
courage" to act. She complains of
initial insomnia, but no weight loss or   Can you make a diagnosis at
diurnal mood change. She has worked   this time? _____
until the present as a waitress.

492

She has no thought disorder and
denies perceptual disturbances and
Schneiderian first rank symptoms.

She cannot concentrate and cannot
properly copy a cross or a key but the
remainder of her cognitive testing is
within normal limits.

An example of construction
apraxia.

Physical examination and laboratory
data are within normal limits. There
is no evidence of coarse brain disease
although she does have some cognitive
dysfunction as you have already observed.

There is no history or evidence of
drug abuse or systemic illness.

Your diagnosis is major depression.

List the criteria:
1. Sad or anxious mood
2. Three of the following (a through f)
   a. early a.m. waking
   b. diurnal mood swing (worse in the a.m.)
   c. greater than 5 pound weight loss in
      3 weeks
   d. psychomotor retardation or agitation
   e. suicidal thoughts or behavior
   f. feelings of guilt, self-reproach,
      hopelessness, worthlessness
3. No coarse brain disease or use of steroids
   or reserpine in the past month, no systemic
   illness known to cause depressive symptoms.

Poor response to items testing cortical function indicates cortical dysfunction. However, the implication of dysfunction does not imply coarse disease.

CASE V

A 27-year-old white woman called the police
and said "I want to kill myself." The police
responded and brought her to see you.

She says she has wanted to kill herself for a
long time. She finds life to be empty,
but has never had "sufficient courage"
to act. She complains of initial insomnia,
but no weight loss or diurnal mood change.
She has worked until the present as a
waitress.

Can you make a diagnosis
at this time? No

493

She makes no eye contact and cries frequently during your examination. Her mood is sad, but occasionally it lifts and she smiles. After talking to you for a while, she says (through her tears) that you may be able to help her. She is physically healthy.

Does she satisfy criteria for a major depression? _____
A minor depression? _____

CASE VI

A 25-year-old white woman comes to see you with the complaint "I feel like driving my car into a telephone pole." She also complains of being unable to walk without aid, of staggering for the past week and of having severe headaches.

Your neurological examination, EEG and cognitive evaluation are all within normal limits.

She also complains of being "depressed," of poor appetite (has lost 2 or 3 pounds), of episodes of insomnia alternating with hypersomnia and, for the past five days, she has been suffering from what her relatives describe as possible "grand mal seizures." Two days prior to seeing you she remained "unconscious" for about 10 minutes. She has no aura and no recollection of these episodes.

If you are a bit enthusiastic and do a CAT-scan, brain scan and lumbar puncture, they too are within normal limits.

She says her staggering is severe and is associated with weakness, nausea and vomiting. She has no other history of possible neurological disease.

She says she has a history of "borderline" hyperthyroidism," but that she doesn't require medication.

She had pancreatitis several years ago and still has abdominal pain and diarrhea. Her physician told her that her pancreatitis led to "secondary hydronephrosis," and she occasionally gets kidney infections from this, manifested by frequency, urgency and some burning on micturition.

A recent IVP was normal. So is the urinalysis you request.

She says she also has had a chronic vaginal discharge, vaginal pruritis and dyspareunia. In the past she had "gonorrhea" and pelvic inflammatory disease which required surgery. She says she has chronic back pain and vaginal burning because of this.

Her pelvic examination shows no pathology.

She makes no eye contact and cries frequently during your examination. Her
mood is sad, but occasionally it lifts and
she smiles. After talking to you for a
while, she says (through her tears) that
you may be able to help her. She is
physically healthy.

Does she satisfy criteria for
a major depression? No (does
not have 3 of 6 criteria)
A minor depression? Yes

CASE VI

A 25-year-old white woman comes to
see you with the complaint "I feel
like driving my car into a telephone
pole." She also complains of being
unable to walk without aid, of staggering for the past week and of having severe headaches.

Your neurological examination,
EEG and cognitive evaluation
are all within normal limits.

She also complains of being "depressed,"
of poor appetite (has lost 2 or 3 pounds),
of episodes of insomnia alternating with
hypersomnia and, for the past five days,
she has been suffering from what her
relatives describe as possible "grand
mal seizures." Two days prior to seeing
you she remained "unconscious" for
about 10 minutes. She has no aura and
no recollection of these episodes.

If you are a bit enthusiastic
and do a CAT-scan, brain
scan and lumbar puncture,
they too are within normal
limits.

She says her staggering is severe and
is associated with weakness, nausea
and vomiting. She has no other
history of possible neurological disease.

She says she has a history of "borderline" hyperthyroidism," but that she
doesn't require medication.

She had pancreatitis several years
ago and still has abdominal pain and
diarrhea. Her physician told her that her
pancreatitis led to "secondary hydronephrosis," and she occasionally gets kidney
infections from this, manifested by frequency, urgency and some burning on
micturition.

A recent IVP was normal.
So is the urinalysis you request.

She says she also has had a chronic vaginal discharge, vaginal pruritis and dyspareunia. In the past she had "gonorrhea" and pelvic inflammatory disease
which required surgery. She says
she has chronic back pain and vaginal
burning because of this.

Her pelvic examination shows
no pathology.

495

She also states that she is allergic to
several medications and has "asthma" which
causes her periodic discomfort characterized
by chest pain, breathing difficulties,
palpitations, dizziness and fearfulness.

Physical examination and other laboratory
data are within normal limits.

Your diagnosis is _____

_____ _____ .

CASE VII

A 41-year-old black man is brought into
the emergency room because of "agitation,"
and because he was "unmanageable" at home.

Your examination reveals him to be in poor
nutrition, unkempt and unclean. His gait
is unsteady and he is restless. He looks
anxious. His breath smells of alcohol.
The patient's affect is increased in _____
and increased in _____ .
His mood is appropriate but he is irritable.
His speech is slurred and on occasion his
thoughts miss the point and some associations do not seem to follow in sequence
(loosening between associations).

This is an example of
_____ speech.

There is no perceptual disturbance
or apophany. There are no first rank
symptoms evident.

List the first rank symptoms
you would look for:

_____
_____
_____
_____
_____

He cannot concentrate.

What tasks would you ask
him to do to determine his
concentrating ability?

_____
_____
_____

Recent memory is impaired.

How would you test for this?

_____
_____

He is disoriented.

Your diagnosis is _____

_____ .

Property							
Compressive strength, rupture or 1% yield, 10^3 lb·in^{-2}	20		20		10–16	28	11.5–16
Elongation at break, %	100–1000	3–6	100–1100	100–700			1–2
Flexural modulus at 23°C, 10^3 lb·in^{-2}	10–100	610	10–350		1000–2500	17	380–450
Flexural strength, rupture or yield, 10^3 lb·in^{-2}	0.7–4.5	19	0.7–9		9–14		8–14
Hardness, Rockwell (or Shore)			(A65–D80)	(A15–A65)	M80–M90		M60–M75
Impact strength (Izod) at 23°C, J·m^{-1}	1334 to flexible	21	No break		13–427	16	13–21
Tensile modulus, 10^3 lb·in^{-2}	10–100		10–350				350–485
Tensile strength at break, 10^3 lb·in^{-2}	0.175–10	10–11	1.5–8.4	0.35–1.0	4–6.5	6–8	5.3–7.9
Tensile yield strength, 10^3 lb·in^{-2}							
Thermal							
Burning rate, mm·min^{-1}		87–93			0–78		
Coefficient of linear thermal expansion, 10^{-6}°C	100–200		100–200	300–800	20–50	30	70–80
Deflection temperature under flexural load (264 lb·in^{-2}), °C	Varies over wide range		Varies over wide range		260	74–100	
Maximum recommended service temperature, °C					371		93
Specific heat, cal·g^{-1}	0.43		0.43				0.3
Thermal conductivity, W·m^{-1}·K^{-1}	0.21		0.07–0.31	0.15–0.31	0.30	0.68	0.09–0.13

TABLE 10-2 Properties of commercial plastics (*continued*)

	Styrenic						
	Polystyrene	Acrylonitrile-butadiene-styrene copolymer					
			Molding				
Properties	Heat-resistant	Extrusion	Heat-resistant	High-impact	Flame-retarded	Platable	20% glass-reinforced
Physical							
Melting temperature, °C							
Crystalline							
Amorphous	110–125	88–120	110–125	100–110	110–125	100–110	
Specific gravity	1.05–1.09	1.02–1.06	1.05–1.08	1.01–1.04	1.16–1.21	1.06–1.07	1.22
Water absorption (24 h), %	0.03–0.12	0.20–0.45	0.20–0.45	0.20–0.45	0.2–0.6		
Dielectric strength, kV · mm^{-1}	20	14–20	14–20	14–20	14–20	16–22	18
Electrical							
Volume (dc) resistivity, ohm-cm							
Dielectric constant (60 Hz)				2.4–5.0			
Dielectric constant (10^6 Hz)				2.4–3.8			
Dissipation (power) factor (60 Hz)				0.003–0.008			
Dissipation factor (10^6 Hz)				0.007–0.015			
Mechanical							
Compressive modulus, 10^3 lb · in^{-2}		150–390	190–440	140–300	130–310		

Compressive strength, rupture or 1% yield, 10^3 lb·in^{-2}	11.5–16	5.2–10	7.2–10	4.5–8	6.5–7.5		14
Elongation at break, %	2–60	20–100	3–20	5–70	5–25		
Flexural modulus at 23°C, 10^3 lb·in^{-2}	340–470	130–420	300–400	250–350	300–400	340–390	710
Flexural strength, rupture or yield, 10^3 lb·in^{-2}	8.9–14	4–14	10–13	8–11	9–14	10.5–11.5	15.5
Hardness, Rockwell (or Shore)	L80–L108	R75–R115	R100–R115	R85–R105	R100–R120	R103–R109	M85
Impact strength (Izod) at 23°C, J·m^{-1}	21–181	133–640	107–347	347–400	160–640	267–283	64
Tensile modulus, 10^3 lb·in^{-2}	320–460	130–380	300–350	230–330	320–400	330–380	740
Tensile strength at break, 10^3 lb·in^{-2}	5–7.8	2.5–8.0	6–7.5	4.8–6.3	5–8	6–6.4	11
Tensile yield strength, 10^3 lb·in^{-2}			5.5–7	4–5.5	4–6		
Thermal							
Burning rate, mm·min^{-1}		1.3		1.3			
Coefficient of linear thermal expansion, 10^{-6}°C	60–70	60–130	60–93	95–110	65–95	47–53	21
Deflection temperature under flexural load (264 lb·in^{-2}), °C	93–120 annealed	77–104 annealed	104–116 annealed	96–102 annealed	90–107 annealed	96–102 annealed	
Maximum recommended service temperature, °C				110			99
Specific heat, cal g^{-1}				0.3–0.4			
Thermal conductivity, W·m^{-1}·K^{-1}			0.19–0.34				

TABLE 10-2 Properties of commercial plastics (*continued*)

| | Styrenic | | | Sulfone | | | |
| | Styrene-acrylonitrile copolymer | | | Polysulfone | | | |
Properties	Unfilled	20% glass-fiber-reinforced	Styrene-butadiene copolymer, high-impact	Unfilled	20% glass-fiber-reinforced	Poly(ether sulfone)	Poly(phenyl sulfone)
Physical							
Melting temperature, °C							
Crystalline							
Amorphous	115–125	115–125	90–110	200	200	230	220
Specific gravity	1.07–1.08	1.22	1.03–1.06	1.24	1.46	1.37	1.29
Water absorption (24 h), %	0.2–0.3	0.15–0.20	0.05–0.10	0.22	0.23	0.43	1.1–1.3 (saturated)
Dielectric strength, kV · mm^{-1}	16–20	20	18	17	17	17	16
Electrical							
Volume (dc) resistivity, ohm-cm				10^{15}			
Dielectric constant (60 Hz)				3.14	3.7		
Dielectric constant (10^6 Hz)				3.26	3.7		
Dissipation (power) factor (60 Hz)				0.004	0.002		
Dissipation factor (10^6 Hz)				0.008	0.009		
Mechanical							
Compressive modulus, 10^3 lb · in^{-2}	530			370			

Compressive strength, rupture of 1% yield, 10^3 lb·in^{-2}	14–17	19	4–9	13.9	22		
Elongation at break, %	1–4	1–2	13–50	50–100	2	30–80	60
Flexural modulus at 23°C, 10^3 lb·in^2	550	100–1100	280–450	390	1000	375	330
Flexural strength, rupture or yield, 10^3 lb·in^{-2}	14–17	20	5.3–9.4	15.4	23	18.7	12.4
Hardness, Rockwell (or Shore)	M80–M90	R122	M10–M68	M69, R120	R123	M88	
Impact strength (Izod) at 23°C, J·m^{-1}	19–27	53	32–192	64	59	85	640
Tensile modulus, 10^3 lb·in^{-2}	400–560	1150–1200	280–465	360	1200	350	310
Tensile strength at break, 10^3 lb·in^{-2}	9–12	15.8–18	3.2–4.9				
Tensile yield strength, 10^3 lb·in^{-2}			2.9–4.9	10.2	17	12.2	10.4
Thermal							
Burning rate, mm·min^{-1}	36–38	38–40	70–101	52–56	25	55	31
Coefficient of linear thermal expansion, 10^{-6}°C							
Deflection temperature under flexural load (264 lb·in^{-2}), °C	88–104	99	74–93	174	182	203	204
Maximum recommended service temperature, °C				149			
Specific heat, cal·g^{-1}							
Thermal conductivity, W·m^{-1}·K^{-1}	0.12	0.26–0.28	0.12–0.21	0.12	0.38	0.14–0.19	

TABLE 10-2 Properties of commercial plastics (*continued*)

Properties	Thermoplastic elastomers				Urea formaldehyde, alpha-cellulose filled	Vinyl — Poly(vinyl chloride) and poly(vinyl acetate)	
	Polyolefin	Polyester	Block copolymers of styrene and butadiene or styrene and isoprene	Block copolymers of styrene and ethylene or styrene and butylene		Rigid	Flexible and unfilled
Physical							
Melting temperature, °C					Thermoset		
Crystalline		168–206					
Amorphous						75–105	75–105
Specific gravity	0.88–0.90	1.17–1.25	0.9–1.2	0.9–1.2	1.47–1.52	1.30–1.58	1.16–1.35
Water absorption (24 h), %	0.01		0.19–0.39		0.4–0.8	0.04–0.4	0.15–0.75
Dielectric strength, kV · mm^{-1}	24–26		16–21		12–16	14–20	12–16
Electrical							
Volume (dc) resistivity, ohm-cm					0.5–5.0	10^{12}–10^{15}	10^{11}–10^{14}
Dielectric constant (60 Hz)					7.7–9.5	3.2–4.0	5.0–9.0
Dielectric constant (10^6 Hz)					6.7–8.0	3.0–4.0	3.0–4.0
Dissipation (power) factor (60 Hz)					0.036–0.043	0.01–0.02	0.03–0.05
Dissipation factor (10^6 Hz)					0.025–0.035	0.006–0.02	0.06–0.1
Mechanical							
Compressive modulus, 10^3 lb · in^{-2}			3.6–120				

Property							
Compressive strength, rupture or 1% yield, 10^3 lb·in^{-2}	150–300	350–450	500–1350	600–800	25–45	8–13	0.9–1.7
Elongation at break, %	1.5–2.0	7–75	4–150	4–100	<1	40–80	200–450
Flexural modulus at 23°C, 10^3 lb·in^{-2}					1300–1600	300–500	300–500
Flexural strength, rupture or yield, 10^3 lb·in^{-2}					10–18	10–16	
Hardness, Rockwell (or Shore)	(A65–A92)	(D40–D72)	(A40–A90)	(A50–A90)	M110–M120	(D65–D95)	(A50–A100)
Impact strength (Izod) at 23°C, J·m^{-1}	No break	208 to no break	No break	No break	13–21	21–1068	Varies over wide range
Tensile modulus, 10^3 lb·in^{-2}		1.1–2.5	0.8–50		1000–1500	350–600	
Tensile strength at break, 10^3 lb·in^{-2}	0.65–2.0	3.7–5.7	0.6–3.0	1–3	5.5–13	6–75	1.5–3.5
Tensile yield strength, 10^3 lb·in^{-2}							
Thermal							
Burning rate, mm·min^{-1}					Self-extinguishing	Self-extinguishing	Slow to self-extinguishing
Coefficient of linear thermal expansion, 10^{-6}°C	130–170		130–137		22–36	50–100	70–250
Deflection temperature under flexural load (264 lb·in^{-2}), °C			<0–49		127–143	60–77	
Maximum recommended service temperature, °C					77	70–74	80–105
Specific heat, cal·g^{-1}					0.6	0.2–0.28	0.36–0.5
Thermal conductivity, W·m^{-1}·K^{-1}	0.19–0.21		0.15		0.30–0.42	0.15–0.21	0.13–0.17

TABLE 10-2 Properties of commerical plastics (*continued*)

Properties	Vinyl					
	Poly(vinyl chloride) and poly(vinyl acetate) Flexible and filled	Poly(vinyl chloride), 15% glass-fiber-reinforced	Poly(vinylidene chloride)	Poly(vinyl formal)	Chlorinated poly(vinyl chloride)	Poly(vinyl butyral), flexible
Physical						
Melting temperature, °C						
Crystalline						
Amorphous	75–105	75–105	210	105	110	49
Specific gravity	1.3–1.7	1.54	1.65–1.72	1.2–1.4	1.49–1.56	1.05
Water absorption (24 h), %	0.5–1.0	0.01	0.1	0.5–3.0	0.02–0.15	1.0–2.0
Dielectric strength, kV · mm^{-1}	9.8–12	24–31	16–24	19		14
Electrical						
Volume (dc) resistivity, ohm-cm			10^{14}–10^{16}			
Dielectric constant (60 Hz)			4.5–6.0			
Dielectric constant (10^6 Hz)						
Dissipation (power) factor (60 Hz)						
Dissipation factor (10^6 Hz)						
Mechanical						
Compressive modulus, 10^3 lb · in^{-2}					335–600	

Property						
Compressive strength, rupture or 1% yield, 10^3 lb · in^{-2}	1.0–1.8	9	2–2.7		9–22	150–450
Elongation at break, %	200–400	2–3	50–250	5–20	4–65	
Flexural modulus at 23°C, 10^3 lb · in^{-2}		750			380–450	
Flexural strength, rupture or yield, 10^3 lb · in^{-2}		13.5	4.2–6.2	17–18	14.5–17	
Hardness, Rockwell (or Shore)	(A50–A100)	R118	M50–M65	M85	R117–R122	A10–A100
Impact strength (Izod) at 23°C, J · m^{-1}	Varies over wide range	53	16–53	43–75	53–299	Varies over wide range
Tensile modulus, 10^3 lb · in^{-2}		870	50–80	350–600	360–475	
Tensile strength at break, 10^3 lb · in^{-2}	1–3.5	9.5	3–5	10–12	7.5–9	0.5–3.0
Tensile yield strength, 10^3 lb · in^{-2}						
Thermal						
Burning rate, mm · min^{-1}			Self-extinguishing			Slow
Coefficient of linear thermal expansion, 10^{-6}°C			190	64	68–78	
Deflection temperature under flexural load (264 lb · in^{-2}), °C		68	54–71	71–77	94–112	
Maximum recommended service temperature, °C			100			
Specific heat, cal · g^{-1}			0.32			
Thermal conductivity, W · m^{-1} · K^{-1}	0.13–0.17		0.13	0.16	0.14	

FORMULAS AND ADVANTAGES OF RUBBERS

Gutta Percha

Gutta percha is a natural polymer of isoprene (3-methyl-1,3-butadiene) in which the configuration around each double bond is *trans*. It is hard and horny and has the following formula:

$$\left[\begin{array}{c} \underset{\underset{CH_2}{|}}{\overset{CH_3}{\overset{|}{C}}} \overset{CH_2}{\underset{CH}{=}} \end{array} \right]_n$$

Natural Rubber

Natural rubber is a polymer of isoprene in which the configuration around each double bond is *cis* (or *Z*):

$$\left[\begin{array}{c} H_3C \\ \diagdown \\ C=CH \\ \diagup \qquad \diagdown \\ -CH_2 \qquad\quad CH_2- \end{array} \right]_n$$

Its principal advantages are high resilience and good abrasion resistance.

Chlorosulfonated Polyethylene

Chlorosulfonated polyethylene is prepared as follows:

$$[-CH_2-CH_2-]_n + HSO_3Cl \;\rightarrow\; \left[\begin{array}{c} -CH_2-CH- \\ | \\ SO_3H \end{array} \right]_n + HCl$$

Cross-linking, which can occur as a result of side reactions, causes an appreciable gel content in the final product.

The polymer can be vulcanized to give a rubber with very good chemical (solvent) resistance, excellent resistance to aging and weathering, and good color retention in sunlight.

Epichlorohydrin

Epichlorohydrin is a product of covulcanization of epichlorohydrin (epoxy) polymers with rubbers, especially *cis*-polybutadiene.

Its advantages include impermeability to air, excellent adhesion to metal, and good resistance to oils, weathering, and low temperature.

Nitrile Rubber (NBR, GRN, Buna N)

Nitrile rubber can be prepared as follows:

$$CH_2=CH-CH=CH_2 + CH_2=CH-CN \;\rightarrow$$
$$\text{2 parts} \qquad\qquad \text{1 part}$$

$$\left[\begin{array}{c} -CH_2-CH=CH-CH_2-CH_2-CH-CH_2-CH=CH-CH_2- \\ | \\ CN \end{array} \right]_n$$

Nitrile rubber is also known as nitrile-butadiene rubber (NBR), government rubber nitrile (GRN), and Buna N.

It possesses resistance to oils up to 120°C and excellent abrasion resistance and adhesion to metal.

Polyacrylate

Polyacrylate has the following formula:

$$\left[\begin{array}{c} -CH_2-CH- \\ | \\ CN \end{array} \right]_n$$

It possesses oil and heat resistance to 175°C and excellent resistance to ozone.

cis-Polybutadiene Rubber (BR)

cis-Polybutadiene is prepared by polymerization of butadiene by mostly 1,4-addition.

$$CH_2=CH-CH=CH_2 \rightarrow [-CH_2-CH=CH-CH_2-]_n$$

The polybutadiene produced is in the Z (or cis) configuration.

cis-Polybutadiene has good abrasion resistance, is useful at low temperature, and has excellent adhesion to metal.

Polychloroprene (Neoprene)

Polychloroprene is prepared as follows:

$$CH_2=CH-\underset{\underset{Cl}{|}}{C}=CH_2 \rightarrow [-CH_2-CH=C(Cl)-CH_2-]_n$$

It has very good weathering characteristics, is resistant to ozone and to oil, and is heat-resistant to 100°C.

Ethylene-Propylene-Diene Rubber (EPDM)

Ethylene-propylene-diene rubber is polymerized from 60 parts ethylene, 40 parts propylene, and a small amount of nonconjugated diene. The nonconjugated diene permits sulfur vulcanization of the polymer instead of using peroxide.

It is a very lightweight rubber and has very good weathering and electrical properties, excellent adhesion, and excellent ozone resistance.

Polyisobutylene (Butyl Rubber)

Polyisobutylene is prepared as follows:

$$\underset{98 \text{ parts}}{H_3C-\underset{\underset{CH_3}{|}}{C}=CH_2} + \underset{2 \text{ parts}}{CH_2=\underset{\underset{CH_3}{|}}{C}-CH=CH_2} \rightarrow \left[\left(-\underset{\underset{CH_3}{|}}{\overset{\overset{CH_3}{|}}{C}}-CH_2- \right)_n -CH_2-\underset{\underset{CH_3}{|}}{C}=CH-CH_2- \right]$$

It possesses excellent ozone resistance, very good weathering and electrical properties, and good heat resistance.

(Z)-Polyisoprene (Synthetic Natural Rubber)

Polymerization of isoprene by 1,4-addition produces polyisoprene that has a *cis* (or *Z*) configuration.

$$\left[\begin{array}{c} H_3C \diagdown \diagup H \\ C=C \\ -CH_2 \diagup \diagdown CH_2- \end{array} \right]_n$$

Polysulfide Rubbers

Polysulfide rubbers are prepared as follows:

$$Cl-R-Cl + Na-S-S-S-S-Na \rightarrow HS[-R-S-S-S-S-]_nR-SH$$

where R can be

$$-CH_2CH_2-, \quad -CH_2CH_2-O-CH_2CH_2-,$$

or

$$-CH_2CH_2-O-CH_2-O-CH_2CH_2-.$$

Polysulfide rubbers possess excellent resistance to weathering and oils and have very good electrical properties.

Poly(vinyl chloride) (PVC)

Poly(vinyl chloride) as previously discussed under "Formulas and Key Properties of Plastic Materials" has the following structures:

$$\left[\begin{array}{c} -CH_2-CH- \\ | \\ Cl \end{array} \right]_n$$

PVC polymer plus special plasticizers are used to produce flexible tubing which has good chemical resistance.

Silicone Rubbers

Silicone rubbers are prepared as follows:

$$\begin{array}{ccccc}
CH_3 & & CH_3 & & \left[\begin{array}{c}CH_3\end{array}\right. \\
| & H_2O & | & polymerize & | \\
Cl-Si-Cl & \xrightarrow{} & HO-Si-OH & \xrightarrow{} & -Si-O- \\
| & & | & & | \\
CH_3 & & CH_3 & & \left. CH_3\right]_n
\end{array}$$

Other groups may replace the methyl groups.

Silicone rubbers have excellent ozone and weathering resistance, good electrical properties, and good adhesion to metal.

Styrene-Butadiene Rubber (GRS, SBR, Buna S)

Styrene-butadiene rubber is prepared from the free-radical copolymerization of one part by weight of styrene and three parts by weight of 1,3-butadiene. The butadiene is incorporated by both 1,4-addition (80%) and 1,2-addition (20%). The configuration around the double bond of the 1,4-adduct is about 80% *trans*. The product is a random copolymer with these general features:

trans-1,4-Adduct   1,2-Adduct   *trans*-1,4-Adduct   Styrene   *cis*-1,4-Adduct

Styrene-butadiene rubber (SBR) is also known as government rubber styrene (GRS) and Buna S.

Urethane

See Table 10-3.

TABLE 10-3 Properties of natural and synthetic rubbers

Rubber	Specific gravity	Durometer hardness (or Shore)	Ultimate elongation % (23°C)	Tensile strength, $lb \cdot in^{-2}$ (23°C)	Service temperature, °C Minimum	Service temperature, °C Maximum
Gutta percha (hard rubber)	1.2–1.95	(65–95)	3–8	4000–10,000	−56	104
Natural rubber (NR)	0.93	20–100	750–850	3000–4500		82
Chlorosulfonated polyethylene	1.10	50–95	100–500	500–3000	−54	121
Epichlorohydrin	1.27	60–90	100–400	1000–2500	−46	121
Fluoroelastomers	1.4–1.95	60–90	100–350	2000–3000	−40	232
Isobutene-isoprene rubber (IIR) [also known as government rubber I(GR-I)]	0.91	(40–70)	750–950	2300–3000		121
Nitrile rubber (butadiene-acrylonitrile rubber) (also known as Buna N and NBR)	1.00	30–100	100–600	500–4000	−54	121
Polyacrylate	1.10	40–100	100–400	1000–2200	−18	149
Polybutadiene rubber (BR)	0.93	30–100	100–700	2500–3000	−62	79–100
Polychloroprene (neoprene)	1.23	20–90	800–1000	2000–3500	−54	121
Poly(ethylene-propylene-diene) (EPDM)	0.85	30–100	100–300	1000–3000	−40	149
Polyisobutylene (butyl rubber)	0.92	30–100	100–700	1000–3000	−54	100
Polyisoprene	0.94	20–100	100–750	2000–3000	−54	79–82
Polysulfide (Thiokol ST)	1.34	20–80	100–400	700–1250	−54	82–100
Poly(vinyl chloride) (Koroseal)	1.32	(80–90)		2400–3000		71
Silicone, high-temperature				700–800		316
Silicone	0.98	20–95	50–800	500–1500	−84	232
Styrene-butadiene rubber (SBR) (also known as Buna S)	0.94	40–100	400–600	1600–3700	−60	107
Urethane	0.85	62–95	100–700	1000–8000	−54	100

CHEMICAL RESISTANCE

TABLE 10-4 Resistance of selected polymers and rubbers to various chemicals at 20°C

The information in this table is intended to be used only as a general guide. The chemical resistance classifications are E = excellent (30 days of exposure causes no damage), G = good (some damage after 30 days), F = fair (exposure may cause crazing, softening, or loss of strength), N = not recommended (immediate damage may occur).

Polymers	Chemical												
	Acids, dilute or weak	Acids, strong and concentrated	Alcohols, aliphatic	Aldehydes	Alkalies, concentrated	Esters	Ethers	Glycols	Hydrocarbons, aliphatic	Hydrocarbons, aromatic	Hydrocarbons, halogenated	Ketones	Oxidizing agents, strong
Acetals	F	N	E	N	N	N	N	G	N	N	N	N	N
Acrylics: poly(methyl methacrylate)	G	N	E	—	N	N	E	E	G	N	N	N	N
Allyls: diallyl phthalate	G	—	—	—	N	—	—	—	E	G	G	N	—
Cellulosics: cellulose-acetate-butyrate and cellulose-acetate-propionate polymers	F	N	N	N	N	N	N	G	F	N	N	N	—
Fluorocarbons	E	E	E	E	E	E	E	E	E	E	E	E	E
Polyamides	N	N	G	E	E	G	—	G	G	F	F	E	E
Polycarbonates	G	G	G	F	N	N	F	G	N	F	F	G	N
Polyesters	G	G	G	—	N	N	N	E	G	F	F	N	N
Poly(methyl pentene)	E	E	E	G	E	G	N	E	F	F	N	N	F
Low-density polyethylene	E	E	E	G	E	G	N	E	F	G	N	F	F
High-density polyethylene	E	E	E	E	E	G	N	E	G	G	N	G	F
Polybutadiene	G	F	E	—	—	—	—	—	—	E	E	E	—

10-65

TABLE 10-4 Resistance of selected polymers and rubbers to various chemicals at 20°C (continued)

	Chemical												
	Acids, dilute or weak	Acids, strong and concentrated	Alcohols, aliphatic	Aldehydes	Alkalies, concentrated	Esters	Ethers	Glycols	Hydrocarbons, aliphatic	Hydrocarbons, aromatic	Hydrocarbons, halogenated	Ketones	Oxidizing agents, strong
Polymers (continued)													
Polypropylene and polyallomer	E	E	E	E	E	G	N	E	G	F	N	G	F
Polystyrene	N	N	E	E	N	N	—	E	N	N	N	N	N
Styrene-acrylonitrile copolymers	—	—	N	—	N	—	—	F	F	—	—	—	—
Styrene-acrylonitrile-butadiene copolymers	—	N	G	—	G	N	—	—	F	N	N	N	—
Sulfones: polysulfone	G	N	F	F	E	N	F	G	F	N	N	N	G
Vinyls: poly(vinyl chloride)	E	G	E	G	G	N	F	F	G	N	N	N	G
Rubbers													
Natural rubber	—	—	E	—	—	N	N	E	N	N	N	N	—
Nitrile rubber	—	—	E	—	—	N	G	E	E	N	N	N	—
Polychloroprene	—	—	E	—	—	N	F	E	F	N	N	N	—
Polyisobutylene	—	—	E	—	—	F	F	E	N	N	N	N	—
Polysulfide rubbers: Thiokol	—	—	E	—	—	E	E	E	E	F	N	N	—
Styrene-butadiene rubber	—	—	E	—	—	N	N	E	N	N	N	N	—

GAS PERMEABILITY

TABLE 10-5A Gas permeability constants ($10^{10}P$) at 25°C for polymers and rubbers

The gas permeability constant P is defined as

$$P = \frac{\text{amount of permeant}}{(\text{area}) \times (\text{time}) \times (\text{driving forced across the film})}$$

The gas permeability constant is the amount of gas expressed in cubic centimeters passed in 1 s through a 1-cm^2 area of film when the pressure across a film thickness of 1 cm is 1 cmHg and the temperature is 25°C. All tabulated values are multiplied by 10^{10} and are in units of seconds^{-1} (centimeters of Hg)$^{-1}$. Other temperatures are indicated by exponents and are expressed in degrees Celsius.

Polymer or rubber	Gas						
	He	N$_2$	H$_2$	O$_2$	CO$_2$	H$_2$O	Other
Cellulose (cellophane)	0.005^{20}	0.003 2	0.006 5	0.002 1	0.004 7	1 900	0.006^{45} (H$_2$S); 0.001 7 (SO$_2$)
Cellulose acetate	13.6^{20}	0.28^{30}	3.5^{20}	0.78^{30}	22.7^{30}	5 500	3.5^{30} (H$_2$S); 17^0 (ethylene oxide); 6.8^{60} (bromomethane)
Cellulose nitrate	6.9	0.12	2.0^{20}	1.95	2.12	6 290	57.1 (NH$_3$); 1.76 (SO$_2$)
Ethyl cellulose	400^{30}	8.4^{30}	87^{20}	26.5^{30}	41.0^{30}	12 000^{20}	705 (NH$_3$); 204 (SO$_2$); 420^0 (ethylene oxide)
Gutta percha		2.17	14.4	6.16	35.4	510	15.7 (CO); 30.1 (CH$_4$); 1.68 (C$_3$H$_8$); 98.9 (C$_2$H$_2$);
Natural rubber		9.43	52.0	23.3	15.3	2 290	550 (CH$_3$C≡CH); 3.59 (SF$_6$)
Nylon 6	0.53^{20}	0.009 5^{30}		0.038^{30}	0.10^{30}	177	0.33^{30} (H$_2$S); 1.2^{20} (NH$_3$); 0.84^{60} (CH$_3$Br)
Nylon 11	1.95^{30}		1.78^{30}		1.00^{40}		0.344^{30} (Ne); 0.189^{40} (Ar);
Poly(acrylonitrile)				0.000 2	0.000 8	300	13.6^{50} (propyne)

TABLE 10-5A Gas permeability constants ($10^{10}P$) at 25°C for polymers and rubbers (*continued*)

Polymer or rubber	Gas						
	He	N_2	H_2	O_2	CO_2	H_2O	Other
Acrylonitrile-styrene copolymer (66:34)				0.048	0.21	2 000	
Poly(1,3-butadiene)		6.42	41.9	19.0	138.0	5 070	
Poly(*cis*-1,4-butadiene)	32.6	19.2					19.2 (Ne); 41.0 (Ar)
Butadiene-acrylonitrile copolymer (80:20)	12.2	1.06	15.9	3.85	30.8		24.8 (C_2H_2); 7.7 (propyne)
Butadiene-styrene copolymer (80:20)	13.4	1.71					5.01 (Ne); 4.49 (Ar)
Butadiene-styrene copolymer (92:8)	22.9	5.11					9.70 (Ne); 12.7 (Ar)
Polychloroprene		1.2	13.6	4.0	25.8		3.79 (Ar); 3.27 (CH_4)
Polyethylene, low-density	4.9	0.969	12.0[30]	2.88	12.6	90	2.88 (CH_4); 6.81 (C_2H_6); 9.43 (C_3H_8); 1.48 (CO); 49^0 (ethylene oxide); 14.4 (propene); 42.2 (propyne); 0.170 (SF_6); 472^{60} (CH_3Br)
Polyethylene, high-density	1.14	0.143	3.0[20]	0.403	0.36	12.0	0.388 (CH_4); 0.590 (C_2H_6); 0.537 (C_3H_8); 0.008 3 (SF_6); 1.69 (Ar); 4.01 (propene)
Poly(ethylene terephthalate)							
Crystalline	1.32	0.006 5		0.035	0.17	130	0.003 2 (CH_4); 0.08^{60} (CH_3Br)
Amorphous	3.28	0.013	3.70[20]	0.059	0.30		0.009 (CH_4)
Poly(ethyl methacrylate)	6.82	0.220		1.15	5.00	3 200	2.98 (Ne); 0.565 (Ar); 0.370 (Kr); 3.83 (H_2S); 0.000 001 65 (SF_6)
Isobutene-isoprene copolymer (98:2)	8.38	0.324	7.20	1.30	5.16	110[38]	
Isoprene-acrylonitrile copolymer (76:24)	7.77	0.181	7.41	0.852	4.32		13.6[50] (C_3H_8)

							Other gases
Isoprene-methacrylonitrile copolymer (76:24)							
Methacrylonitrile-styrene-butadiene copolymer (88:7:5)		0.596	13.6	2.34	14.1	600	
Poly(methylpentene)	101	7.83	136	32.0	92.6	51	
Polypropylene	38^{20}	0.44^{30}	41^{20}	2.3^{30}; 0.004 8	9.2^{30}; 0.014		0.33^{20} (H_2S); 9.2^{20} (NH_3)
Silicone rubber, 10% filler	233^{0}	227^{0}	464^{0}	489^{0}	3 240	$43\,000^{35}$	191^{0} (Ne); 550^{0} (Ar); $1\,020^{0}$ (Kr); $2\,550^{0}$ (Xe); $19\,000^{0}$ (butane)
Polystyrene	18.7	0.788	23.3	2.63	10.5	1 200	15.7 (NO_2); 37.5 (N_2O_4)
Poly(tetrafluoroethylene)	6.8^{20}	1.4	9.8	4.2	11.7		1.2^{0} (ethylene oxide); 4.6^{60} (CH_3Br)
Poly(trifluoroethylene)		0.003	0.94^{20}	0.025^{40}	0.048^{40}	0.29	
Poly(vinyl acetate)	12.6^{30}		89^{30}	0.50^{30}			2.64^{30} (Ne); 0.19^{30} (Ar); 0.078^{30} (Kr); 0.050^{30} (CH_4)
Poly(vinyl alcohol)	0.001^{30}	$<0.001^{14}$	0.009	0.008 9	0.001^{23}		0.007 (H_2S); 0.002^{0} (ethylene oxide)
Poly(vinyl chloride)	2.05	0.011 8	1.70	0.045 3	0.157	275	3.92 (Ne); 0.011 5 (Ar); 0.028 6 (CH_4)
Poly(vinylidene chloride)	0.31^{34}	$0.000\,94^{30}$		$0.005\,3^{30}$	0.03^{30}	0.5	0.03^{30} (H_2S); 0.008^{60} (CH_3Br)

TABLE 10-5B Vapor permeability constants ($10^{10}P$) at 35°C for polymers

All tabulated values are multiplied by 10^{10} and are in units of seconds^{-1} (centimeters of Hg)$^{-1}$.

Polymer	Vapor				
	Benzene	Hexane	Carbon tetrachloride	Ethanol	Ethyl acetate
Cellulose	1.4	0.912	0.836	85.8	13.4
Cellulose acetate	512	2.80	3.74	2 980	3 595
Poly(acrylonitrile)	2.61	1.59	1.47	0	1.34
Polyethylene, low-density	5 300	2 910	3 810	55.9	513
Polystyrene	10 600		6 820	0	soluble
Poly(vinyl alcohol)	3.58	2.34	1.61	32.7	2.53

FATS, OILS, AND WAXES

TABLE 10-6 Constants of fats and oils

Fat or oil	Solidification point, °C	Specific gravity (15°C/15°C)	Refractive index	Acid value	Saponification value	Iodine value
		Animal origin				
Butterfat	20–23	$0.91^{40°C}_{15°C}$	1.455	0.5–35	210–230	26–38
Chicken fat	21–27	0.924		1.2	193–205	66–72
Cod-liver oil	–3	0.92–0.93	$0.925^{25°C}$	5.6	171–189	137–166
Deer fat		0.96–0.97		0.8–5.3	195–200	26–36

Dolphin	−3 to +5	0.91–0.93		2–12	203 (body); 290 (jaw)	127 (body); 33 (jaw)

Goat butter	22–24	$0.91\text{–}0.94^{38°C}$			233–236	25–37
Goose fat		0.92–0.93		0.6	191–193	58–67
Herring oil		0.92–0.94	$0.900^{60°C}$	1.8–44	170–194	102–149
Horse fat	20–45	0.92–0.93		0–2.4	195–200	75–86
Human fat	15	0.903	1.460		193–200	57–73
Lard oil	−2 to +4	0.913–0.915	1.462	0.1–2.5	193–198	63–79
Lard oil, fatty tissue	27–30	0.93–0.94	1.462	0.5–0.8	195–203	47–67
Menhaden oil	−5	0.92–0.93	$1.465^{60°C}$	3–12	189–193	148–185
Neat's-foot oil	−2 to +10	0.91–0.92	$1.464^{25°C}$	0.1–0.6	193–199	58–75
Porpoise, body oil	−16	0.926		1.2	203	127
Rabbit fat	17–23	0.93–0.94		1.4–7.2	199–203	70–100
Sardine oil	20–22	0.92–0.93	$1.466^{60°C}$	4–25	188–196	130–152
Seal	3	0.915–0.926		1.9–40	188–196	130–152
Shark		0.916–0.919			157–164	115–139
Sperm oil	15.5	0.878–0.884		13	120–137	80–84
Tallow, beef	31–38	˃ 0.895		0.25	196–200	35–42
Tallow, mutton	32–41	0.937–0.953	$1.457^{40°C}$	2–14	195–196	48–61
Whale oil	−2 to 0	0.917–0.924	$1.460^{60°C}$	1.9	160–202	90–146

Plant origin

Acorn	−10	0.916			199	100
Almond	−20 to −15	0.914–0.921	$1.443^{60°C}$	0.5–3.5	183–208	93–103
Babassu oil	22–26	$0.893^{60°C}$			247	16
Beechnut oil	−17	0.922			191–196	97–111
Castor oil	−18 to −17	0.960–0.967	1.477	0.1–0.8	175–183	84
Chaulmoogra oil, USP	<−25	$0.950^{25°C}$			196–213	98–110
Chinese vegetable tallow	24–34	0.918–0.922		2.4	179–206	23–41
Cocoa butter	21.5–23	0.964–0.974	$1.457^{40°C}$	1.1–1.9	193–195	33–42
Coconut oil	14–22	0.926	$1.449^{40°C}$	2.5–10	153–262	6–10
Corn (maize) oil	−20 to −10	0.921–0.928	$1.473^{40°C}$	1.4–2.0	187–193	111–128

TABLE 10-6 Constants of fats and oils (continued)

Fat or oil	Solidification point, °C	Specific gravity (15°C/15°C)	Refractive index	Acid value	Saponification value	Iodine value
		Plant origin (continued)				
Cottonseed oil	−13 to +12	0.918$^{25°C}_{25°C}$	1.474$^{40°C}$	0.6–0.9	194–196	103–111
Hazelnut oil	−18 to −17	0.917			191–197	87
Hemp-seed oil	−28 to −15	0.928–0.934	1.478$^{25°C}$	0.45	190–195	145–162
Linseed oil	−27 to −19	0.930–0.938	1.475$^{40°C}$	1–3.5	188–195	175–202
Mustard, black, oil	16	0.918–0.921	1.462$^{40°C}$	5.7–7.3	173–175	99–110
Neem oil	−3	0.917	1.471$^{40°C}$		195	71
Niger-seed oil		0.925			190	129
Oiticica oil		0.974$^{25°C}$				140–180
Olive oil	−6	0.914–0.918	1.468$^{40°C}$	0.3–1.0	185–196	79–88
Palm oil	35–42	0.915	1.458$^{40°C}$	10	200–205	49–59
Palm kernel oil	24	0.918–0.925	1.457$^{40°C}$	0.3–0.6	220–231	26–32
Peanut oil	3	0.917–0.926	1.469$^{40°C}$	0.8	186–194	88–98
Perilla oil		0.930–0.937	1.481$^{25°C}$		188–194	185–206
Pistachio-nut oil	−10 to −5	0.913–0.919			191	83–87
Poppy-seed oil	−18 to −16	0.924–0.926	1.469$^{40°C}$	2.5	193–195	128–141
Pumpkin-seed oil	−15	0.923–0.925			188–193	121–130
Rapeseed oil	−10	0.913–0.917	1.471$^{40°C}$	0.36–1.0	168–179	94–105
Safflower oil	−18 to −13	0.925–0.928	1.462$^{60°C}$	0.6	188–203	122–141
Sesame oil	−6 to −4	0.919$^{25°C}_{25°C}$	1.465$^{40°C}$	9.8	188–193	103–117
Soybean oil	−16 to −10	0.924–0.927	1.473$^{40°C}$	0.3–1.8	189–194	122–134
Sunflower-seed oil	−17	0.924–0.926	1.469$^{40°C}$	11.2	188–193	129–136
Tung oil	−2.5	0.94–0.95	1.517$^{25°C}$	2	190–197	163–171
White-mustard-seed oil	−16 to −8	0.912–0.916		5.4	171–174	94–98
Wheat-germ oil						125

TABLE 10-7   Constants of Waxes

Wax	Melting point, °C	Specific gravity (15°C/15°C)	Refractive index	Acid value	Saponification value	Iodine value
Bamboo leaf	79–80	$0.961^{25°C}$	$1.436^{80°C}$	14–15	43–44	7.8
Bayberry (myrtle)	47–49	0.99		3–4	205–212	4–9.5
Beeswax, ordinary	62–66	0.95–0.97	1.44–$1.48^{40°C}$	17–21	88–100	8–11
Beeswax, East Indian	61–67	0.95–0.97	$1.44^{40°C}$	5–10.5	87–117	4–10.5
Beeswax, white, USP	61–69	0.95–0.98	1.45–$1.47^{65°C}$	17–24	90–96	7–11
Candelilla	73–77	0.98–0.99	1.45–$1.46^{85°C}$	19–24	55–64	14–20
Cape berry	40–45	1.01	$1.45^{45°C}$	2.5–4.0	211–215	0.5–2.5
Caranda	80–85	0.99–1.00		5.0–9.5	64–79	8–9
Carnauba, No. 1 yellow	86–88	0.99–1.00		1.5–2.5	75–86	
Carnauba, No. 3, crude	86–90	0.99–1.01		3.0–8.5	75–89	
Carnauba, No. 3, refined	86–89	0.96–0.97	$1.47^{40°C}$	3.0–5.0	76–85	7–13.5
Castor oil, hydrogenated	83–88	0.98–$0.99^{20°C}$		1.0–5.0	177–181	2.5–8.5
Chinese insect	80–85	0.95–0.97	$1.46^{40°C}$	2–9	78–93	1.0–2.5
Cotton	68–71	0.96		32	71	25
Cranberry	207–218	0.97–0.98		42–59	131–134	44–53
Esparto	75–79	0.985–0.995		22–27	58–73	7–15
Flax	61–70	0.91–0–0.99		17–48	37–102	22–29
Japan	49–56	0.97–1.00		4–15	210–235	4–15
Jojoba	11–12	0.86–$0.90^{25°C}$	$1.465^{25°C}$	0.2–0.6	92–95	82–88
Microcrystalline, amber	64–91	0.91–0.94	1.42–$1.45^{80°C}$	0	0	0
Microcrystalline, white	71–89	0.93–0.94	$1.441^{80°C}$	0	0	0
Montan, crude	76–86	1.01–$1.02^{25°C}$		22–31	59–92	14–18
Montan, refined	77–84	1.02–1.04		23–45	72–115	10–14
Ouricury	86–89	0.99–1.01		12–19	88–96	6.9–7.8
Ozokerite	56–82	0.90–1.00		0	0	4–8
Palm	74–86	0.99–1.05		5–11	64–104	9–17

TABLE 10-7 Constants of Waxes (continued)

Wax	Melting point, °C	Specific gravity (15°C/15°C)	Refractive index	Acid value	Saponification value	Iodine value
Paraffin, American	49–63	0.896–0.925	$1.44-1.48^{80°C}$	0	0	0
Shellac	79–82	0.97–0.98		12–24	64–83	6–9
Sisal hemp	74–81	1.007–1.010		16–19	56–58	28–29
Spermaceti	41–49	0.905–0.960	$1.51^{25°C}$	0.5–3.0	121–135	2.5–8.5
Sugarcane, refined	76–82	0.96–0.98	$1.48^{40°C}$	8–23	55–70	13–29
Wool	38–40	0.97		6–22	82–130	15–47

SECTION 11
MISCELLANEOUS

PHYSICAL CONSTANTS

TABLE 11-1 Fundamental physical constants

Source: E. R. Cohen and B. N. Taylor, *J. Phys. Chem. Ref. Data,* **2**(4):663 (1973).

A. Defined values

Name of unit	Symbol	Definition
		SI base units
Meter (metre) (preferred spelling in U.S. is meter)	m	1 650 763.73 wavelengths in vacuum of the orange-red line of the spectrum of krypton-86
Kilogram	kg	Mass of a cylinder of platinum-iridium alloy kept at Paris
Second	s	Duration of 9 192 631 770 cycles of the radiation associated with a specified transition of the cesium atom
Ampere	A	Magnitude of the current that, when flowing through each of two long parallel wires separated by one meter in free space, results in a force between the two wires 2×10^{-7} newton for each meter of length
Kelvin (degree Kelvin)	K	Defined in the thermodynamic scale by assigning 273.16 K to the triple point of water (freezing point, 273.15 K = 0°C)
Candela	cd	Luminous intensity of 1/600 000 of a square meter of a radiating cavity at the temperature of freezing platinum (2042 K)
Mole	mol	Amount of substance which contains as many specified entities (molecules, atoms, ions, electrons, photons, etc.) as there are atoms of carbon-12 in exactly 0.012 kg of that nuclide
		Supplementary SI units
Radian	rad	The plane angle between two radii of a circle which cut off on the circumference an arc equal in length to the radius
Steradian	sr	The solid angle which, having its vertex in the center of a sphere, cuts off an area of the surface of the sphere equal to that of a square with sides of length equal to the radius of the sphere

B. Derived SI units

Quantity and symbol	Name of SI unit	Symbol and definition
Capacitance (electric), C	farad	$F = C \cdot V^{-1}$
Charge (electric), quantity of electricity, Q	coulomb	$C = A \cdot s$
Conductance (electric), $G(=1/R)$	siemens	$S = \Omega^{-1}$
Energy, work, quantity of heat, H	joule	$J = kg \cdot m^2 \cdot s^{-2}$

TABLE 11-1   Fundamental physical constants (*continued*)

Quantity and symbol	Name of SI unit	Symbol and definition
Force	newton	$N = kg \cdot m \cdot s^{-2}$
Frequency	hertz	$Hz = s^{-1}$
Illuminance, illumination	lux	$lx = lm \cdot m^{-2}$
Inductance, L	henry	$H = \Omega \cdot s$
Luminous flux	lumen	$lm = cd \cdot sr$
Magnetic flux	weber	$Wb = V \cdot s$
Magnetic flux density	tesla	$T = Wb \cdot m^{-2}$
Potential difference, E	volt	$V = kg \cdot m^2 \cdot s^{-3} \cdot A^{-1} = J \cdot A^{-1} \cdot s^{-1}$
Power, radiant flux	watt	$W = kg \cdot m^2 \cdot s^{-3} = J \cdot s^{-1}$
Pressure, stress	pascal	$Pa = N \cdot m^{-2} = kg \cdot m^{-1} \cdot s^{-2}$
Resistance (electric), R	ohm	$\Omega = V \cdot A^{-1} = kg \cdot m^2 \cdot s^{-3} \cdot A^{-2}$

C. Recommended Consistent Values of Constants

The digits in parentheses following a numerical value represent the standard deviation of that value in terms of the final listed digits.

Constant	Symbol and value
Anomalous electron moment correction	$(\mu_e/\mu_0) - 1 = 1.159\ 615(15) \times 10^{-3}$
Atomic mass unit	$u = (10^{-3}\ kg \cdot mol^{-1})/N_A = 1.660\ 566(9) \times 10^{-27}\ kg$
Avogadro constant	$N_A = 6.022\ 045(31) \times 10^{23}\ mol^{-1}$
Bohr magneton	$\mu_B = e\hbar/2m_ec = 9.274\ 078(36) \times 10^{-24}\ J \cdot T^{-1}$
Bohr radius	$a_0 = \alpha/4\pi R_\infty = 0.529\ 177\ 06(44) \times 10^{-10}\ m$
Boltzmann constant	$k = R/N_A = 1.380\ 662(44) \times 10^{-23}\ J \cdot K^{-1}$
Charge-to-mass ratio for electron	$e/m_e = 1.758\ 805(5) \times 10^{11}\ C \cdot kg^{-1}$
Compton wavelength of electron	$\lambda_c = \alpha^2/2R_\alpha = 2.426\ 309(4) \times 10^{-12}\ m$
	$\lambdabar_c = \lambda_c/2\pi = \alpha a_0 = 3.861\ 591(6) \times 10^{-13}\ m$
Compton wavelength of neutron	$\lambda_{c,n} = h/m_nc = 1.319\ 591(2) \times 10^{-15}\ m$
Compton wavelength of proton	$\lambda_{c,p} = h/m_pc = 1.321\ 410(2) \times 10^{-15}\ m$
Diamagnetic shielding factor, spherical H_2O molecule	$1 + \sigma(H_2O) = 1.000\ 025\ 64(7)$
Electron g-factor	$g_e/2 = \mu_e/\mu_B = 1.001\ 159\ 657(4)$
Electron magnetic moment	$\mu_e = 9.284\ 832(36) \times 10^{-24}\ J \cdot T^{-1}$
Electron radius (classical)	$\alpha\lambdabar_c = \mu_0e^2/4\pi m_e = r_e = 2.817\ 938(7) \times 10^{-15}\ m$
Electron rest mass	$m_e = 0.910\ 953(5) \times 10^{-30}\ kg$
	$= 5.485\ 803(2) \times 10^{-4}\ u$
Elementary charge	$e = 1.602\ 189(5) \times 10^{-19}\ C$
Faraday constant	$N_Ae = F = 9.648\ 456(27) \times 10^4\ C \cdot mol^{-1}$
Fine structure constant	$\mu_0ce^2/2h = \alpha = 0.007\ 297\ 351(6)$
	$1/\alpha = 1.370\ 360(1)$
First radiation constant	$2\pi hc^2 = c_1 = 3.741\ 83(2) \times 10^{-16}\ W \cdot m^2$
Gas constant (molar)	$R = P_0V_m/T_0 = 8.314\ 41(26)\ J \cdot mol^{-1} \cdot K^{-1}$
	$= 82.0568(26)\ cm^3 \cdot atm \cdot mol^{-1} \cdot K^{-1}$
	$= 1.987\ 19(6)\ cal \cdot mol^{-1} \cdot K^{-1}$
Gravitational constant	$G = 6.672(4) \times 10^{-11}\ N \cdot m^2 \cdot kg^{-2}$

Constant	Symbol and value
Gyromagnetic ratio of proton (uncorrected for diamagnetism of H_2O)	$\gamma_p = 2.675\ 199(8) \times 10^8\ \text{s}^{-1} \cdot \text{T}^{-1}$
	$\gamma'_p = 675\ 130(8) \times 10^8\ \text{s}^{-1} \cdot \text{T}^{-1}$
Josephson frequency-voltage ratio	$2e/h = 4.835\ 939(13) \times 10^{14}\ \text{Hz} \cdot \text{V}^{-1}$
Magnetic flux quantum	$\Phi_0 = h/2e = 2.067\ 851(5) \times 10^{-15}\ \text{Wb}$
Molar standard volume, ideal gas	$V_m = RT_0/P_0 = 0.022\ 413\ 8(7)\ \text{m}^3 \cdot \text{mol}^{-1}$
Muon g-factor	$e\hbar/2m_\mu c = g_\mu/2 = 1.001\ 166\ 16(31)$
Muon magnetic moment	$\mu_\mu = 4.490\ 474(18) \times 10^{-26}\ \text{J} \cdot \text{T}^{-1}$
Muon rest mass	$m_\mu = 1.883\ 566(11) \times 10^{-28}\ \text{kg}$
Neutron rest mass	$m_n = 1.674\ 954(9) \times 10^{-27}\ \text{kg}$
Normal volume, perfect gas	$V_0 = 2.241\ 36(30) \times 10^4\ \text{cm}^3 \cdot \text{mol}^{-1}$
Nuclear magneton	$\mu_N = e\hbar/2m_p c = 5.050\ 824(20) \times 10^{-27}\ \text{J} \cdot \text{T}^{-1}$
Permeability of vacuum	$\mu_0 = 4\pi \times 10^{-7}\ \text{H} \cdot \text{m}^{-1}$
Permittivity of vacuum	$\varepsilon_0 = (\mu_0 c^2)^{-1} = 8.854\ 187\ 82(7) \times 10^{-12}\ \text{F} \cdot \text{m}^{-1}$
Planck constant	$h = 6.626\ 176(36) \times 10^{-34}\ \text{J} \cdot \text{s}$
	$\hbar = h/2\pi = 1.054\ 589(6) \times 10^{-34}\ \text{J} \cdot \text{s}$
Proton magnetic moment:	$\mu_p = 1.410\ 617(5) \times 10^{-26}\ \text{J} \cdot \text{T}^{-1}$
In Bohr magnetons	$\mu_p/\mu_B = 1.521\ 032\ 209(16) \times 10^{-3}$
In nuclear magnetons	$\mu_p/\mu_N = 2.792\ 845\ 6(11)$
Proton rest mass	$m_p = 1.672\ 649(9) \times 10^{-27}\ \text{kg}$
Quantum-charge ratio	$h/e = 4.135\ 701(11) \times 10^{-15}\ \text{J} \cdot \text{Hz}^{-1} \cdot \text{C}^{-1}$
Quantum of circulation	$h/m_e = 7.273\ 89(1) \times 10^{-4}\ \text{J} \cdot \text{s} \cdot \text{kg}^{-1}$
Ratio, electron to proton magnetic moments	$\mu_e/\mu_p = 6.582\ 106\ 88(7) \times 10^2$
Ratio, kxu (Siegbahn) to angstrom	$= 1.000\ 020\ 5(56)$
Ratio, muon moment to proton moment	$\mu_\mu/\mu_p = 3.183\ 340(7)$
Rydberg constant	$R_\infty = 1.097\ 373\ 18(8) \times 10^7\ \text{m}^{-1}$
Second radiation constant	$c_2 = hc/k = 1.438\ 786(45) \times 10^{-2}\ \text{m} \cdot \text{K}$
Speed of light in vacuum	$c = 2.997\ 924\ 58(12) \times 10^8\ \text{m} \cdot \text{s}^{-1}$
Stefan–Boltzmann constant	$\sigma = (\pi^2/60)k^4/\hbar^3 c^2 = 5.670\ 3(7) \times 10^{-8}\ \text{W} \cdot \text{m}^{-2} \cdot \text{K}^{-4}$
Thomson cross section	$\sigma_e = 8\pi r_e^2/3 = 6.652\ 448(33) \times 10^{-28}\ \text{m}^2$
Voltage-wavelength product	$V\lambda = 1.239\ 852(3) \times 10^{-6}\ \text{eV} \cdot \text{m}$
Wien displacement constant	$b = 0.289\ 78(4)\ \text{cm} \cdot \text{K}$
Zeeman splitting constant	$\mu_B/hc = 4.668\ 58(4) \times 10^{-5}\ \text{cm}^{-1} \cdot \text{G}^{-1}$
Energy equivalents:	
1 atomic mass unit	$u = 931.501\ 6(26)\ \text{MeV}$
1 proton mass	$m_v = 938.279\ 6(27)\ \text{MeV}$
1 neutron mass	$m_n = 939.573\ 1(27)\ \text{MeV}$
1 muon mass	$m_\mu = 105.659\ 48(35)\ \text{MeV}$
1 electron mass	$m_e = 0.511\ 003\ 4(14)\ \text{MeV}$
1 electronvolt	$1\ \text{eV}/k = 1.160\ 450(36) \times 10^4\ \text{K}$
	$1\ \text{eV}/hc = 8.065\ 479(21) \times 10^3\ \text{cm}^{-1}$
	$1\ \text{eV}/h = 2.417\ 970(6) \times 10^{14}\ \text{Hz}$

GREEK ALPHABET

TABLE 11-2   Greek alphabet

Capital letter	Lowercase letter	Letter name	Capital letter	Lowercase letter	Letter name
A	α	Alpha	N	ν	Nu
B	β	Beta	Ξ	ξ	Xi
Γ	γ	Gamma	O	o	Omicron
Δ	δ	Delta	Π	π	Pi
E	ε	Epsilon	P	ρ	Rho
Z	ζ	Zeta	Σ	σ	Sigma
Ḣ	η	Eta	T	τ	Tau
Θ	θ	Theta	Y	υ	Upsilon
I	ι	Iota	Φ	ϕ	Phi
K	κ	Kappa	X	χ	Chi
Λ	λ	Lambda	Ψ	ψ	Psi
M	μ	Mu	Ω	ω	Omega

PREFIXES

TABLE 11-3   Prefixes for naming multiples and submultiples of units

For example: 10^{-9} gram is one nanogram, or 1 ng.

Factor	Prefix	Symbol	Factor	Prefix	Symbol
10^{12}	tera	T	10^{-2}	centi	c
10^{9}	giga	G	10^{-3}	milli	m
10^{6}	mega	M	10^{-6}	micro	μ
10^{3}	kilo	k	10^{-9}	nano	n
10^{2}	hecto	h	10^{-12}	pico	p
10	deka	da	10^{-15}	femto	f
10^{-1}	deci	d	10^{-18}	atto	a

TABLE 11-4   Numerical prefixes

Number	Prefix	Number	Prefix	Number	Prefix
$\frac{1}{2}$	hemi	6	hexa	13	trideca
1	mono	7	hepta	14	tetradeca
$1\frac{1}{2}$	sesqui	8	octa	15	pentadeca
2	di or bi	9	nona	16	hexadeca
3	tri	10	deca	17	heptadeca
4	tetra	11	undeca	18	octadeca
5	penta	12	dodeca	19	nonadeca

TABLE 11-4   Numerical prefixes (*continued*)

Number	Prefix	Number	Prefix	Number	Prefix
20	icosa	34	tetratriaconta	48	octatetraconta
21	henicosa	35	pentatriaconta	49	nonatetraconta
22	docosa	36	hexatriaconta	50	pentaconta
23	tricosa	37	heptatriaconta	51	henpentaconta
24	tetracosa	38	octatriaconta	52	dopentaconta
25	pentacosa	39	nonatriaconta	53	tripentaconta
26	hexacosa	40	tetraconta	54	tetrapentaconta
27	heptacosa	41	hentetraconta	55	pentapentaconta
28	octacosa	42	dotetraconta	56	hexapentaconta
29	nonacosa	43	tritetraconta	57	heptapentaconta
30	triaconta	44	tetratetraconta	58	octapentaconta
31	hentriaconta	45	pentatetraconta	59	monapentaconta
32	dotriaconta	46	hexatetraconta	60	hexaconta
33	tritriaconta	47	heptatetraconta		

TRANSFORMATIONS

TABLE 11-5   Conversion formulas for solutions having concentrations expressed in various ways

Abbreviations Used in the Table

wt %, weight percent of solute
MW_1, molecular weight of solute
MW_2, molecular weight of solvent
d, density of solution $(g \cdot mL^{-1})$

m, molality
M, molarity
n, mole fraction
G, grams of solute per liter of solution

To obtain	From	Compute
molarity	weight per cent of solute	$M = \dfrac{10d(\text{wt }\%)}{MW_1}$
molarity	molality	$M = \dfrac{1000\,dm}{1000 + (MW_1)m}$
molarity	grams of solute per liter of solution	$M = \dfrac{G}{MW_1}$
molarity	mole fraction	$M = \dfrac{1000\,dn}{n(NW_1) + MW_2(1 - n)}$
mole fraction	weight per cent of solute	$n = \dfrac{(\text{wt }\%)/MW_1}{(\text{wt }\%)/MW_1 + (100 - \text{wt }\%)MW_2}$
mole fraction	molality	$n = \dfrac{(MW_2)m}{(MW_2)m + 1000}$
mole fraction	molarity	$n = \dfrac{M(MW_2)}{M(MW_2 - MW_1) + 1000\,d}$

TABLE 11-5 Conversion formulas for solutions having concentrations expressed in various ways (*continued*)

To obtain	From	Compute
mole fraction	grams of solute per liter of solution	$n = \dfrac{G(MW_2)}{G(MW_2 - MW_1) + 1000d(MW_1)}$
weight percent of solute	mole fraction	$wt\% = \dfrac{100n(MW_1)}{n(MW_1) + MW_2(1 - n)}$
weight percent of solute	grams of solute per liter of solution	$wt\% = \dfrac{G}{10d}$
weight percent of solute	molarity	$wt\% = \dfrac{M(MW_1)}{10d}$
weight percent of solute	molality	$wt\% = \dfrac{100m(MW_1)}{1000 + m(MW_1)}$
molality	molarity	$m = \dfrac{1000M}{1000d - M(MW_1)}$
molality	grams of solute per liter of solution	$m = \dfrac{1000G}{MW_1(1000d - G)}$
molality	weight percent of solute	$m = \dfrac{1000(wt\%)}{MW_1(100 - wt\%)}$
molality	mole fraction	$m = \dfrac{1000n}{MW_2 - n(MW_2)}$

TABLE 11-6 Conversion factors

The data have been compared with the *International Standard ISO* 31 (1979-80) and the *American Society for Testing and Materials Standard for Metric Practice E* 380-79. Relations which are exact are indicated by an asterisk (*). Factors in parentheses are also exact.

To convert	Into	Multiply by
ampere per square centimeter	ampere per square inch*	6.451 6
ampere-hour	coulomb*	3 600
ampere-turn	gilbert	1.256 637
angstrom	meter*	1×10^{-10}
	nanometer*	0.1
apostib	candela per square meter	0.318 309 9(1π)
	lambert*	1×10^{-4}
atmosphere	bar*	1.013 25
	inch of mercury	29.921 26
	millimeter of mercury*	760
	millimeter of water	$1.033\ 227 \times 10^4$
	newton per square meter*	$1.013\ 25 \times 10^5$
	pascal*	$1.013\ 25 \times 10^5$
	torr*	760

TABLE 11-6 Conversion factors (*continued*)

To convert	Into	Multiply by
bar	atmosphere	0.986 923
	dyne per square centimeter*	1×10^6
	millimeter of mercury	750.062
	pascal	1×10^5
barn	square meter*	1×10^{-28}
barrel (petroleum)	gallon (British)	34.972 3
	gallon (U.S.)*	42
	liter	158.987
barrel (U.S., dry)	bushel (U.S.)	3.281 22
	liter	115.627 1
barrel (U.S., liquid)	gallon (U.S.)	31.5
	liter	119.240 5
becquerel	curie*	2.7×10^{-11}
British thermal unit (Btu)	calorie	251.996
	joule	1 055.056
	kilowatt-hour	$2.930\ 71 \times 10^{-4}$
	liter-atmosphere	10.412 6
bushel (U.S.)	barrel (U.S., dry)	0.304 765
	cubic foot	1.244 456
	cubic inch*	2 150.42
	gallon (U.S.)	9.309 18
	liter	35.239.07
	pint (U.S., dry)	64
	quart (U.S., dry)	32
calorie	Btu	0.003 968 320
	joule*	4.186 8
	liter-atmosphere	0.041 320 5
calorie (thermochemical)	joule*	4.184
calorie per minute	watt*	0.069 78
calorie per second	watt*	4.186 8
candela	Hefner unit	1.11
	lumen per steradian*	1
candela per square centimer	candela per square foot*	929.303 4
	lambert	$3.141\ 593(\pi)$
carat (metric)	gram*	0.2
Celsius (Centigrade) temperature scale, °C	Fahrenheit temperature scale, °F	$\frac{9}{5}°C + 32 = °F$
centimeter	foot	0.032 808 4
	inch	0.393 700 8
	mil	393.700 8
centimeter of mercury	pascal	1 333.22
centimeter per second	foot per second	0.032 808 4

TABLE 11-6   Conversion factors (*continued*)

To convert	Into	Multiply by
centimeter-dyne	erg*	1
	joule*	1×10^{-7}
centipoise	pascal-second*	0.001
centistokes	square meter per second*	1×10^{-6}
coulomb	ampere-second*	1
cubic centimeter	cubic foot	$3.531\ 47 \times 10^{-5}$
	liter*	0.001
	ounce (U.S., fluid)	0.033 814 02
	quart (U.S., dry)	$9.080\ 83 \times 10^{-4}$
	quart (U.S., liquid)	0.001 056 688
cubic centimeter per second	liter per hour*	3.6
curie	becquerel*	3.7×10^{10}
cycle per second	hertz*	1
day (mean solar)	hour*	24
	minute*	1 440
	second	8.64×10^{4}
Debye unit	coulomb-meter	$3.335\ 64 \times 10^{-30}$
decibel	neper	0.115 129 255
degree (angle)	circumference	0.002 777 78(1/360)
	minute (angle)*	60
	quadrant	0.011 111 1(1/90)
	radian	$0.017\ 453\ 29(\pi/180)$
degree Celcius (Centigrade) (temperature difference), °C	degree Fahrenheit, °F*	1.8
	degree Rankine*	1.8
	kelvin*	1
dram (apothecaries or troy)	dram (avoirdupois)	2.194 285 7
dram (avoirdupois)	grain*	27.343 75
	gram	1.771 845 2
	ounce (avoirdupois)	0.062 5(1/16)
dram (U.S., fluid)	cubic centimeter	3.696 691 2
	ounce (U.S., fluid)*	0.125(1/8)
	pint (U.S., liquid)*	0.007 812 5(1/128)
dyne	kilogram-force	$1.019\ 716 \times 10^{-6}$
	newton*	1×10^{-5}
dyne per square centimeter	bar*	1×10^{-6}
	millimeter of mercury	$7.500\ 617 \times 10^{-4}$
	pascal	0.1
dyne-centimeter	erg*	1
	joule*	1×10^{-7}
	newton-meter*	1×10^{-7}

TABLE 11-6   Conversion factors (*continued*)

To convert	Into	Multiply by
dyne-second per square centimer	poise*	1
	pascal-second	0.1
electronvolt	erg	$1.602\,19 \times 10^{-12}$
	joule	$1.602\,19 \times 10^{-19}$
em	millimeter	4.217 52
erg	dyne-centimeter*	1
	joule*	1×10^{-7}
	watt-hour	$2.777\,78 \times 10^{-11}$
Fahrenheit temperature, °F	Celsius temperature, °C	$\frac{5}{9}(°F - 32) = °C$
fathom	foot*	6
fermi	meter*	1×10^{-15}
foot	centimeter*	30.48
	inch	12
foot-candle	lumen per square foot*	1
	lumen per square meter	10.763 9
foot-lambert	candela per square centimeter	$3.426\,26 \times 10^{-4}$
	candela per square foot	0.318 309 9
	lambert	0.001 076 39
gallon (British, imperial)	gallon (U.S.)	1.200 95
	liter*	4.546 09
gallon (U.S.)	liter	3.785 412
	ounce (U.S., fluid)*	128
	pint (U.S., liquid)*	8
gauss	tesla*	1×10^{-4}
	weber per square meter	1×10^{-4}
gilbert	ampere-turn	0.795 775
grain	milligram*	64.798 91
gram	carat (metric)*	5
	grain	15.432 358
	ounce (avoirdupois)	0.035 273 962
	ounce (troy)	0.032 150 747
	pound	0.002 204 622 6
	ton (metric)	1×10^{-6}
gram-force	dyne*	980.665
	newton*	0.009 806 65
gram-force per square centimeter	pascal*	98.066 5
gram-force-centimeter	joule*	$9.806\,65 \times 10^{-5}$
Hefner unit	candela	0.9
hertz	cycles per second*	1

TABLE 11-6   Conversion factors (*continued*)

To convert	Into	Multiply by
hour (mean solar)	minute*	60
	second	3 600
inch	centimeter*	2.54
	foot	0.083 333 3(1/12)
	mil*	1 000
	millimeter*	25.4
joule	Btu	$9.478\ 170 \times 10^{-4}$
	calorie	0.238 845 9
	erg*	1×10^{7}
	liter-atmosphere	0.009 869 233
	newton-meter*	1
	watt-hour	$2.777\ 78 \times 10^{-4}(1/3600)$
kelvin temperature scale, K	Celsius scale, °C	°C + 273.1 = K
kilocalorie per second	kilowatt*	4.186 8
kilogram	ounce (avoirdupois)	35.273 963
	ounce (troy)	32.150 747
	pound	2.204 622 6
	ton (long)	$9.842\ 065\ 3 \times 10^{-4}$
	ton (metric)	0.001
	ton (short)	0.001 102 311 3
kilometer	foot	3 280.840
	light-year	$1.057\ 02 \times 10^{-13}$
	mile (statute)	0.621 371 192
kilowatt	Btu per hour	3 412.14
	horsepower (metric)	1.359 62
	joule per hour*	3.6×10^{-6}
	kilocalorie per hour	859.845
knot	foot per minute	101.268 6
	meter per minute	30.866 7
	mile (nautical) per hour*	1
	mile (statute) per hour	1.150 78
lambert	candela per square centimeter	0.318 310
liter	cubic centimeter*	1 000
	cubic decimeter*	1
	cubic inch	61.023 74
	gallon (U.S.)	0.264 172 1
	ounce (U.S., fluid)	33.814 02
	pint (U.S., liquid)	2.113 376
	quart (U.S., liquid)	1.056 688
liter per minute	gallon (U.S.) per hour	15.850 3
liter-atmosphere	Btu	0.096 037 6
	calorie	24.201 1
	joule*	101.325

TABLE 11-6 Conversion factors (*continued*)

To convert	Into	Multiply by
lumen per square centimeter	lux*	1×10^4
lux	lumen per square meter*	1
maxwell	weber*	1×10^{-8}
megohm	ohm*	1×10^6
meter	angstrom*	1×10^{10}
	foot	3.280 839 895
mho (ohm^{-1})	siemens*	1
micrometer (micron)	angstrom	1×10^4
	millimeter*	0.001
mil	inch*	0.001
	millimeter*	0.025 4
mile (statute)	foot*	5.280
	furlong*	8
	kilometer*	1.609 344
	mile (nautical)	0.868 976
milligram per assay ton	milligram per kilogram	34.285 714
	ounce (troy) per ton (short)*	1
milliliter	cubic centimeter*	1
millimeter	inch	0.039 370 8
millimeter of mercury	atmosphere	0.001 315 789(1/760)
	dyne per square centimeter	1 333.224
	pascal	133.322 4
	torr*	1
minute (angle)	circumference	$4.629\ 63 \times 10^{-5}$
	degree (angle)	0.016 666 7(1/60)
	radian	$2.908\ 88 \times 10^{-4}$
	second (angle)*	60
minute	day	$6.944\ 444 \times 10^{-4}$
	hour	0.016 666 7(1/60)
	second*	60
newton	dyne*	1×10^5
newton per square centimeter	pascal*	1×10^4
oersted	ampere per meter	79.577 5
ounce (avoirdupois)	dram*	16
	grain*	437.5
	gram*	28.349 523 125
	ounce (troy)	0.911 458 33
	pound*	0.062 5(1/16)
ounce (U.S., fluid)	cubic centimeter	29.573 530
	gallon (U.S.)*	0.007 812 5(1/128)
	milliliter	29.573 530

TABLE 11-6 Conversion factors (*continued*)

To convert	Into	Multiply by
	pint (U.S., liquid)*	0.062 5(1/16)
	quart (U.S., liquid)*	0.031 25(1/32)
parsec	kilometer	$3.085\ 68 \times 10^{13}$
part per million	gram per ton (metric)*	1
	milligram per kilogram*	1
pascal	bar*	1×10^{-5}
	dyne per square centimeter*	10
	inch of mercury	$2.953\ 00 \times 19^{-4}$
	millimeter of mercury	$7.500\ 62 \times 10^{-3}$
	newton per square meter*	1
pascal-second	poise*	10
pica (printer's)	point*	12
pint (U.S., liquid)	cubic centimeter	473.176 5
point (printer's, U.S.)	millimeter*	0.351 459 8
poise	pascal-second*	0.1
pound	dram*	256
	grain*	7 000
	gram*	453.592 37
	ounce (avoirdupois)*	16
	ton (long)	$4.462\ 285\ 7 \times 10^{-4}$
	ton (metric)*	$4.535\ 923\ 7 \times 10^{-4}$
	ton (short)*	$5 \times 10^{-4}(1/2000)$
poundal	gram-force	14.098 1
	newton	0.138 255
proof (U.S.)	percent alcohol by volume*	0.5
quart (U.S., dry)	cubic centimeter	1 101.221
	cubic foot	0.038 889 25
	pint (U.S., dry)	2
quart (U.S., liquid)	gallon (U.S.)*	0.25
	liter	0.946 353
	ounce (U.S., fluid)*	32
	pint (U.S., liquid)*	2
radian	degree (angle)	57.295 780
	minute (angle)	3.437.75
	revolution	0.159 155
ream	quire*	20
	sheet	480 or 500
revolution	degree (angle)*	360
revolution per minute	radian per second	0.140 720
roentgen	coulomb per kilogram*	2.58×10^{-4}
second (angle)	degree	$2.777\ 78 \times 10^{-4}$
	radian	$4.848\ 137 \times 10^{-6}$

TABLE 11-6   Conversion factors (*continued*)

To convert	Into	Multiply by
siemens	mho (ohm^{-1})*	1
steradian	sphere	0.079 577 5
	spherical right angle	0.636 620
stokes	square meter per second*	1×10^{-4}
tablespoon (metric)	cubic centimeter*	15
teaspoon (metric)	cubic centimeter*	5
tesla	weber per square meter*	1
ton (long)	kilogram*	1 016.046 908 8
	pound*	2 240
	ton (metric)	1.016 046 9
	ton (short)*	1.12
torr	millimeter of mercury	1
	pascal	133.322 4
volt-second	weber*	1
watt	Btu per hour	3.412 14
	calorie per second	0.238 846
	erg per second*	1×10^7
	joule per second*	1
weber	maxwell*	1×10^8
X unit	meter	$1.002\ 02 \times 10^{-13}$

STATISTICS

TABLE 11-7   Values of *t*

Source: Perry, Chilton, and Kirkpatrick, *Chemical Engineers' Handbook*, 4th ed., McGraw-Hill, New York (1963).

df	$t_{.60}$	$t_{.70}$	$t_{.80}$	$t_{.90}$	$t_{.95}$	$t_{.975}$	$t_{.99}$	$t_{.995}$
1	0.325	0.727	1.376	3.078	6.314	12.706	31.821	63.657
2	0.289	0.617	1.061	1.886	2.920	4.303	6.965	9.925
3	0.277	0.584	0.978	1.638	2.353	3.182	4.541	5.841
4	0.271	0.569	0.941	1.533	2.132	2.776	3.747	4.604
5	0.267	0.559	0.920	1.476	2.015	2.571	3.365	4.032
6	0.265	0.553	0.906	1.440	1.943	2.447	3.143	3.707
7	0.263	0.549	0.896	1.415	1.895	2.365	2.998	3.499
8	0.262	0.546	0.889	1.397	1.860	2.306	2.896	3.355
9	0.261	0.543	0.883	1.383	1.833	2.262	2.821	3.250
10	0.260	0.542	0.879	1.372	1.812	2.228	2.764	3.169

TABLE 11-7 Values of *t* (*continued*)

df	$t_{.60}$	$t_{.70}$	$t_{.80}$	$t_{.90}$	$t_{.95}$	$t_{.975}$	$t_{.99}$	$t_{.995}$
11	0.260	0.540	0.876	1.363	1.796	2.201	2.718	3.106
12	0.259	0.539	0.873	1.356	1.782	2.179	2.681	3.055
13	0.259	0.538	0.870	1.350	1.771	2.160	2.650	3.012
14	0.258	0.537	0.868	1.345	1.761	2.145	2.624	2.977
15	0.258	0.536	0.866	1.341	1.753	2.131	2.602	2.947
16	0.258	0.535	0.865	1.337	1.746	2.120	2.583	2.921
17	0.257	0.534	0.863	1.333	1.740	2.110	2.567	2.898
18	0.257	0.534	0.862	1.330	1.734	2.101	2.552	2.878
19	0.257	0.533	0.861	1.328	1.729	2.093	2.539	2.861
20	0.257	0.533	0.860	1.325	1.725	2.086	2.528	2.845
21	0.257	0.532	0.859	1.323	1.721	2.080	2.518	2.831
22	0.256	0.532	0.858	1.321	1.717	2.074	2.508	2.819
23	0.256	0.532	0.858	1.319	1.714	2.069	2.500	2.807
24	0.256	0.531	0.857	1.318	1.711	2.064	2.492	2.797
25	0.256	0.531	0.856	1.316	1.708	2.060	2.485	2.787
26	0.256	0.531	0.856	1.315	1.706	2.056	2.479	2.799
27	0.256	0.531	0.855	1.314	1.703	2.052	2.473	2.771
28	0.256	0.530	0.855	1.313	1.701	2.048	2.467	2.763
29	0.256	0.530	0.854	1.311	1.699	2.045	2.462	2.756
30	0.256	0.530	0.854	1.310	1.697	2.042	2.457	2.750
40	0.255	0.529	0.851	1.303	1.684	2.021	2.423	2.704
60	0.254	0.527	0.848	1.296	1.671	2.000	2.390	2.660
120	0.254	0.526	0.845	1.289	1.658	1.980	2.358	2.617
∞	0.253	0.524	0.842	1.282	1.645	1.960	2.326	2.576
df*	$-t_{.40}$	$-t_{.30}$	$-t_{.20}$	$-t_{.10}$	$-t_{.05}$	$-t_{.025}$	$-t_{.01}$	$-t_{.006}$

* When the table is read from the foot, the table values should be prefixed with a negative sign. Interpolation should be performed using the reciprocals of the degrees of freedom.

INDEX

She also states that she is allergic to
several medications and has "asthma" which
causes her periodic discomfort characterized
by chest pain, breathing difficulties,
palpitations, dizziness and fearfulness.

Physical examination and other laboratory
data are within normal limits.

Your diagnosis is definite Briquet's Syndrome.

CASE VII

A 41-year-old black man is brought into
the emergency room because of "agitation,"
and because he was "unmanageable" at home.

Your examination reveals him to be in poor
nutrition, unkempt and unclean. His gait
is unsteady and he is restless. He looks
anxious. His breath smells of alcohol.
The patient's affect is increased
in range and increased in intensity.
His mood is appropriate but he is irritable.
His speech is slurred and on occasion his
thoughts miss the point and some assoc-   This is an example of ramb-
iations do not seem to follow in sequence   ling speech.
(loosening between associations).

There is no perceptual disturbance or   List the first-rank symptoms
apophany. There are no first-rank   you would look for:
symptoms evident.   1. Phonemes (complete aud-
                                                 itory hallucinations)
                                             2. Thought broadcasting
                                             3. Experiences of influence
                                             4. Experiences of alienation
                                             5. Delusional perceptions

He cannot concentrate.   What tasks would you ask him
                                             to do to determine his con-
                                             centrating ability?
                                             1. Serial 7's
                                             2. Word "world" spelled
                                                 backwards
                                             3. Numbers repeated forward
                                                 and backwards

Recent memory is impaired.   How would you test for this?
                                             remembering 4 words after
                                             5 minutes.

He is disoriented.   Your diagnosis is (delirium)
                                             alcohol intoxication.

CASE VIII

An 18-year-old black man comes
to see you because "I don't feel
right."

He complains of periodic "anxiety"
followed by short periods (60-90 seconds)
for which he does not remember the details, but is told he becomes "blank"
and then smacks his lips and "flops"
his arms. After these episodes he feels
tired and has a headache.

He has a history of head injury.
Physical examination and routine laboratory
data are within normal limits.

What other specialized diagnostic tests do you think
might be helpful?

_____

What is the most likely diagnosis?

_____
_____

CASE IX

A 25-year-old white woman comes to
see you because "I think I am going
to kill my mother."

She states she has been having recurrent
thoughts of wanting to strangle her
mother for the past three years. She
says these thoughts frighten her and
are "stupid" but she can't help herself.
Most recently she has also had thoughts,
persistent and unwanted, that she
should throw liquids (water, milk, cold
coffee) at peoples' faces. She always
feels mortified afterwards. Yesterday,
when thinking about strangling her
mother, she actually raised her hand.
She became frightened and decided to
come and see you.

Besides a mild decrease in range of affect
and some physiological signs of anxiety,
her mental status is within normal limits.

Physical examination and laboratory data
are also within normal limits.

What is the most likely diagnosis?

_____
_____

498

CASE VIII

An 18-year-old black man comes to see you because "I don't feel right."

He complains of periodic "anxiety" followed by short periods (60-90 seconds) for which he does not remember the details, but is told he becomes "blank" and then smacks his lips and "flops" his arms. After these episodes he feels tired and has a headache.

He has a history of head injury. Physical examination and routine laboratory data are within normal limits.

What other specialized diagnostic tests do you think might be helpful?
electroencephalogram

What is the most likely diagnosis?
psychomotor epilepsy (temporal lobe)

CASE IX

A 25-year-old white woman comes to see you because "I think I am going to kill my mother."

She states she has been having recurrent thoughts of wanting to strangle her mother for the past three years. She says these thoughts frighten her and are "stupid" but she can't help herself. Most recently she has also had thoughts, persistent and unwanted, that she should throw liquids (water, milk, cold coffee) at peoples' faces. She always feels mortified afterwards. Yesterday, when thinking about strangling her mother, she actually raised her hand. She became frightened and decided to come and see you.

Besides a mild decrease in range of affect and some physiological signs of anxiety, her mental status is within normal limits.

Physical examination and laboratory data are also within normal limits.

What is the most likely diagnosis?
Obsessive Compulsive Disorder

499

References

1. Abrams, R., Taylor, M.A.: Catatonia: Prediction of Response to Somatic Treatments. Am. J. Psychiat. 134:78-80, 1977.
2. Abrams, R., Taylor, M.A.: Differential EEG Abnormalities in Affective Disorder and Schizophrenia. Arch. Gen. Psychiat. 36: 1355-1358, 1979.
3. Abrams, R., Taylor, M.A.: Mania and Schizo-affective Disorder, Manic Type: A Comparison. Am. J. Psychiat. 133:1445-1447, 1976.
4. Abrams, R., Redfield, J., Taylor, M.A.: Neuropsychological Dysfunction Compared in Schizophrenia, Affective Disorder and Coarse Brain Disease. Biol. Psychiat., in press.
5. Abrams, R., Taylor, M.A., Gaztanaga, P.: Paranoid Schizophrenia and Manic-Depressive Illness: A Phenomenologic Family History and Treatment Response Study. Arch. Gen. Psychiat. 31:640-642, 1974.
6. Abrams, R., Taylor, M.A.: Unipolar and Bipolar Depression. Am. J. Psychiat. 137: 1084-1087, 1980.
7. Abrams, R., Taylor, M.A.: Unipolar and Bipolar Depressive Illness: Phenomenology and Response to ECT. Arch. Gen. Psychiat. 30:320-321, 1974.
8. Abrams, R., Taylor, M.A.: Unipolar Mania - A Preliminary Report. Arch. Gen. Psychiat. 30:441-443, 1974.
9. Abrams, R., Taylor, M.A., Hayman, M.A., Krishna, N.R.: Unipolar Mania Revisited. J. Affective Disorder 1:59-68, 1979.
10. Alberti, G.: Rilievi Catamnestici sulle Psicosi Maniacodepressive. Riv. Sper. Freniat. 87:909-995, 1963.
11. Alexander, M.P., Stuss, D.T., Benson, D.F.: Capgras Syndrome: A Reduplicative Phenomenon. Neurol. 29:334-339, 1979.
12. Almy, G.L., Taylor, M.A.: Lithium Retention in Mania. Arch. Gen. Psychiat. 29:232-234, 1973.
13. American Psychiatric Association: Diagnostic and Statistical Manual of Mental Disorders (3rd Ed.). DSM-III, Washington, D.C., American Psychiatric Association, 1980.
14. Arkonac, O., Guze, S.B.: A Family Study of Hysteria. N. E. J. M. 268:239-242, 1963.
15. Bailey, M.B., Haberman, P., Alksne, H.: The Epidemiology fo Alcoholism in an Urban Residential Area. Quart. J. Stud. Alcohol 26:19-40, 1965.
16. Bear, D.M., Fedio, P.: Quantitative Analysis of Interictal Behavior in Temporal Lobe Epilepsy. Arch. Neurol. 34:454-467, 1977.

17. Benton, A., Van Allen, M.: Prosopagnosia and Facial Discrimination. J. Neurol. Sci. 15:167-172, 1972.
18. Bleuler, M.: Psychotische Belastung von Korperlich Kranken. Z. Ges Neurol. Psychiat. 142:780, 1932.
19. Blumer, D.: Neuropsychiatric Aspects of Psychomotor and Other Forms of Epilepsy, in Livingston, S. (Ed.) Comprehensive Management of Epilepsy in Infancy, Childhood and Adolescence, Springfield, Ill., C.C. Thomas, 1971, pp. 486-497.
20. Blumer, D.: Temporal Lobe Epilepsy and its Psychiatric Significance, in Benson, D.F., Blumer, D. Psychiatric Aspects of Neurologic Disease, New York, Grune & Stratton, 1975, pp. 171-198.
21. Blumer, D., Benson, D.F.: Personality Changes with Frontal and Temporal Lobe Lesions, in Benson, D.F., Blumer, D. (Eds.) Psychiatric Aspects of Neurologic Disease, New York, Grune & Stratton, 1975, pp. 151-170.
22. Brown, F.W.: Heredity in the Psychoneuroses. Proc. Roy. Soc. Med. 35:785-790, 1942.
23. Cahalan, D., Cisin, I.H., Crossley, H.M.: American Drinking Practices: A National Survey of Behavior and Attitudes. Monograph No. 6, New Brunswick, New Jersey, Rutgers Center of Alcoholic Studies, 1969.
24. Carlson, G.A., Goodwin, R.K.: The States of Mania, Arch. Gen. Psychiat. 28:221-228, 1973.
25. Carpenter, W.T., Jr., Strauss, J.S., Bartko, J.J.: An Approach to the Diagnosis and Understanding of Schizophrenia I. Use of Signs and Symptoms for the Identification of Schizophrenic Patients. Schizophrenia Bulletin, Issue 11, 37-49, 1974.
26. Carroll, B.J., Curtes, G.C., Mendels, J.: Neuroendocrine Regulation in Depression II. Discrimination of Depressed from Non-depressed Patients. Arch. Gen. Psychiat. 33:1051-1-58, 1976.
27. Chatel, J.C., Peele, R.: A Centennial Review of Neurasthenia. Am. J. Psychiat. 126:1404-1413, 1970.
28. Chodoff, P., Lyones, H.: Hysteria: The Hysterical Personality and Hysterical Conversion. Am. J. Psychiat. 114:734-740, 1958.
29. Christiansen, K.O.: Crime in a Danish Twin Population. Acta Genet. Med. Gemellol, 19:323-326, 1970.
30. Clayton, P.J., Rodin, L., Winokur, G.: Family History Studies III. Schizo-affective Disorder, Clinical and Genetic Factors Including a One- to Two-year Follow-up. Compr. Psychiat. 9:31-49, 1968.
31. Cleckley, H.: The Mask of Sanity. St. Louis, C.V. Mosby, 1950.
32. Cloninger, C.R., Guze, S.B.: Psychiatric Illness in the Families of Female Criminals: A Study of 288 First-Degree Relatives. Brit. J. Psychiat. 122:697,703, 1973.
33. Cloninger, C.R., Guze, S.B.: Psychiatric Illness and Female Criminality: The Role of Sociopathy and Hysteria in the Antisocial Woman. Am. J. Psychiat. 127:303-311, 1970.
34. Cohen, M.E., Badal, D.W., Kilpatrick, A., et al.: The High Familial Prevalence of Neurocirculatory Asthenia (Anxiety Neurosis, Effort Syndrome) Am. J. Hum. Genet. 3:126-158, 1951.
35. Cohen, M.E., White, P.: Life Situation, Emotions and Neurocirculatory Asthenia (Anxiety Neurosis, Neuroasthenia, Effort Syndrome). Ass. Res. Nerv. Dis. Proc. 29:832-869, 1950.
36. Cohen, M.E., Allen, M.G., Pollin, W., et al.: Relationship of Schizo-affective Psychosis to Manic-Depressive Psychosis and Schizophrenia: Findings in 15,909 Veteran Twin Pairs. Arch. Gen. Psychiat. 26:539-546, 1972.
37. The Committee on Nomenclature and Statistics of the American Psychiatric Association, Diagnostic and Statistical Manual of Mental Disorders, 2nd Edition (DSM-II), Washington D.C., American Psychiatric Association, 1968.

38. Cooper, J.E., Kendell, R.E., Gurland, B.J., et al.: Cross-National Study of Diagnosis of the Mental Disorders: Some Results from the First Comparative Investigation. Am. J. Psychiat. (Suppl.) 125:25-29, 1969.
39. Craft, M.: Ten Studies into Psychopathic Personality. Bristol, John Wright and Sons, Inc., 1965.
40. Critchley, M.: The Parietal Lobes. New York, Hafner Press, 1953.
41. Crowe, R.R.: The Adopted Offspring of Women Criminal Offenders. Arch. Gen. Psychiat. 27:600-603, 1972.
42. Davidson, K., Bagley, C.R.: Schizophrenic-like Psychoses Associated with Organic Disorders, in Herrington, R.N. (Ed.) Current Problems in Neuropsychiatry: Schizophrenia, Epilepsy, The Temporal Lobe. Brit. J. Psychiatry Special Publication #4, Ashford, Kent, Headley Bros. Ltd. 1969, pp. 113-184.
43. Detre, T.P., Jarecki, H.G.: Modern Psychiatric Treatment. Philadelphia, J.B. Lippincott, Co., 1971, pp. 396-455.
44. Dunner, D.L., Fleiss, J.L., Fieve, R.R.: The Course of Development of Mania in Patients with Recurrent Depression, Am. J. Psychiat. 133:905-908, 1976.
45. Engel, G.L.: Delirium, in Freedman, A.M., Kaplan, H.I. (Eds.) Comprehensive Textbook of Psychiatry, Baltimire, The Williams & Wilkins Co., 1967.
46. Engle, G.L., Romano, J.: Delirium, A Syndrome of Cerebral Insufficiency. J. Chronic Dis. 9:260-277, 1959.
47. Eysenck, H.J., Rachman, S.: The Causes and Cures of Neurosis. San Diego, R.R. Knapp, 1965.
48. Eysenck, H.J.: The Classification of Depressive Illness. Brit. J. Psychiat. 117:241-250, 1970.
49. Farley, J., Woodruff, R.A., Jr., Guze, S.B.: The Prevalence of Hysteria and Conversion Symptoms. Brit. J. Psychiat. 114:1121-1125, 1968.
50. Feighner, J.P., Robins, E., Guze, S.B., et al.: Diagnostic Criteria for Use in Psychiatric Research. Arch. Gen. Psychiat. 29:57-63, 1972.
51. Flor-Henry, P.: Lateralized Temporal-Limbic Dysfunction and Psychopathology. Annals N.Y. A.S. 280:777-797, 1976.
52. Flor-Henry, P.: Psychosis and Temporal Lobe Epilepsy. A Controlled Investigation. Epilepsia 10:363-395, 1969.
53. Forrest, A.D., Fraser, R.H., Priest, R.G.: Environmental Factors in Depressive Illness. Brit. J. Psychiat. 111:243-253, 1965.
54. Fremming, K.: The Expectation of Mental Infirmity in the Sample of the Danish Population, in Occasional Papers of Eugenics, #7, London, Cassell, 1951.
55. Fremming, K.: Sygdomsrisikoen for Sindslideleser og Andre Sjaeledige Abnormtilstande i den danske Gennemsontsbefolkning. Copenhagen, Ejnar Munksgaard, 1947.
56. Gastuat, H., Vigouroux, M.: Electro-clinical correlations in 500 Cases of Psychomotor Seizures, in Baldwin, M., Bailey, P. (Eds.) Temporal Lobe Epilepsy, Springfield, Ill., C.C. Thomas, 1958.
57. Gerstmann, J.: Some Notes on the Gerstmann-Syndrome. Neurology 7:866-869, 1957.
58. Geschwind, N.: The Clinical Setting of Aggression in Temporal Lobe Epilepsy, in Fields, W.S., Sweet, W.H. (Eds.) The Neurobiology of Violence St. Louis, Warren H. Green, 1975, pp. 273-281.
59. Gittleson, N.L.: The Phenomenology of Obsessions in Depressive Psychosis. Brit. J. Psychiat. 112:261-264, 1966.
60. Goodwin, D.W., Crane, J.B., Guze, S.B.: Alcoholic "Blackouts": A Review and Clinical Study of 100 Alcoholics. Am. J. Psychiat. 126:191-198, 1969.

61. Goodwin, D.W., Guze, S.B., Robins, E.: Follow-up Studies in Obsessional Neurosis. Arch. Gen. Psychiat. 20:182-187, 1969.
62. Gurzelier, J., Flor-Henry, P. (Eds.) Hemisphere Asymmetries of Function in Psychopathology. New York, MacMillan, Amsterdam, Elsevier/North Holland Biomedical Press, 1979.
63. Guze, S.B., Goodwin, D.W., Crane, J.B.: Criminality and Psychiatric Disorders. Arch. Gen. Psychiat. 20:583-591, 1969.
64. Guze, S.B.: Criminality and Psychiatric Disorders. New York, Oxford University Press, 1976.
65. Guze, S.B., Goodwin, D.W., Crane, J.B.: Criminal Recidivism and Psychiatric Illness. Am. J. Psychiat. 127:832-835, 1970.
66. Guze, S.B.: The Diagnosis of Hysteria: What are we Trying to Do? Am. J. Psychiat. 24:491-498, 1967.
67. Guze, S.B., Woodruff, R.A., Jr., Clayton, P.J.: Hysteria and Antisocial Behavior: Further Evidence of an Association. Am. J. Psychiat. 127:957-960, 1971.
68. Guze, S.B., Perley, M.J.: Observations on the Natural History of Hysteria. Am. J. Psychiat. 119:960-965, 1963.
69. Guze, S.B., Wolfgrom, E.D., McKinney, J.K., Cantwell, D.P.: Psychiatric Illness in the Families of Convicted Criminals. A Study of 519 First-Degree Relatives. Dis. Nerv. Syst. 28:651-659, 1967.
70. Guze, S.B.: The Role of Follow-up Studies: Their Contribution to Diagnostic Classification as Applied to Hysteria. Semin. Psychiat. 2:392-402, 1970.
71. Guze, S.B., Woodruff, R.A., Clayton, P.J.: A Study of Conversion Symptoms in Psychiatric Outpatients. Am. J. Psychiat. 128:643-646, 1971.
72. Guze, S.B., Robins, E.: Suicide and Primary Affective Disorders. Brit. J. Psychiat. 117:437-438, 1970.
73. Guze, S.B.: The Validity and Significance of the Clinical Diagnosis of Hysteria (Briquet's Syndrome). Am. J. Psychiat. 132:138-141, 1975.
74. Hamilton, M., White, J.M.: Factors Related to Outcome of Depression Treated with ECT. J. Ment. Sci. 106:1031-1041, 1960.
75. Hayman, M., Abrams, R.: Capgras' Syndrome and Cerebral Dysfunction. Brit. J. Psychiat. 130:68-71, 1977.
76. Hays, P.: Etiological Factors in Manic-Depressive Psychosis. Arch. Gen. Psychiat. 33:1187-1188, 1976.
77. Hecaen, H., Albert, M.L.: Disorders of Mental Functioning Related to Frontal Lobe Pathology, in Benson, D.F., Blumer, D. (Eds.), Psychiatric Aspects of Neurologic Disease, New York, Grune & Stratton, 1975, pp. 137-149.
78. Helgason, T.: Epidemiology of Mental Disorders in Iceland. A Psychiatric and Demographic Investigation of 5395 Icelanders. Acta. Psychiat. Scand. 40:Suppl. 173, 1964.
79. Ingram, I.M.: Obsessional Illness in Mental Hospital Patients. J. Ment. Sci. 107:382-402, 1961.
80. Inouye, E.: Similar and Dissimilar Manifestations of Obsessive-Compulsive Neuroses in Monozygotic Twins. Am. J. Psychiat. 121:1171-1175, 1965.
81. Jellinek, E.M.: The Disease Concept of Alcoholism. New Haven, Hillhouse Press, 1960.
82. Jellinek, E.M.: Phases of Alcohol Addiction. Quart. J. Stud. Alcohol 13:673-684, 1952.
83. Kaplan, H.I.: Current Psychodynamic Concepts in Psychomatic Medicine, in Pasnau, R.O. (Ed.), Consultation-Liaison Psychiatry, New York, Grune & Stratton, 1975, pp. 33-46.
84. Kennard, M.: The EEG in Schizophrenia, in Wilson, W.P. (Ed.), Applications of Electroencephalography in Psychiatry, Durham, Duke University Press, 1965, pp. 168-184.

503

85.   Kiloh, L.G., Garside, R.F.: The Independence of Neurotic and Endogenous Depression. Brit. J. Psychiat. 109:451-463, 1963.
86.   Kinglen, E.: Obsessional Neurotics: A Long-Term Follow-up. Brit. J. Psychiat. 111:709-722, 1965.
87.   Koehler, K., Seminario, I.: "First Rank" Schizophrenia and Research Diagnosable Schizophrenic and Affective Illness. Compr. Psychiat. 19: 401-406, 1978.
88.   Kraepelin, E.: Manic-Depressive Insanity and Paranoia. New York, Arno Press, 1976.
89.   Kramer, M.: Cross-National Study of Diagnosis of the Mental Disorders Origin of the Problem. Am. J. Psychiat. (Suppl) 125:1-11, 1969.
90.   Krishna, N.R., Taylor, M.A., Abrams, R.: Response to Lithium Carbonate. Biol. Psychiat. 13:601-6-6, 1978.
91.   Lader, M., Marks, I.: Clinical Anxiety. New York, Grune & Stratton, 1971.
92.   Leonhard, K.: Aufteilung der endogenen Psychosen, 2nd Edition, Berlin, Akademie, Verlag, 1959.
93.   Lewis, A.J.: Problems of Obsessional Illness. Proc. Roy. Soc. Med. 29:325-336, 1936.
94.   Lief, A. (Ed.): Fundamental Conceptions of Dementia Praecox, The Commonsense Psychiatry of Dr. Adolf Meyer: 52 Selected Papers. New York, Arno Press 1973, pp. 184-192.
95.   Liskow, P.I., Clayton, P., Woodruff, R., et al.: Briquet's Syndrome, Hysterical Personality and the MMPI. Am. J. Psychiat. 134:1134-1139, 1977
96.   Lipkins, L.M., Dyrud, J., Meyer, G.G.: The Many Faces of Mania. Arch. Gen. Psychiat. 22:262-267, 1970.
97.   Lunden, W.A.: Statistics on Delinquents and Delinquency. Springfield, Ill., C.C. Thomas, 1964.
98.   Lundquist, G.: Prognosis and Course in Manic-Depressive Psychoses. Acta Psychiat. Neurol. Suppl. 35, 1945.
99.   Luria, A.: The Working Brain: An Introduction to Neuropsychology. New York, Basic Books, 1973.
100. Luxenberger, H.: Demographiscle und Psychiatrische Untersuchungen in der Engeren Biologischen Familie von Paralytikerehegatten. Z. Ges. Neurol. Psychiat. 112:331, 1928.
101. Maddocks, P.D.: A Five-Year Follow-up of Untreated Psychopaths. Brit. J. Psychiat. 116:511-515, 1970.
102. Marks, I.M.: Agoraphobic Syndrome (Phobic Anxiety State), Arch. Gen. Psychiat. 25:538-553, 1970.
103. Marks, I.M.: The Classification of Phobic Disorders. Brit. J. Psychiat 116:377-386, 1970.
104. Marks, I.M.: Fears and Phobias. London, Heinemann Medical, 1969.
105. Marks, I.M.: Phobic Disorders Four Years After Treatment: A Prospective Follow-up. Brit. J. Psychiat. 118:683-689, 1971.
106. McCabe, M.S., Fowler, J.S., Cadoret, R.J., et al.: Familial Differences in Schizophrenics with Good and Poor Prognosis. Psychol. Med. 1: 326-332, 1971.
107. Meadows, J.: The Anatomic Basis of Prosopagnosia. J. Neurol. Neurosurg. Psychiat. 37:489-501, 1974.
108. Mendelson, W., Johnson, N., Stewart, M.A.: Hyperactive Children as Teenagers: A Follow-up Study. J. Nerv. Ment. Dis. 153:273-279, 1971.
109. Morrison, J.R.: Catatonia: Retarded and Excited Types. Arch. Gen. Psychiat. 28:39-41, 1973.
110. Morrison, J.R., Clancy, J., Crowe, R. et al.: The Iowa 500 I: Diagnostic Validity in Mania, Depression and Schizophrenia. Arch. Gen. Psychiat. 27:457-461, 1972.

111.   Morse, R.M., Liten, E.M.: Post-Operative Delirium: A Study of Etiologic Factors. Am. J. Pshchat. 126:388-395, 1969.
112.   Nielsen, J.: Gerstmann's Syndrome: Finger Agnosia, Agraphia, Comparison of Right and Left and Acalculia. Arch. Neurol. Psychiat. 39:536-560, 1938.
113.   Pemberton, D.A.: A Comparison of the Outcome of Treatment in Female and Male Alcoholics. Brit. J. Psychiat. 113:367-373, 1967.
114.   Perley, M.J., Guze, S.B.: Hysteria - The Stability and Usefulness of Clinical Criteria: A Quantitative Study Based on a Follow-up Period of 6-8 Years in 39 Patients. N. Engl. J. Med. 266:421-426, 1962.
115.   Pincus, J.H., Tucker, G.J.: Behavioral Neurology, 2nd Edition, New York, Oxford University Press, 1978.
116.   Pitts, F.N., Jr.: The Biochemistry of Anxiety. Sci. Am. 220:69-75, 1969.
117.   Pitts, F.N., Jr., McClure, J.N., Jr.: Lactate Metabolism in Anxiety Neurosis. N. Engl. J. Med. 277:1329-1336, 1967.
118.   Pollitt, J.: Natural History of Obsessional States: A Study of 150 Cases. Brit. Med. J. 1:194-198, 1957.
119.   Pope, H.G., Jr., Lipinski, J.F., Jr.: Diagnosis in Schizophrenia and Manic-Depressive Illness: A Reassessment of the Specificity of "Schizophrenic" Symptoms in Light of Current Research. Arch. Gen. Psychiat. 35:811-828, 1978.
120.   Prichard, J.C.: A Treatise on Insanity and Other Disorders Affecting the Mind. London, Sherwood, Gilbert & Piper, 1835.
121.   Purtell, J.J., Robins, E., Cohen, M.E.: Observations on the Clinical Aspects of Hysteria: A Quantitative Study of 50 Patients in 156 Control Subjects. J.A.M.A. 146:902-909, 1951.
122.   Rachman, S.: Phobias: Their Nature and Control, Springfield, Ill., C.C. Thomas, 1968.
123.   Rake, R.H.: Life Stress and Illness, in Pasnau, R.O. (Ed.), Consultation-Liaison Psychiatry, New York, Grune & Stratton, 1975, pp. 47-59.
124.   Robins, L.N.: Deviant Children Grown Up. Baltimore, The Williams & Wilkins Co., 1966.
125.   Robins, L.N., Murphy, G.E., Breckenridge, M.B.: Drinking Behavior of Young Negro Men. Quart. J. Stud. Alcohol. 29:657-684, 1968.
126.   Rose, J.T.: Reactive and Endogenous Depressions. Response to ECT. Brit. J. Psychiat. 109:212-217, 1963.
127.   Rosenberg, C.M.: Familial Aspects of Obsessional Neurosis. Brit. J. Psychiat. 113:405-413, 1967.
128.   Roth, M.: The Phenomenology of Depressive States. Can. Psychiat. Assoc. J. (Suppl) 4:532-553, 1959.
129.   Roth, M.: The Phobic-Anxiety-Depersonalization Syndrome. Proc. Roy. Soc. Med. 52:587, 1959.
130.   Rubin, R.T.: Mind-Brain-Body Interaction: Elucidation of Psychosomatic Intervening Variables, in Pasnau, R.O. (Ed.), Consultation-Liaison Psychiatry, New York, Grune & Stratton, 1975, pp. 73-85.
131.   Sadoun, R., Lolli, G., Silverman, M.: Drinking in French Culture, Monographs of the Rutger's Center of Alcohol Studies No. 5, New Haven, College and University Press, 1965.
132.   Schlesser, M.A., Winokur, G., Sherman, B.M.: Genetic Subtypes of Unipolar Primary Depressive Illness Distinguished by Hypothalamic-Pituitary-Adrenal Axis Activity. Lancet 1:739-741, 1979.
133.   Schnieder, K.: Psychopathic Personalities. London, Cassell, 1958.
134.   Schulsinger, F.: Psychopathy, Heredity and Environment. Int. J. Ment. Health 1:190-206, 1972.
135.   Selye, H.: The Physiology and Pathology of Exposure to Stress. Montreal, Acta, Inc., 1950.

505

136. Shagass, C., Naiman, J., Mihalik, J.M.: An Objective Test Which Differentiates Between Neurotic and Psychotic Depression. Arch. Neurol. Psychiat. 75:461-471, 1956.
137. Shields, J.: Heredity and Psychological Abnormality, in Eysenck, J.H. (Ed.), Handbook of Abnormal Psychology, San Diego, California, R.R. Knapp 1963, pp. 541-603.
138. Sjogren, T.: Genetic-Statistical and Psychiatric Investigations of a West Swedish Population. Acta. Pshchiat. Neurol. Suppl. 52, 1948.
139. Slaby, A.E., Wyatt, R.J.: Dementia in the Presenium. Springfield, Ill., C.C. Thomas, 1974.
140. Slater, B., Shields, J.: Genetical Aspects of Anxiety. Brit. J. Psychiat. Special Publication No. 3. Studies of Anxiety, Ashford, Kent, Headley Bros. Ltd. 1969, pp. 62-71.
141. Slater, E., Cowie, V.: The Genetics of Mental Disorders, London, Oxford University Press, 1971, pp. 72-74.
142. Slater, E.: The Incidence of Mental Disorder. Ann. Eugenics 6:172, 1935.
143. Slater, E., Roth, M.: Mayer-Gross Clinical Psychiatry, 3rd Edition, Baltimore, The Williams & Wilkins Co., 1969.
144. Slater, E., Beard, A.W.: The Schizophrenic-like Psychoses of Epilepsy Brit. J. Psychiat. 109:95-150, 1963.
145. Snaith, R.P.: A Clinical Investigation of Phobias. Brit. J. Psychiat. 114:673-698, 1968.
146. Sovner, R.D., McHugh, P.R.: Bipolar Course in Schizo-affective Illness. Biol. Psychiat. 11:195-204, 1976.
147. Spitzer, R.L., Endicott, J., Robins, E.: Research Diagnostic Criteria (RDC) for a Selected Group of Functional Disorders. NIMH Clinical Research Branch Collaborative Program on the Psychobiology of Depression. Washington, D.C. 1975.
148. Stern, R.S., Cobb, J.P.: Phenomenology of Obsessive-Compulsive Neurosis. Brit. J. Psychiat. 132:233-239, 1978.
149. Sutherland, J.M., Tait, H.: The Epilepsies: Modern Diagnosis and Treatment Edinburgh, E. & S. Livingstone Ltd. 1969.
150. Taylor, M.A., Abrams, R.: Acute Mania: A Clinical and Genetic Study of Responders and Non-Responders to Treatments. Arch. Gen. Psychiat. 32:863-865, 1975.
151. Taylor, M.A., Abrams, R., Hayman, M.: The Classification of Affective Disorder: A Reassessment of the Bipolar-Unipolar Dichotomy I.: A Clinical, Laboratory and Family Study. J. Affective Dis. 2:95-109, 1980.
152. Taylor, M.A., Abrams, R.: A Critique of the "St. Louis" Psychiatric Research Criteria for Schizophrenia. Am. J. Psychiat. 132:1276-1280, 1973.
153. Taylor, M.A., Greenspan, B., Abrams, R.: Lateralized Neuropsychological Dysfunction in Affective Disorders and Schizophrenia. Am. J. Psychiat. 136: 1031-1034, 1979.
154. Taylor, M.A., Abrams, R., Gaztanaga, P.: Manic-Depressive Illness and Acute Schizophrenia, A Clinical, Family History and Treatment Response Study. Am. J. Psychiat. 131:678-682, 1974.
155. Taylor, M.A., Abrams, R.: Manic-Depressive Illness and "Good Prognosis" Schizophrenia. Am. J. Psychiat. 132:741-742, 1975.
156. Taylor, M.A., Abrams, R., Gaztanaga, P.: Manic-Depressive Illness and Schizophrenia: A Partial Validation of Research Diagnostic Criteria Utilizing Neuropsychological Testing. Compr. Psychiat. 16:91-96, 1975.
157. Taylor, M.A., Abrams, R.: The Phenomenology of Mania: A New Look at Some Old Patients. Arch. Gen. Psychiat. 29:520-522, 1973.

158. Taylor, M.A., Abrams, R.: The Prevalence and Importance of Catatonia in the Manic-Phase of Manic-Depressive Illness. Arch. Gen. Psychiat. 34: 1223-1225, 1977.
159. Taylor, M.A., Abrams, R.: The Prevalence of Schizophrenia: A Reassessment Using Modern Diagnostic Criteria. Am. J. Psychiat. 135:945-948, 1978.
160. Tsuang, M.T., Woolson, R.F.: Excess Mortality in Schizophrenia and Affective Disorders: Do Suicides and Accidental Deaths Solely Account for this Excess? Arch. Gen. Psychiat. 35:1181-1185, 1978.
161. Tsuang, M.T., Dempsey, G.M., Dvoredsky, A., et al.: A Family History Study of Schizo-affective Disorder. Biol. Psychiat. 12:331-338, 1977.
162. Tsuang, M.T., Woolson, R.F.: Mortality in Patients with Schizophrenia, Mania, Depression and Surgical Conditions, A Comparison with General Population Mortality. Brit. J. Psychiat. 130:162-166, 1977.
163. Tsuang, M.T., Dempsey, G.M., Rauscher, R.: A Study of "Atypical" Schizophrenia: Comparison with Schizophrenia and Affective Disorder by Sex, Age of Admission, Precipitant, Outcome and Family History. Arch. Gen. Psychiat. 33:1157-1160, 1976.
164. Tucker, G.T., Detre, T., Harrow, M., et al. Behavior and Symptoms of Psychiatric Patients and the Electroencephalogram. Arch. Gen. Psychiat. 12:278-286, 1965.
165. Tyrer, P., Steinberg, D.: Symptomatic Treatment of Agoraphobia and Social Phobias: A Follow-up Study. Brit. J. Psychiat. 127:163-168, 1975.
166. U.S. Department of Health, Education and Welfare, National Institute of Mental Health: Mental Health Statistical Note 138. Washington, D.C., U.S. Government Printing Office, 1977.
167. Vianna, U.: The Electroencephalogram in Schizophrenia. Brit. J. Psychiat. Spec. Pub. No. 10, Ashford, Kent, Headley Bros. Ltd., 1975, pp. 54-58.
168. Weinstein, E., Kahn, R.: Denial of Illness: Symbolic and Physiological Aspects. Springfield, Ill., C.C. Thomas, 1955.
169. Wells, C.E.: Chronic Brain Disease: An Overview. Am. J. Psychiat. 135:1-12, 1978.
170. Wells, C.E.: Delirium and Dementia, in Abram, H.S. (Ed.), Basic Psychiatry for the Primary Care Physician. Boston, Little Brown & Co., 1976.
171. Wells, C.E.: Dementia. Philadelphia, F.A. Davis & Co., 1971.
172. Welner, A., Welner, Z., Fishman, R.: The Group of Schizo-affective and Related Psychoses: IV. A Family Study. Compr. Psychiat. 20:21-26, 1979.
173. Welner, A., Cronghan, J.L., Fishman, R. et al.: The Group of Schizo-affective and Related Psychoses: A Follow-up Study. Compr. Psychiat. 18:413-422, 1977.
174. Wheeler, E.O., White, P.D., Reed, E.W., Cohen, M.E.: Familial Incidence of Neurocirculatory Asthenia (Anxiety Neurosis, Effort Syndrome). J. Clin. Invest. 27:562, 1948.
175. Wheeler, E.O., White, P.D., Reed, E.W., Cohen, M.E.: Neurocirculatory Asthenia (Anxiety Neurosis, Effort Syndrome, Neurasthenia). J.A.M.A. 142:878-889, 1950.
176. Winokur, G., Morrison, J.: The Iowa 500: Follow-up of 225 Depressives. Brit. J. Psychiat. 123:543-548, 1973.
177. Winokur, G., Clayton, P.J., Reich, T.: Manic-Depressive Illness. St. Louis, C.V. Mosby, 1969.
178. Woodruff, R.A., Goodwin, D.W., Guze, S.B.: Psychiatric Diagnosis. New York, Oxford University Press, 1974, p. 6.

179.   Woerner, P.I., Guze, S.B.: A Family and Marital Study of Hysteria. Brit. J. Psychiat. 114:161-168, 1968.
180.   Woodruff, R.A., Jr., Clayton, P.J., Guze, S.B.: Hysteria, Studies of Diagnosis, Outcome and Prevalence. J.A.M.A. 215:425-428, 1971.
181.   Woodruff, R.A., Jr., Guze, S.B., Clayton, P.J.: The Medical and Psychiatric Implications of Antisocial Personality (Sociopathy). Dis. Nerv. Syst. 32:712-714, 1971.